Modern Trends in
Forensic Medicine

Modern Trends in

Forensic Medicine—3

Edited by

A. Keith Mant
M.D.(PATH.), F.R.C.PATH.

*Head of Department
of Forensic Medicine,
Guy's Hospital
Medical School;
Senior Lecturer in
Forensic Medicine,
King's College Hospital
Medical School, London*

Butterworths

ENGLAND: BUTTERWORTH & CO. (PUBLISHERS) LTD.
               LONDON: 88 Kingsway, WC2B 6AB

AUSTRALIA: BUTTERWORTHS PTY. LTD.
               SYDNEY: 586 Pacific Highway 2067
               MELBOURNE: 343 Little Collins Street, 3000
               BRISBANE: 240 Queen Street, 4000

CANADA: BUTTERWORTH & CO. (CANADA) LTD.
               TORONTO: 14 Curity Avenue, 374

NEW ZEALAND: BUTTERWORTHS OF NEW ZEALAND LTD.
               WELLINGTON: 26–28 Waring Taylor Street, 1

SOUTH AFRICA: BUTTERWORTH & CO. (SOUTH AFRICA) (PTY.) LTD.
               DURBAN: 152–154 Gale Street

Suggested U.D.C. Number: 340.6
Suggested Additional Number: 61: 34

©

ISBN 0 407 29202 0

Printed in Great Britain by
Bell & Bain Ltd.
Glasgow

Contents

Page

PREFACE ix

Chapter

1. COT DEATHS 1
   Michael M. Lyons, M.D., *Associate Professor in the Department of Pathology, New Jersey College of Medicine and Dentistry, Newark; Associate Research Professor in the Department of Forensic Medicine and Pathology, New York University Medical School*

2. CHILD ABUSE—THE BATTERED BABY 19
   Keith Simpson, M.A.(Oxon.), M.D.(Path.), M.D.(Ghent), F.R.C.P.(Lond.), F.R.C.Path., D.M.J., *Emeritus Professor of Forensic Medicine in the University of London at Guy's Hospital Medical School*

3. NEWER TECHNIQUES IN PATERNITY BLOOD GROUPING . 43
   Alan Grant, M.A., M.D., F.R.C.Path., *Lecturer in Forensic Serology in the University of London at Guy's Hospital Medical School*

   and

   Ian D. Bradbrook, B.Sc., *Research Assistant, Department of Forensic Medicine, Guy's Hospital Medical School*

4. THE HISTOPATHOLOGY OF WOUNDS 64
   Peter Pullar, M.D., M.R.C.Path., D.M.J., *Consultant Pathologist, Wessex Department of Forensic Medicine, Winchester; Lecturer in Forensic Medicine in the University of London at Guy's Hospital Medical School and at Southampton University*

CONTENTS

Chapter *Page*

5. THE PATHOLOGIST'S ROLE AND MODERN SCIENTIFIC
    TECHNIQUES AT THE SCENE OF THE CRIME . . . 93
    A. Keith Mant, M.D.(Path.), F.R.C.Path., *Head of
    Department of Forensic Medicine, Guy's Hospital Medical
    School; Senior Lecturer in Forensic Medicine, King's
    College Hospital Medical School, London*

6. FIREARMS INJURIES 120
    William Q. Sturner, B.S., M.D., D.M.J., *Medical Examiner,
    Dallas County; Assistant Professor of Pathology, University
    of Texas Southwestern Medical School at Dallas*
                                and
    Charles S. Petty, B.S., M.S., M.D., *Chief Medical
    Examiner, Dallas County; Professor of Forensic Sciences
    and Pathology, University of Texas Southwestern Medical
    School at Dallas*

7. THE INVESTIGATION OF INJURIES IN ROAD TRAFFIC
    ACCIDENTS 139
    E. Grattan, B.A., M.B., B.Ch., F.R.C.S., *Principal Scienti-
    fic Officer, Transport and Road Research Laboratory
    (formerly Road Research Laboratory), Crowthorne, Berk-
    shire*

    J. G. Wall, B.Sc., *Principal Scientific Officer, Transport and
    Road Research Laboratory, Crowthorne, Berkshire*
                                and
    J. A. Hobbs, *Scientific Officer, Transport and Road Re-
    search Laboratory, Crowthorne, Berkshire*

8. INVESTIGATION OF MASS DISASTER 170
    Peter J. Stevens, O.B.E., M.D., F.R.C.Path., D.C.P.,
    D.T.M.&H., *Consultant Pathologist, Regional Plastic
    Surgery and Jaw Injuries Centre, Queen Victoria Hospital,
    East Grinstead; Honorary Senior Lecturer in Pathology of
    Trauma, London Hospital Medical College*

9. RECENT IMPROVEMENTS IN ESTIMATING STATURE, SEX, AGE
    AND RACE FROM SKELETAL REMAINS 193
    T. D. Stewart, M.D., *Anthropologist Emeritus, Department
    of Anthropology, National Museum of Natural History,
    Smithsonian Institution, Washington, D.C.*

Chapter *Page*

10. MODERN TOXICOLOGY AND IDENTIFICATION TECHNIQUES . 212
    A. S. Curry, M.A., Ph.D., F.R.I.C., F.R.C.Path., *Director
    of the Home Office Central Research Establishment,
    Aldermaston, Berkshire*

11. RECOMMENDED CHANGES IN DEATH CERTIFICATION,
    CREMATION REGULATIONS, AND CORONERS' PROCEDURE   248
    David M. Paul, M.R.C.S., L.R.C.P., D.A., D.M.J.(Clin.),
    *Her Majesty's Coroner to the City of London and to the
    Northern District of Greater London; Honorary Lecturer
    in Court Practice and Clinical Forensic Medicine, Guy's
    Hospital Medical School; Honorary Lecturer in Clinical
    Forensic Medicine, St. Bartholomew's Hospital Medical
    College*

INDEX 295

Preface

The application of modern scientific techniques to forensic medicine has advanced this discipline of law enforcement so rapidly in the last decade that the selection of material for the Third Series of Modern Trends has been no sinecure. An attempt has been made to approach the task on a broad front and yet at the same time to avoid subject matter covered in the last series. The first two series had a wide circulation in North America and this has been recognized by the inclusion of three chapters by eminent experts working in the United States. The subjects selected for this Third Series are weighted towards traumatology.

Dr. Lyons, who has spent several years investigating 'cot deaths', has reviewed the current theories and research, and Professor Simpson's chapter on the 'battered baby' follows as the natural sequel.

William Sturner and Charles Petty have written about firearm wounds inflicted by modern weapons and ammunition; Mr. Grattan upon the current trends in road accident investigation; and Dr. Peter Stevens upon the investigation of mass disaster: three subjects of increasing importance to forensic pathologists. By general demand there is a chapter on the scientific investigation of the scene of crime.

Dr. Peter Pullar has reviewed the modern techniques of wound dating and Dr. Alan Curry has dealt with the latest techniques available to the toxicologist. Dr. Alan Grant and Mr. Ian Bradbrook have covered the advances in blood grouping techniques and their application in paternity cases.

Dr. Dale Stewart, formerly Chief Physical Anthropologist at the Smithsonian Institution, has reviewed the trends in skeletal ageing techniques which have become current since the First Series 20 years ago.

Finally, Dr. David Paul has reviewed the long-awaited Brodrick Committee Report.

I am most grateful to Professor Keith Simpson for his valuable advice and assistance in the compilation of this volume.

A.K.M.

A*

1 Cot Deaths

SUDDEN DEATH IN INFANCY SYNDROME

MICHAEL M. LYONS

INTRODUCTION

Cot deaths—or crib deaths as they are called in the United States—are medico-legally classified as *sudden unexpected natural deaths in infants*. They are also referred to as the *sudden death syndrome in infants*. All terms call attention to the various aspects of the entity and the last especially marks the concept of diverse conditions presenting in a similar fashion. Because of their unexplained aetiology and mechanism of death, and because the vast majority in all series do die in a bed or a cot, they will be called cot deaths in this review.

The general incidence of cot deaths is difficult to ascertain with exactitude. As will be discussed, the socio-economic setting in which they are most common will vary from one region to another and accordingly in respective countries. In round figures it has been held accountable for approximately 1,100 deaths per year in Great Britain and an estimated 25,000 deaths per year in the USA (Valdes-Dapena, 1963). A current evaluation on culled vital statistical records would place the incidence at between 7,000 and 10,000. Epidemiologically and relative to the general incidence of cot deaths, one study noted that between 28 days and one year of life, there are 6 deaths per 1,000 live born children. Of these 6 deaths, 3 are attributable to cot deaths (Steele, Kraus and Langworth, 1967). Undoubtedly cot deaths are world-wide in occurrence but they take on greater prominence in those areas where infectious disease and nutritional disorders in children are controlled. The significance of this incidence is heightened when it is realized that most of the cases cluster between six weeks and six months of age.

There have been numerous papers and several reviews on cot deaths since the mid-1940s. The condition was known to clinicians and pathologists before that period, but the relatively recent dramatic control of infectious disease in Great Britain and the USA must account for the increased general awareness of cot deaths in these countries. The past 25 years have been marked by a sharper delineation of the condition. This has been attended by the disproving or lack of corroboration of certain findings, the application of new and varied diagnostic laboratory procedures with generally negative results and the partial testing of various hypotheses. All this has essentially amounted to 'clearing the air'.

The purpose of this review is to present the current state of information on cot deaths considering the data as such and balancing this against the hypotheses that have been or are now being offered. The references cited will be either to previous reviews or to those articles that document the evolving consensus. No attempt is made to cite all the available literature. To facilitate the presentation, the material will be handled under specific headings.

Between 1964 and 1967, Doctors Milton Helpern, John Devlin and myself carried out an investigation of 141 cot deaths at the Office of the Chief Medical Examiner of the City of New York. Since then, we have pursued special areas of study, all relative to cot death. These past and current investigations, plus our shared knowledge of the entity, constitute our personal experience. It should be noted that these 141 cot deaths constitute approximately 16 per cent of the paediatric (under 14 years of age) forensic cases seen over a $2\frac{1}{2}$ year period. Approximately 100 cot death cases are handled each year by the Office of the Chief Medical Examiner of New York City.

COT DEATH CASE PROCEDURE

This category is placed first to emphasize that the final conclusion that a particular case is a cot death is by a diagnosis by exclusion. The scene should be visited and the family interviewed. In this manner, the prior general health of the dead infant can be ascertained and the data relative to trauma, infectious disease (infant, family, neighbourhood) or previous explained or unexplained infant or paediatric death noted. These are all important to the forensic and/or public health problem of overwhelming sepsis, battered child, suffocation (circumstances, rolling over case?) and unsuspected accidental traumatic death. A complete autopsy is performed on all cases. Histology is obtained on all tissue with particular reference to the respiratory tree. It was our procedure to perform certain routine bacterial and viral isolations on all cases, but as these were generally unrewarding we now simply obtain a bacterial culture on blood, lung and then any additional studies as would be indicated by the case. Radiographs of the skeletal system can be rewarding, if not critical, when the problem of minimal trauma is present and the question of a battered child is entertained. When all this is done and non-cot death cases sorted out before the autopsy, there will still be a definitive (non-cot) cause of death found in approximately 15 per cent of the clinically considered cot deaths. Two points are herein worthy of consideration. First, when the clinical data are not obtained casually, the proper evaluation of what is a cot death will be seriously compounded. Secondly, there is a point of view among some informed observers that when the clinical setting is well documented and the physician (pathologist or otherwise) is familiar with the entity, then an autopsy is not essential to the final diagnosis of cot death. In this instance, one would have labelled about 85 per cent of the deaths correctly, but would not know whether a particular case was or was not a cot death.

SEX INCIDENCE

There is general agreement as to a male preponderance with percentages of 55–62 per cent (Valdes-Dapena, 1963) and 56 per cent (Steele and Langworth, 1966) from larger series and similar figures from smaller series. Of our 141 cases, 88 were male (62 per cent) and 53 female (38 per cent). No reason has been advanced for this sex ratio. A roughly similar sex ratio has been noted for death due to congenital heart disease in the first year of life.

AGE INCIDENCE

Most workers agree that cot deaths occur in the first six months of life. Valdes-Dapena (1963) notes that few cases occur before three weeks or after six months of age, and that there is a relative peak between two and four months. Johnstone and Lowy (1966) record a case-age span of four days to two years. Table 1 indicates our data and three pertinent age span summations. The concordance of age data from these and other studies would appear to establish this aspect of cot deaths as proved. Its special significance is in suggesting a pathophysiological mechanism or situation unique to this age range. This uniqueness may, however, merely be the time required for a prior biological 'trauma' and its reaction to reach a fatal termination seemingly unattended by any prodromata. As such, it has been the partial or complete background against which the hypotheses were developed based on serum globulin levels (Spain, Bradess and Greenblatt, 1954), fatal viral infection with antigen–antibody com-

3

TABLE 1

Occurrence of Cot Deaths by Age

Age in months	Number		
First	18	2 weeks+ : 6	3 weeks+ : 11
Second	28	4–6 weeks+ : 10	6 weeks+ : 18
Third	24		
Fourth	28		
Fifth	13		
Sixth	10		
Seventh	5		
Eighth	3		
Ninth	2		
Tenth	0		
Eleventh	0		
Twelfth	2		
1 Year	3		
1 Year+	5	15 months, 18 months, 2 years, 3 years	
	141		
Birth to 6 months	121—86%		
6 weeks to 6 months	91—65%		
6 weeks to 4 months	70—50%		

plex 'disease' in infancy (Gunther, 1966) and cow's milk hypersensitivity with fatal anaphylactic reaction (Parish *et al.*, 1960). The age pattern has been used as a telling argument against suffocation as a mechanism of death, the impression being that such a mechanism would be more apt to occur in the younger infant (Judge, 1953).

The occurrence of five cases over the age of one year calls attention to the particular problem of whether such cases are cot deaths, and the general problem of unexpected and pathologically unexplained deaths in relatively healthy people of any age.

SEASON

There is an excess of cases in the winter in those countries or regions having a temperate climate. This is described as more frequently in winter (Valdes-Dapena, 1963), an excess in winter (Carpenter and Shaddick, 1965), infrequent in summer and commonest in winter (Johnstone and Lowy, 1966), and a winter peak (Gunther, 1966). Brisbane, Australia, has a sub-tropical climate and cases studied there showed no seasonal incidence, but a tendency to occur in groups (O'Reilly and Whiley, 1967). Clustering of cases on a single day was noted in a Canadian study. Furthermore, this individual day cluster occurred throughout the year and in different localities. Those instances of case clustering on a single day in the December–March period are associated with a sharp drop in temperature from low to lower (Steele, Kraus and Langworth, 1967). New York City has a temperate climate, but autumn tends to be milder and spring quite variable though generally inclement and cool to cold. This is particularly true of March. The figures are tabulated by the month for the two year period from September 1964 to September 1966 (Table 2). Grouped by whatever preference, there is seen to be a high

TABLE 2

Monthly Incidence of Cot Deaths:
September 1964 to August 1966

Month	Number of cases
January	9
February	10
March	17
April	15
May	7
June	7
July	3
August	1
September	4
October	3
November	12
December	12

plateau from November to April and a decided decreased incidence in the summer months. This increased 'winter' incidence is not due to a larger number of children at risk. It has generally been the basis for the infectious disease aetiology concept. One investigator has offered the concept of a relationship between a preceding winter (first trimester of pregnancy) maternal disease with a subsequent viral antigen–antibody fatal mechanism in the cot death infant in the subsequent winter (Gunther, 1966).

TIME OF DEATH

Over 90 per cent of our cases died sometime between the early evening hours of one day and the late morning hours of the next.

Because of the indeterminate nature of when death took place, it is not possible to be more exact. Close questioning of many parents who checked their child during the night reveals their inability to be certain if it was alive at these intermediate times. Most often the infant was found dead when the parents went to awaken it for the morning feeding. There are such a fair number of cases with a documented time of death sprinkled throughout the bedtime period to suggest that death occurs at all times with a moderate preponderance in the early morning hours (midnight to 4 am). These general findings are similar to other studies (Valdes-Dapena, 1963; Stowens, 1966). The time interval of death has been recorded in 11 out of 66 cases (Steele, Kraus and Langworth, 1967). This must be a minimum percentage, since these deaths are quiet and do not announce themselves and are therefore noted and hence recordable only when the parent discovers the dead infant.

MATERNAL FACTORS

Steele and Langworth (1966) noted a lower maternal age for the first pregnancy, a higher incidence of maternal smoking, a higher incidence in the cot death child of a birth weight under 2,500 g and a gestation period under 37 weeks. Stowens (1966) states that the condition is more common in premature infants. One study found that a higher percentage of SUD mothers were college-educated than the percentage at large (Steele, Kraus and Langworth, 1967). The many diverse elements of income, ethnic minority problems and housing conditions render judgment difficult in our estimation, but one investigator has summed up these and other factors and described it as a lower standard of mothering (Banks, 1966). While there may be some validity to this general remark, our experience has been that the cot death infant is generally well developed, well nourished and shows no signs of physical abuse or neglect. These statements do not contradict one another, but in either case, no light is shed on the problem.

SOCIO-ECONOMIC STATUS

The definition of social class and/or economic group is difficult in anything but general terms. We have relied upon the determination of the ethnic group, the apparent family income and the physical make-up of the living quarters. Valdes-Dapena (1963) found cot deaths four times more common in non-Caucasians and generally in a lower income group. Carpenter and Shaddick (1965), using the criterion of the social class of the chief wage earner, found it to be lower in the cot death case. They also noted that there were more persons per room in cot death cases. Fifty-six per cent of our cases were Negroes and 25 per cent were Puerto Rican. In general, these cases came from ghetto areas and very often from the poorer districts. However, approximately 30 per cent of our cases came from middle class and better homes, Caucasian and non-Caucasian.

PREMONITORY SYMPTOMS AND MODE OF DEATH

The pattern of a relatively healthy, well-developed and well-nourished child being found dead in bed or baby carriage by a parent or other member of the family is monotonously repeated in the cot death cases. A very small number are found in a terminal state and then rushed to a nearby municipal hospital. Most of these infants are dead on arrival, or die almost immediately after arrival. When one questions these parents, the possibility of the infant being in fact dead upon discovery in bed and then being rushed in desperation to a hospital becomes very real. A small number of cases are observed to die. These deaths sometimes occur in the mother's arms. Observation as used here does not strictly mean visualization of the moment of death, but rather that the infant was noticed to have become dead while in the presence of adults. We have two such cases, and Johnstone and Lowy (1966) comment on twelve. They are similar in all respects to the 'classic' cot death and we so classify them. They afford added evidence that cot deaths are unattended by any unusual terminal signs or symptoms. These cases suggest a relatively rapid terminal event, although this is strictly an unproved point for cot deaths as a whole. There are, however, a large number of classic cases in which the child has died within an hour of having last been checked and found alive and normal.

These children are invariably healthy prior to death (Valdes-Dapena, 1963). Several investigators have noticed the presence of a preceding upper respiratory infection (URI) (Johnstone and Lowy, 1966) and one study showed a two-fold increase of URI in cot death cases over a matched living controlled series (Carpenter and Shaddick, 1965). These symptoms have been regarded as insignificant and certainly not such as would herald an overwhelming infection (Banks, 1966). An overwhelming infection is postulated because of the dramatic life-to-death turn of events clinically and the general negative autopsy evidence of an infectious process. However, Gunther (1966) has noted in a sudden death study in twins that, whereas 42 per cent had recent symptoms, the autopsy in these cases

7

was still negative. Our experience is in accordance with Banks' remarks, in that we have not discerned any significant recent signs or symptoms in the cot death cases. This data does not lend itself to proper quantification as it is subjective, retrospective and in many cases involves questioning parents who are emotionally confused by the mysterious death of a healthy child.

PATHOLOGY: GROSS AND MICROSCOPIC

Valdes-Dapena (1963) notes that, on autopsy with subsequent indicated laboratory investigations, a cause of death is found in 16 per cent of cot death cases. In 5 per cent of cases the basic lesion is demonstrable on gross examination. We have found 7 gross lesions in our 141 cases (5 per cent): 4 of these were cardiac (2 transpositions of the great vessels, neonatal myocarditis, endocardial fibro-elastosis) and 3 primarily infectious (bilateral adrenal haemorrhages in meningococcaemia, bilateral purulent otitis media and an acute laryngo-tracheo-bronchitis). Questioning of the parents of the 7 children did elucidate a variety of minimal symptoms, all generally referable to the respiratory tract and/or poor feeding, but all in no way dramatically different from the histories of many other autopsy-negative cot death cases.

Grossly, one category which must be borne in mind is the battered child in whom there is no external evidence of trauma on careful examination. It should be emphasized here that clinical histories in these cases are often purposely confabulated and that many times the injury is of a blunt force type and may escape external detection (Luke, Lyons and Devlin, 1967).

A number of investigators have noted a variety of histological changes at autopsy. Pulmonary changes have consisted of upper respiratory tract inflammation (Valdes-Dapena, 1963; Handforth, 1959), intra-alveolar large mononuclear cells with an explosive desquamation of bronchial epithelial cells (Gunther, 1966) and mild diffuse alveolar over-distension accompanied by pulmonary oedema with a 15 per cent incidence of petechiae (Stowens, 1966). We have seen all these changes, alone or in combination, and generally minimal in degree, in a distinct minority of our cases. The data does not allow for quantification and affords no pertinent positive information. No morphological basis for any presumptive or definitive diagnosis, such as bronchiolitis, laryngospasm, laryngitis (Huntington and Jarzynka, 1962), croup or interstitial pneumonitis is seen. Stowens (1966) comments that in cot death cases there is a decrease in the number of eosinophils in the thymus, a retention of infantile characteristics by the thymus and a diffuse swelling of the arterioles in many organs manifested by a thickened vascular wall. We do not find any of these changes in our cases.

The further question of thymic change is raised by the proposition of status thymicolymphaticus and/or a deranged thymic–adrenal mechanism. We agree with Stowens (1966) that the thymus weights are relative to the general health, cause of death and rapidity of death in a child. We have a small number of sudden traumatic death cases in the cot death age range. These control cases have thymus weights no different from those found in our cot death cases. The adrenals were part of an investigation we conducted on cot deaths (Lyons, Devlin and Helpern, 1967). Adrenal glands were removed at autopsy, stripped of all fat and weighed immediately on an analytical balance. Matched against controls, there was no significant difference of wet weights between the two sets. Status thymicolymphaticus remains a controversial issue. Whether one believes such a condition exists, we note the stated morphological definition as a large thymus, small adrenals and lymph nodes, hypoplasia of the aorta, generalized thinness and 'fragility' of blood vessels with particular reference to cerebral vessels and a smooth 'marble like' skin. We have never seen this constellation of findings in our cot death cases. The lymph nodes and spleens will of course show a difference in follicular structure from the mature histological state until after the third or fourth month. In short, we find no morphological evidence to incriminate the thymus in cot death cases.

We find no evidence for gastric aspiration. Although not uncommonly found, it is invariably limited to the larynx and upper trachea, has no mechanical obstructive features, is associated with no gross microscopic inflammatory response and is regarded as agonal. It has been determined that gastric contents can move from the stomach to the trachea in the post-mortem period.

Cardiac pathologists have demonstrated no myocardial cell lesion but have presented equivocal data on conduction system changes (Fraggott, Lynas and Marshall, 1968; Davies, 1968; James, 1968). It has been claimed that the neonate heart has an increased sensitivity to norepinephrine due to an under-developed sympathetic system, and further, that the AV node allows a more rapid propagation of the impulse to the ventricle and could be responsible for ventricular fibrillation (Davies, 1968). James (1968) has described resorptive changes in the left portion of the His bundle and the left margin of the AV node. These changes were, however, present in some controlled cases. It is now becoming clearer that there is a structural remodelling of the conduction system in the infant heart.

9

When in childhood this process is completed and whether there are functionally unstable states is not known. Haemorrhage and degeneration have been described in cardiac ganglia and nerves and endothelial proliferation noted in the sinus node artery (James, 1968). This data is difficult to evaluate, but it would seem that considerably more information is needed on the transient and fatal or otherwise arrhythmias in the cot death age period of the infant. This should be coupled with an extensive analysis of the conduction system in the first year of life, both in cot death cases and normal controls. The hypotheses that some cot deaths are caused by inherited conduction anomalies has not been proved.

Cardiac electrolyte imbalances have been described and refuted in cot death cases (Fraggott, Lynas and Marshall, 1968). Particular attention has been given to calcium. Adult human studies (myocardial infarction, arrhythmias) and considerable animal experiments have documented the production of fatal arrhythmias by various electrolyte disturbances. The nature and rôle of any one or more of the essential elements in sudden fatal cardiac arrhythmia and/or cardiac power failure is a field of active current investigation in human cardiology. Although, as stated, no positive data has been advanced in cot death cases, no large specific study has been done to allow a definite answer to this question.

One study advanced data that the parathyroids are absent in cot death cases. Other studies have not corroborated this finding. The demonstration of fusion of parathyroids to thymus in cot deaths has now also been noted in otherwise explained infant deaths. It is apparently a structural variant and presumably has no significance.

Nasopharyngeal obstruction, coupled with obligatory mouth breathing in a given infant, has been claimed as a cause of cot death. The infant, when placed in such a position or situation wherein it cannot breathe through its mouth, would suffocate. The nasopharyngeal abnormality can be studied either by gross inspection or by radiography. The findings have not been uniformly corroborated and the arguments against suffocation are likewise valid here. It has been noted that, with the development of adenoidal (and tonsillar) tissue sufficient to impede posterior nasopharyngeal air passage, children can develop a hypoventilation syndrome. This occurs in a somewhat older paediatric group and generally associates with a clinical picture and some structural evidence of pulmonary hypertension. Whether it does occur in any of the cot death cases without overt signs of pathology is not known.

Beckwith has described a focal area of fibrinoid necrosis in the vocal cords. The change occurs at a point halfway between the arytenoid cartilages and the apex of the laryngeal lumen anteriorly. The hypothesis would revolve around a fatal laryngospasm and can include a URI, sleep and constitutional autonomic reactivity. Laryngospasm, like fatal cardiac arrhythmia, has been used as a mechanism of death relative to this lesion, as well as other lesions described in the laryngo-tracheobronchial tree. The presence and incidence of the laryngeal lesion has varied considerably in certain studies, and a comparable related matched control series is not available. Whether the lesion is simply produced by crying has not been clarified.

Acute epiglottitis is now a well recognized paediatric entity. With emergency roentgenological evaluation, it is being diagnosed and treated effectively. It has not been documented as a cause of cot death.

Cervical spine epidural haemorrhage, minimal to moderate in amount, has been reported in cot death cases. This has been seen by other investigators and ourselves in a minority of such cases. We have seen similar haemorrhage in controlled studies (and also in certain adult cases) and have presumed it to be secondary or agonal. There are no underlying spinal cord changes nor any overlying pathology of the vertebrae or its ligaments.

Many individual studies note a single new pathological finding, e.g. in one-third of cot death cases there is an unexplained colloid depletion of the thyroid follicles. Since I find it impossible to evaluate the separate and generally uncorroborated findings, and since merely to list them in summary fashion would more likely confuse than enlighten, I am not considering such data in this article.

VIRUS ISOLATION

In general, most studies have not recovered a virus. Johnstone and Lowy (1966) were unable to culture a virus in 47 cases. Valdes-Dapena (1963) notes a similar pattern, whereas one investigation (Gold et al., 1961) found enteroviruses in 12 of 48 cases. Parish et al. (1964) cultured fresh autopsy cot death tissues in 8 cases with negative results. Such a procedure avoids the indeterminate deleterious effect of freezing known to kill the respiratory syncytial virus of epidemic infantile bronchiolitis and quite probably other viruses. We have recovered one pathogenic virus (Coxsackie), several polio viruses in the ileum and otherwise a completely negative result in 110 cases. All our tissues were frozen. It would seem clear by now that with 'standard' virus isolation procedures the results in cot death cases will be uniformly negative.

BACTERIA

Valdes-Dapena (1963) states that bacteriological studies are essentially negative and, furthermore, that when a presumed pathogen is isolated from post-mortem tissue, the absence of an inflammatory reaction raises the question of significance. Whether this latter finding can be gainsaid under the heading of overwhelming sepsis is unanswered if not unanswerable. Johnstone and Lowy (1966), on the other hand, found a bacterial pathogen in 37 out of 56 cases, the offender being usually a *Pneumococcus, Klebsiella pneumoniae*, or *Staphylococcus pyogenes*. These were pure or predominant cultures. A relevant problem is the fact that many cot deaths take place sometime in the night between the last evening feeding (generally between 7 and 10 pm) and their discovery sometime around 8 am the next day. Accordingly, there is the problem of post-mortem bacterial overgrowth, and particularly if there has been terminal or agonal tracheal aspiration of gastric contents.

We recovered a presumed pathogenic organism in 13 cases: 6 were from the lung (*Klebsiella* type 1 and type 2, Haemolytic *Staphylococcus*, 2 *Staphylococcus aureus* coagulase +, and *Pneumococcus* type 1–33); 3 were from a purulent otitis media (type 3 *Pneumococcus, Staphylococcus aureus* coagulase +, and *Streptococcus viridans*) and 4 were from the stool with positive liver and spleen in two of these (3 *E. coli* serotype 0127 and 1 *E. coli* serotype 0111). These were either pure cultures or predominant organism growth. We consider them basically pathogenic organisms, although the question of disease production for the *E. coli* organisms is debatable. Except for the otitis media cases, there was a minimal to no inflammatory response. In many other cases, the problem of obvious post-mortem bacterial overgrowth, with particular reference to the lung, made interpretation of laboratory data impossible.

SERUM GAMMA GLOBULIN

In 1954 Spain stated that the serum gamma globulins in three cot deaths were lower (0·150, 0·180 and 0·183 g/100 ml) than in two control cases (0·5 and 0·6 g/100 ml). This was an exceedingly attractive piece of data, as it demarcated an unusually low gamma globulin for cot deaths in the period of known physiological hypogammaglobulinaemia. Several studies (Valdes-Dapena, Eichman and Ziskin, 1963; Coe and Hartman, 1960) have now appeared, however, which deal with a considerably larger number of cases. Valdes-Dapena,

Eichman and Ziskin, in the largest studied group, noted a mean serum gamma globulin level of 0.665 ± 0.04 g per cent in cot deaths as opposed to 0.595 ± 0.07 in normal living control infants. These studies have been concerned only with gamma-G, but subsequent studies demonstrated normal levels of serum gamma-A and gamma-M (Balduzzi, Vaughan and Greendyke, 1968). The infant's gamma-G (Rosen and Janeway, 1964) is almost exclusively derived from the mother, and, until approximately the third month, the infant's lymphoid system is generally under-developed as regards plasma cells, and does not make any appreciable gamma-G. The infant can make gamma-A and gamma-M. This level of gamma-G partially explains the high incidence of Gram negative infections in children under three months of age. Recent studies have demonstrated an elevation of IgG and IgM in 15 per cent of cot death cases (Balduzzi, Vaughan and Greendyke, 1968). IgM increases have now been well demonstrated in the neonate and young infant as diagnostic data of an *in utero* foetal response to a maternal infection. No data is available on IgA in tissue.

SUFFOCATION

Suffocation was the generally presumed cause of many cot deaths until the early 1940s. The better delineation of the condition has, to a large extent, negated this cause. The age incidence with the relative peak in the third to fourth month and the preponderance of cases being over six weeks of age argues against suffocation (Judge, 1953).

Woolley (1945) demonstrated that infants will all respond to an experimentally contrived smothering by rolling over and continuing to breathe well. We have seen cases of suffocation in infants with the use of plastic mattress covers and objects sucked into, or placed in, the mouth of the infant. In either instance, the airway is mechanically blocked by the offending material being trapped in the mouth and pharynx. We have also had cases where infants were suffocated by sleeping parents rolling over and lying on them when they are in the same bed. Although the number of petechiae, external and visceral in distribution and particularly in the conjunctivae, usually attend the infant suffocation case, we have had many such cases with no conjunctival petechiae and a few with absent visceral petechiae. Handforth (1959) produced temporary respiratory obstruction in rats which then caused fatal apnoea. This, plus the finding of minimal upper respiratory tract inflammation in 12 autopsied cot deaths and

13

a seasonal incidence similar to croup and/or laryngeal spasm, led him to postulate a similar mechanism in cot death cases.

We find no evidence in our cases for mechanical asphyxiation.

HYPERSENSITIVITY

Hypersensitivity to milk in particular, or to viruses, bacteria or other foreign proteins, became an important consideration as an aetiology and/or mechanism of death with the paper of Parish *et al.* in 1960. The cow's milk hypersensitivity proposal is based on the contention that (1) cot death infants are invariably bottle-fed; (2) there is a higher level of serum antibodies to milk protein in cot death cases; (3) cow's milk can be demonstrated in the cot death case lung; (4) the mechanism of death would be anaphylactic and hence sudden, unexpected and apparently natural; and (5) there is an animal model that re-creates the proposed aetiology, mechanism and mode of death. Cot death infants are invariably bottle-fed. The data does not lend itself well to summary, but can be brought into focus by the fact that, in one study (Carpenter and Shaddick, 1965), in only 4 cases out of 1,090 was a breast-feed the last feed before death in a cot death case. Matched control living cases were breast-fed longer than cot death cases, but here we are dealing with statistical patterns. There were cot death cases that were breast-fed for the first two or three weeks and then shifted to bottle. The level of serum antibodies to cow's milk protein in cot deaths and varied control cases remains unresolved. Parish *et al.* (1960) found a slightly higher titre in 24 cot deaths, as compared to 286 normal children. Subsequently, Johnstone and Lowy (1966) and Gold and Adelson (1964) found no significant difference between their cot death and control series. Gold and Adelson in addition found no difference in antibody titres between well babies on cow's milk or on a mother's milk.

Parish *et al.* (1964), in later work, demonstrated the presence of cow's milk protein in the lung of 25 out of 60 cot deaths, and only 8 out of 25 normal control. The problem of non-specific and non-deleterious aspiration of gastric contents by any infant beclouds these findings. Guinea pigs sensitized to cow's milk were challenged by Parish with cot deaths' gastric contents. The material was placed in the tracheo-bronchial tree of the lightly anaesthetized animal and produced a quiet death in 15 of 19 animals. There was no reaction in unsensitized animals. A later prototype baboon experiment conducted along these lines was essentially negative. The meaning of all this data, contradictory or otherwise, is difficult to discern. The guinea pig experiment remains as a provocative piece of information, but the entire area remains currently unsettled.

14

Hypersensitivity, although postulated to involve any foreign protein, has concerned itself strictly with cow's milk. Gunther (1966) has, however, proposed an antigen–antibody complex as the agent of biological trauma in cot deaths. The rôle of these complexes is now well recognized in several human diseases. Studies on rubella infections occurring in pregnancy have demonstrated the presence of fresh virus in the serum and/or tissues of the infant. The viral antigen may then be involved in a complex in the reactive infant. The position is speculative, but the bases are relatively recent and no data has been collected in this area in cot death cases.

MISCELLANEOUS SPECULATION

Valdes-Dapena (1963) mentioned a hypersensitive vagal reflex triggered by a minimal laryngitis and promoting pulmonary oedema and/or cardiac arrest. Porter (1966) postulated a subclinical amino acid disorder, coupled with an immature neonatal liver and an overwhelming of the body with exogenous proteins. We studied the adrenals (Lyons, Devlin and Helpern, 1967), measuring their wet weight and cholesterol and cortisol content. This was based on the presumption of a pathological exaggeration of the adrenal diurnal rhythm. Data, though suggestive, was not definitive.

PARTICULAR FORENSIC ASPECTS

Depending upon the thoroughness with which clinical data is gathered, the forensic pathologist will be able to distinguish the presumed cot death case from the case that appears different or unusual. In our experience, we have encountered few unnatural death cases among our presumed cot death cases. Suffocation (rolling over cases), as previously noted, can sometimes be impossible of detection at an autopsy and the evolving clinical history has supplied the answer in most instances. Blunt force trauma to the infant's abdomen with minimal external bruising can be missed in the absence of an autopsy. X-rays may or may not demonstrate old or fresh fractures of different ages. Accidental trauma in the context of this review would only mean head trauma with subdural haematoma or cerebral contusion. The infant, when he falls from a moderate height (cot, bed, dresser), generally lands on his head and hence such localized injury occurs. Depending upon the parents' concern, the incident may be overlooked or forgotten. For whatever reasons, although we have seen such cases in general, they have not presented in a cot death setting. Accidental poisoning is a distinct possibility as the infant becomes mobile. We have not detected gross evidence of a toxic compound, nor, on a small number of random cot death studies, have we chemically detected any toxic compound. A general unknown toxicological investigation of a certain number of these cases would appear a necessary study. Homicide, whether by poisoning or suffocation, has not been a factor in our studies nor in the literature in general. Neonatocide and infanticide have been studied with particular attention to the mother's mental status. This entire area, relative to the cot death cases, has been virtually unexplored. No one would consider it a major entity, but the fact of its occurrence and incidence in the sudden unexplained death in children should be defined.

SUMMARY AND CONCLUSION

Valdes-Dapena and Stone in the United States and Banks in Great Britain are representative of the numerous investigators who have gathered together previous material and made additional individual contributions concerning cot deaths. We have added our current experience to this data and, in general, note a concordance of findings in all the larger series of cases. The conclusions then, as stated, are based on the integration of these previous studies and our own.

Cot deaths are a major cause of death in infants in the first six months of life. Adequate circumstantial investigation and complete pathological study will provide a cause of death in 10–15 per cent of cases. The male preponderance, the age spread of six weeks to six months, the time of death in the evening, the apparent quiet mode of death, and the 'lower' socio-economic standard of the family are attested to in all major studies. Less striking, but generally agreed upon, is the seasonal incidence in the colder months, an age incidence peak of three to four months, and certain maternal and gestation data which are principally prematurity and bottle feeding.

Hypersensitivity to cow's milk protein is the only cause of death that has been proposed and partially supported by human and animal experimental data. The hypothesis has been critically contended and the issue is unsettled. Fatal cardiac arrhythmias or power failure, a sudden fatal respiratory event, overwhelming infectious process with or without emphasis on shock (endotoxic?), these and several other lesser hypotheses are basically unproved at the moment. Whether more intensive microbiological investigation will provide an aetiological agent is a moot point.

The forensic pathologist must be well aware of cot death cases. In larger jurisdictions where a fair number of such cases will be seen the problem is not to overlook the conditions that may pass for it. Where a smaller number of forensic cases are seen, and consequently few cot death cases handled, the forensic pathologist must substantiate the diagnosis. The enigma of a 'healthy' infant dying in this way must be explained to the parents and to the authorities. This 'clearing of the air' will dispel considerable grief and misgiving on the part of the parents, and will prevent unduly provocative investigations or other actions on the part of the law enforcement agencies.

This review has attempted a balanced presentation of the data and speculations and the conclusions that relate to them. Two salient points emerge. First, the routine approach or handling of cot death cases has probably yielded all the practical information that it can. New data toward the resolution of the overall problem must relate to a better knowledge of the normal for this period of life, and this, by necessity, must entail a wider approach involving multiple medical and/or scientific disciplines. Secondly, it is now obvious that cot death as an entity is emerging as a major cause of death in the paediatric age group and deserves considerably more attention.

REFERENCES

Balduzzi, P. C., Vaughan, J. H. and Greendyke, R. M. (1968). 'Immunoglobin levels in sudden unexpected death in infants.' *J. Pediat*, **72**, 689.

Banks, A. L. (1966). 'Enquiry into sudden death in infancy.' *Can. J. publ. Hlth.*, **57**, 328.

Carpenter, R. G. and Shaddick, C. W. (1965). 'Rôle of infection, suffocation and bottle feeding in cot death.' *Br. J. prev. soc. Med.*, **19**, 1.

Coe, J. I. and Hartman, E. E. (1960). 'Sudden, unexpected death in infancy.' *J. Am. med. Ass.*, **56**, 786.

Dawes, G. (1968). 'Sudden death in babies: physiology of the fetus and newborn.' *Am. J. Cardiol.*, **22**, 469.

Fraggott, P., Lynas, M. A. and Marshall, T. K. (1968). 'Sudden death in babies: epidemiology.' *Am. J. Cardiol.*, **22**, 457.

Gold, E. and Adelson, L. (1964). 'The rôle of antibody to cow's milk proteins in the sudden death syndrome.' *Pediatrics, Springfield*, **33**, 541.

— Carver, D. H., Heineberg, H., Adelson, L. and Robbins, F. C. (1961). 'Viral infection: a possible cause of sudden, unexpected death in infants.' *New Engl. J. Med.*, **264**, 53.

Gunther, M. (1966). 'Cot deaths: anaphylactic reaction after uterine infection as potential cause.' *Lancet*, **1**, 912.

Huntington, R. W. and Jarzynka, J. J. (1962). 'Sudden and unexpected death in infancy with special reference to the so-called crib death.' *Am. J. clin. Path.*, **38**, 637.

James, T. (1968). 'Sudden death in babies: new observations in the heart.' *Am. J. Cardiol.*, **22**, 479.

Johnstone, J. M. and Lowy, H. S. (1966). 'Rôle of infection in cot deaths.' *Br. med. J.*, **1**, 706.

Judge, J. D. (1953). 'Sudden and unexpected death in infancy.' *Postgrad. Med.*, **14**, 79.

Luke, J. L., Lyons, M. M. and Devlin, J. F. (1967). 'Pediatric forensic pathology. 1: Death by homicide.' *J. forens. Sci.*, **12**, 421.

Lyons, M. M., Devlin, J. F. and Helpern, M. (1967). 'Adrenal studies in crib death: preliminary report.' Paper presented at VII Congress of International Academy of Legal Medicine and Social Medicine, Budapest.

Handforth, C. R. (1959). 'Sudden, unexpected deaths in infants.' *Can. med. Ass. J.*, **80**, 872.

O'Reilly, M. J. J. and Whiley, M. K. (1967). 'Cot deaths in Brisbane.' *Med. J. Aust.*, **2**, 1084.

Parish, W. E., Barrett, A. M., Coombs, R. R. A., Gunther, M. and Camps, F. (1960). 'Hypersensitivity to milk and sudden death in infancy.' *Lancet*, **2**, 1106.

— Richards, C. B., France, N. E. and Coombs, R. R. A. (1964). 'Further investigations on the hypothesis that some cases of cot death are due to a modified anaphylactic reaction to cow's milk.' *Int. Archs. Allergy appl. Immun.*, **24**, 215.

Porter, A. M. W. (1966). 'Unexpected cot deaths.' *Lancet*, **1**, 914.

Rosen, F. S. and Janeway, C. A. (1964). 'Immunological competence of the newborn infant.' *Pediatrics, Springfield*, **33**, 159.

Spain, D. M., Bradess, V. A. and Greenblatt, I. J. (1954). 'Possible factor in sudden and unexpected death during infancy.' *J. Am. med. Ass.*, **156**, 246.

Steele, R. and Langworth, J. T. (1966). 'The relationship of antenatal and postnatal factors to sudden unexpected death in infancy.' *Can. med. Ass. J.*, **94**, 1165.

— Kraus, A. and Langworth, J. (1967). 'Sudden, unexpected death in infancy in Ontario: Parts I and II.' *Can. J. publ. Hlth.*, **58**, 359.

Stowens, D. (1966). *Pediatric Pathology*. 2nd Edn. Baltimore: Williams and Wilkins.

Valdes-Dapena, M. A. (1963). 'Sudden and unexpected death in infants.' *Pediat. Clins. N. Am.*, **10**, 693.

— Eichman, M. F. and Ziskin, L. (1963). 'Sudden and unexpected death in infants I: Gamma globulin levels in the serum.' *J. Pediat.*, **63**, 290.

Wooley, P. V. (1945). 'Mechanical suffocation during infancy.' *J. Pediat.*, **26**, 579.

2 Child Abuse—The Battered Baby

KEITH SIMPSON

INTRODUCTION

Children have been killed at birth, neglected, starved or abandoned, chastised with cruelty, even to death, for as long as history is recorded. The Schools of Sumer, five thousand years ago, had 'a man in charge of the whip', Romans beat their boys with the ferule, and Eton's headmaster of Elizabethan times was noted for scourging his pupils with 'four apple twigs'. Lady Abergane beat her child of seven and threw it so violently to the ground that its skull was fractured and it died. It was not until the European reformers such as John Colet of St. Paul's School, Roger L'Estrange, with his 'The Children's Petition', John Frank with his eighteenth century laws curbing the punishment of children, and the NSPCC foundation in 1859, that uncivilized savagery of children was itself punished. Nevertheless, cruelty to infants remained a blot on nineteenth century social progress. The more strange, therefore, that when Caffey stumbled across the syndrome to which his name became attached in 1946, he missed its real significance: as a paediatric radiologist he was diverted from the real issue to thoughts of bone fragility. It was left to Silverman (1953) to define the frankly traumatic nature of the subdural haematoma and long bone deformities of Caffey, and to Wooley and Evans (1955) to establish the wilful cruelty that these injuries reflected. What had been a comparatively uncommon eponymous episode became a major paediatric, social and medico-legal problem.

Henry Kempe, who coined the electric phrase 'the battered child syndrome', awakened both American and European schools to the grave dangers to which thousands of infants were exposed—and the alarming frequency with which children at risk, gravely hurt, even dead, were mistakenly regarded as accidentally injured. The American Academy of Paediatrics' national survey in 1961 and the statistics disclosed by the American Humane Society—662 cases in one year in the USA alone—finally defined the problem as a major concern of

19

doctors and society. Statistical studies of infant death in the first decade show clearly that though cases of wilful baby battering did of course occur prior to Caffey's observations, it was not a common scourge until after World War II. The British Paediatric Association did not publish a general warning memorandum until 1966, following the interest aroused by the English reports of cases, from the first by Griffiths and Moynahan in 1963; but pathologists whose records go back prior to 1945/46 will find occasional child murder cases which fit the current conception of the 'battered baby'. These were indeed few as compared with the stream that started to flow in the post-war period, and has continued unabated.

FREQUENCY

Statistics seldom reveal the whole substance of any problem, and those for criminal offences fall notably short of real totals. A very large number of cases of child abuse remain unrevealed because the victim has no way of communicating its misery even to the doctor. Only the ugly scum of the severely injured or the dead can be counted. Even then the evasive lying that is a feature of the syndrome, the skilled assistance in legal representation given by counsel whose duty it is—if they are willing to undertake it—to present their client's case in as favourable a light as possible, and the disinclination of the Crown to prosecute suspect parents or guardians in the absence of some corroborative or circumstantial evidence in support of the medical findings, make it all too likely that the facts will never become statistics. Magistrates are notoriously difficult to convince that such cruelty can possibly exist—faced as they are with ordinary-looking parents denying any knowledge of wilful violence and eager to proffer alternative accidental explanations.

Children's departments and pathologists may well despair of any prosecution, far less a conviction for frank criminal violence when the case rests wholly on the medical evidence.

It is quite clear, however, that the offence of wilful child abuse amounting to 'baby battering' is very common indeed. Many cases of fractured skull or ribs, subdural bleeding, transient blindness or permanent brain damage of obscure origin, have their roots in violence at the hands of parent or guardian, and surveys in Canada, the USA and in England, have brought to light much of the hidden mass of this classic syndrome. Kempe (1971) estimated that 3 in every 1,000 children suffered serious injury, both in the United Kingdom and USA, from 'parent bashing'. His most careful survey of English experience during 1970 also estimated that only 5 per cent of all cases known to social agencies, doctors and hospitals ever reach Court.

Estimates based on the 1964–66 surveys of 14 USA state statistics (the first years of legislation on reporting of infant abuse) suggested that a rate of 36·7 per million was a likely figure. In the USA population of 195 million, the annual incidence of child abuse would thus total 7,158 reported incidents. These were based on the Brandel's University (Massachusetts) definition of child abuse: 'Non-accidental physical attack or physical injury including minimal as well as fatal injury, inflicted upon children by person caring for them' (Gill, 1968).

The study figures in the USA have always shown that high population density is accompanied by a high rate of incidence, and the same feature emerges from the smaller English studies (RSPCC, 1969; Cameron, 1970). For instance, the regional distribution reported by the National Opinion Research Centre of Chicago University was as shown in Table 1.

TABLE 1

	1960 census		NORC survey 1965	
New England	10·5	5·8	3	6·25
Middle Atlantic	34·3	19·1	11	22·92
E. North Central	36·3	20·1	13	27·08
W. North Central	15·4	8·6	4	8·33
South Atlantic	26·1	14·4	0	0·00
E. South Central	12·1	6·7	4	8·33
W. South Central	17·0	9·5	4	8·33
Mountain	7·0	3·9	2	4·17
Pacific	21·4	11·9	3	6·25
Unknown	—	—	—	—

In the USA a survey of 71 hospitals in a one-year period revealed records of 302 cases, of which 33 died and 85 suffered permanent brain damage. Another survey by 77 district attorneys reported 447 cases in one year, of which 45 died and 29 had permanent brain damage. As in trauma and in poisoning statistics in general, about one in ten hospitalized cases dies: no one can calculate the unreported —indeed undiscoverable—baby batterings that occur secretly at home. The NSPCC in England note, in an account in 1969 of 78 children under four suffering serious physical abuse, that 35,000 of 37,000 infant cases investigated by them each year never come to police or court notice.

Sex Incidence

Sex distribution studies have consistently shown a rather higher incidence among boys. Simons and Downs of the Columbia University School in a 1966 Public Health Survey, the NORC (1965) and a Press Survey in America, all reported boy victims in 53–54 per cent of all incidents, reaching (Press Survey) 59·2 per cent boys in fatal cases.

Age Incidence

Age distribution varies in survey studies a little more and particularly in the statistics of pathologists (reporting only fatalities). The bigger studies of de Francis (1963) (662 cases of a Press Survey) showing 56 per cent under 4 years of age, and of Simons and Downs (313 New York children) showing 28 per cent under 1 year, 41 per cent 1–5 years, 23 per cent 5–10 years, and 8 per cent 10 or over, reflect common experience. 'About 25 per cent are under one year, and 55 per cent five years: less than 20 per cent are over five years', is a quotation that is easy to remember and not far from general experience. The peak incidence of all cases is in the region of two to five years—and of fatal cases up to one to two years, reflecting the lethal gravity of serious injury in the infant. Hospital studies, and in particular pathologists' statistics, are weighted too much on fatalities to reflect the overall incidence.

Race Incidence

Race has not been studied so extensively, though where proportionate population incidences is known (the statistics of Schloesser, 1964), the figures are not significant. Whites, coloureds and mixed races all have their similar problems, and it is social and educational rather than racial conditions that engender violence.

The Perpetrator

The perpetrator has been more extensively studied by the socioeconomist. About 80 per cent of children reported in the NORC survey were living with their parents, and about half of the cases occurred in families of two or three children (60 per cent have one or two children). Wedlock or not seems to have little significance.

The peak age of perpetrator is around 25. De Francis' series of 662 cases gave a peak at 26 years. Simons and Downs' New York City study of 313 children showed:

Under 20	9·2 per cent
20 to 25	26·6 per cent
26 to 35	25·6 per cent
36 and over	6·8 per cent
Age not reported	31·8 per cent

Fathers tend to be a year or two older. Mothers causing fatal injury involve younger children—they are more often left alone with them.

Socio-economic studies have consistently shown the perpetrator to be more frequently in the lower education/income bracket. The NORC study showed 56·25 per cent to be 'poor', 39·58 per cent were comfortable: some 65 per cent were self-supporting. The offence is, however, to be watched for in all income groups; the plain fact is that a better education and higher income are bound to change the attitude of mind and tend to defer pressures and frustration.

More studies in parenthood loading and mother–child (or father–child) relationships against the general family background are needed. Mothers of low intelligence with increasing family and domestic strain, whose husbands have little time or inclination to support them, may well deserve sympathetic treatment. The psychiatric studies of Steele and Pollock (1968) accept the use of terms like 'immature', 'demanding', 'impulsive', 'sado-masochistic' and the like, but urge a seeking of some consistent behaviour pattern. Some parents are undoubtedly cold, schizophrenic types, but the majority are venting spleen in a frustrated sense of righteousness and an aggressive demand for discipline. The stupid, resistant, crying or dirty infant must be slapped down and corrected, and when restraint is not exercised the danger of battering is bound to arise. Of course all cases do not fit into categories: an Oxford student beat a neighbour's child to death during a voluntary baby-watching session because its crying interfered with his viewing a favourite television programme—no more.

CLINICAL DATA

It is remarkable that such a very well defined entity as the battered baby syndrome should ever escape clinical detection, but it commonly does. A certain unwillingness on the part of the family doctor to suspect parents of callous brutality towards their children, a lowering of the threshold of suspicion that is constantly necessary for the well-being of children, especially of homes in which there is domestic friction, and two classical features of the syndrome—delay in reporting symptoms and signs of hurt, and deliberately misleading explanations for the injuries—tend to divert the family doctor from the real issue.

The five classic features of the syndrome are:

(1) obscure illness or 'unexplained' injury in infants of up to four or five years—from six or eight weeks, due to . . .

23

(2) repeated abuse, physical hurt, over a period of weeks or months by . . .

(3) either or both parents, guardian or baby-sitter, who . . .

(4) fail to report or delay reporting the incidents, and who, when they do . . .

(5) mislead, indeed deliberately deceive, the nurse, doctor, NSPCC, Health or Children's Department over the cause.

There is, of course, an emotional or psychiatric stage on which these features are set, and a relationship between perpetrator and victim that needs close attention. The marital and socio-economic atmosphere is also well defined: unstable marriage, over-crowding in urban areas of middle and lower class, the struggle for security and a standard of living with the greater content it brings. Family size, the position of the victim among other siblings, race, colour and religion have little part to play. The family at risk is, indeed, a problem for the close attentions of the family doctor, his consultants in the hospital, the Children's Department, welfare and social workers, besides the pathologist and the police.

Caffey, who was himself deceived in his discovery of the syndrome in 1946 into thoughts of bone dysplasia, calcium metabolism defects and blood dyscrasia, only later recognized the real substances of his 'run' of bone injury and subdural bleeding. It was Silverman, another paediatric radiologist, then Wooley and Evans (1955), Griffiths and Moynahan (1963) in England, and a Memorandum by the British Paediatric Society in 1966 that successively delineated the real problem. The expressive words 'battered baby' were finally coined by Kempe, co-author of the only authoritative book on the subject (Helfer and Kempe, 1968).

These authors found no cause for disagreement over a single clinical item.

The children were almost all (*vide supra*) in the first, second or third year, tailing off in the fourth and fifth. Boys were slightly predominant.

The parents were mostly in their early twenties, with females predominant (if only by a little margin) over the first year and males later. Guardians might be any age.

Illegitimacy, race and religion meant little. Marital discord produced conditions of risk; drunkenness, sexual promiscuity, criminal tendencies less.

Intellectual inadequacy, immaturity, emotional instability mattered more than frank psychotic disturbances.

Overcrowding and chronic socio-economic problems might well engender an explosive situation. A minor irritation like wetting the pants may cause a sudden loss of control.

Gibbens and Walker (1956) were of the opinion that parents who had themselves had cold, unemotive parents or had been rejected, tended to be less affectionate or even frankly hostile to their own children. Phrases such as a 'defect in child maturing relationships', and also of parents 'whose stability needed a sense of mastery over their children' and of 'rigid unrelaxing discipline', have been used. Every family doctor must recognize such family groups, and it is his awareness that the infants in such homes are 'at risk' that any prospect of prevention arises.

In assessing the clinical history—the duty, after all, of the pathologist as much as the family doctor or paediatrician—an alert sensitivity to the possibility of battering, caution over evasive explanations, and a thorough clinical examination are vital. A total skeletal x-ray must be done, and an expert radiologist must read the films, for pulled epiphyses are easily overlooked. Blood dyscrasias and disorders like the Ehlers–Danlos syndrome, leukaemia, rickets and scurvy, osteogenesis imperfecta and infantile cortical hyperostosis—differentiated largely by its involvement of the mandible (unaffected in battering)—must all the excluded. It would, however, require a particular clinical blindness to overlook or misdiagnose the ordinary features of repeated battering. Mothers (or fathers) may speak of infants 'always coming out in bruises', 'falling about the place', 'pulling the furniture' on to themselves, banging their little heads or rolling into the fire, getting crushed in loving arms by a trip over a mat or a fall downstairs whilst carrying the baby—these are the very details the doctor (and the pathologist) must assess for themselves. Is this an acceptable explanation for that injury? Is this convulsion or that coma due to intracranial damage—whether or not there is something visible externally? Does the succession and timing of signs described by the parent date in accord with the physical changes found—and the x-ray dating? Parents may flush when asked to explain rib injuries some six weeks ago and a blow in the mouth that split the lips (inside) and wasn't mentioned, though it is by now some days old. Doctors and pathologists alike are pursuing enquiries in the hope of getting at the real facts: a child's safety may depend on their accuracy and skill.

THE INJURIES

Head Injuries

The original observations of Caffey in 1946 and of Silverman in 1953—both radiologists—were naturally concerned mainly with fractures and epiphyseal separations due to snatchings at arms or legs. It is true that Caffey, in the very first instance, drew attention to subdural haematoma, but the classical encysted lesion of adult life is rarely seen, and Caffey was unaware of the more common and sinister patchy subdural bleedings, cortical contusions and retinal haemorrhages that accompany violent shaking of the head, blows from the hand or fist, or throwing against upholstered furniture that may leave no skin marks.

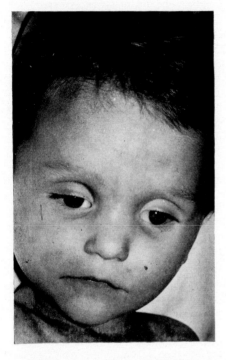

Figure 1. Typical minor injury —sole indication of severe brain contusions with subdural bleeding

Retinal and subhyaloid haemorrhages, the cause of blindness that is, fortunately, more often transient, have been described by Bodian (1964), Harcourt and Hopkins (1971) and Mushin (1971) in connection with child abuse, and Turner's work on optic nerve injury from blows on the head was at once brought to mind (1943).

It is true that Holzel and Tobin (1967) have described both retinal haemorrhages and subdural bleeding in picornavirus infections, and in a type II echo virus infection that occurred whilst in hospital care, but as Gilkes and Mann (1967) have reminded paediatricians, it is only when the history and a full examination and x-ray reveal

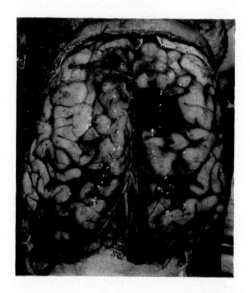

Figure 2. Surface contusions and patchy subdural bleeding

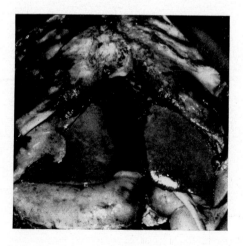

Figure 3. Characteristic liver split under bruised rib margins

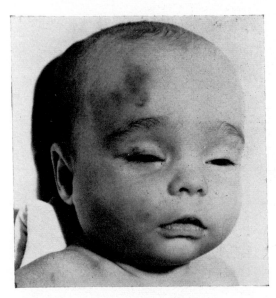

Figure 4. Surface bruising of the right brow, sole external indication of the head injury shown in Figure 5

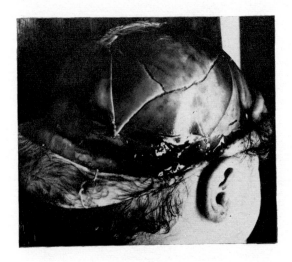

Figure 5. Heavy skull battering causing comminuted, partly depressed fracture of skull and brain injury, with intracranial bleeding

no hint of injury that such a cause may be accepted. Griffith and Dodge (1968) found abnormal electro-encephalograms in some cases of mild head injury.

Scalp bruising is more common than splitting and may easily be overlooked in coloured children or under the hair. The face is a classical area for multiple bruises, and brow, cheeks, mouth and neck are often blotchy with lesions of varying date. The lips are often bruised or split on their under surfaces against the teeth—a lesion

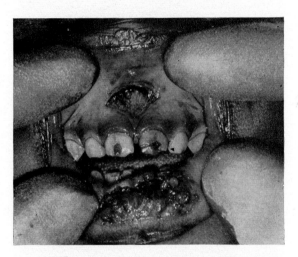

Figure 6. Characteristic lip bruises—often seen only on inspection of the reverse aspects—with mucosal and fraenum splits causing mouth bleeding

easily missed if not kept in mind. Teeth are seldom dislodged and the jaws rarely broken (Tate, 1971).

Excuses are often made for finger marks on the neck and bruised or split lips. 'I must have steadied the face by holding the neck' under the jaw or across the cheeks, and the lips 'must have got bruised (or split) when I was giving mouth-to-mouth'. It would indeed require rough handling and frenetic mouth-to-mouth pressure—but the excuse is a handy one for the lawyer who is doing his best to disturb the medical evidence. It must be resisted firmly. The reply 'I would indeed be surprised if that were the explanation' is a start, and may be followed by the remark that if this explanation were true, the hospitals and clinics receiving infants would have far more cases of split lips than they do. It is unfortunate that the paediatrician and the pathologist have to adopt such an intransigent attitude but it is induced by the support counsel gives to his clients' explanations, however ill-founded.

Multiple bruises all over the body from rough handling or beating or kicking or throwing the infant about are common: they, too, vary

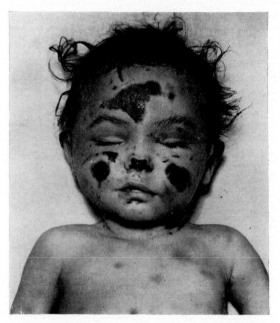

Figure 7. Facial injuries caused by beating with a belt studded with brass ornaments. Further body bruises (R. vs Ptolemy)

in date. Several of varying date should therefore be microscoped in proof.

The Ehlers–Danlos syndrome, sometimes invoked by the defence, is an inherited familiar disorder of the tissues similar to Marfan's syndrome and Hurler's syndrome types of lesion. Characteristic thin hyperpigmented scars are to be seen in the skin, and the large majority of cases do not come to light until well after the first decade. Only 3 in a series of 27 reported by Barabas in 1967 were under ten. The introduction by counsel of a suggestion of this disease being responsible for 'easy bruising' or tissue ruptures is almost certain to be a 'try-on', in the hope that the paediatrician or pathologist will not have thought of it—or possibly not even have heard of it.

The skull may show local depressed fractures where a weapon such as the heel of a shoe, the toe (from kicking), a piece of crockery, a baby's bottle or a piece of furniture, a fireside coal shovel, a broom or hammer—all seen in medico-legal autopsy experience—have been put to use. The shape of the depressed area may be significant and should be photographed to scale or kept at autopsy for later comparison. The skin is often grazed or split from a local impact. Linear or stellate fractures, more often in the temporal or parietal areas,

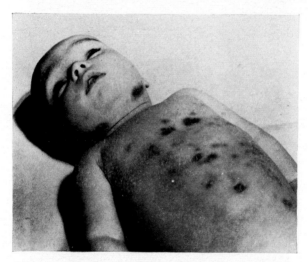

Figure 8. Multiple body bruises and 'steadying' finger marks under the lower jaw for head battering (R. vs Dean)

are the result of banging against flatter, unyielding surfaces like furniture, the wall or the floor, and squashing from side to side with symmetrical fracture when the head is already on the floor. These are particularly difficult to deny, being consistent with a trip over a mat and fall to the floor, or a 'fall downstairs with the baby in my arms', or when 'the wardrobe fell over on it', or 'the pram was tipped over by the other children', etc. The scalp is seldom grazed or split, merely bruised.

Intracranial bleeding is nearly always subdural, patchy and asymmetrical; extradural bleeding is rare in infancy. The cerebrospinal fluid is blood-stained and associated brain damage is usual. The statistics quoted in an earlier section show how common permanent brain damage is.

31

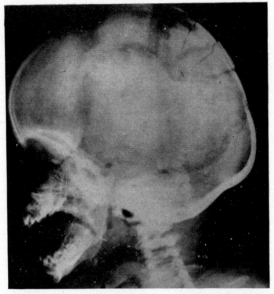

Figure 9. Skull battering on floor, with multiple fractures shattering the vault

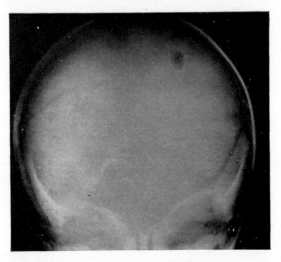

Figure 10. Side-to-side fractures by crushing impact on floor —often 'explained' as due to fall downstairs with child in arms

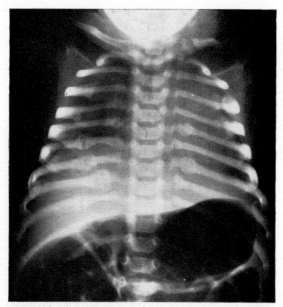

Figure 11. Characteristic rib fractures of varying dates from two cases; (lower) cleared by removal of soft parts at autopsy

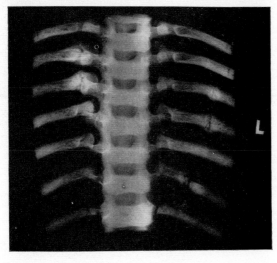

Rib Injuries

Neck and spinal injury is rare, and the pelvis is seldom found injured, but fractured ribs are classical. They are best revealed by x-ray (before or after death) and are most commonly located at the back of the chest, near the angles. The radiologist can often separate several dates of rib injury from the progress of callus formation, and histological examination to support this may be undertaken, though seldom necessary.

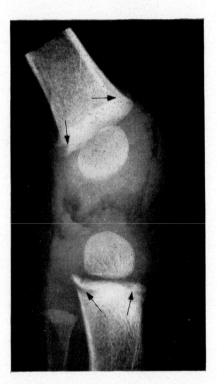

Figure 12. Detachments of epiphyses around the knee joint, and a periosteal 'lift,' part-healed

[Reproduced by courtesy of Dr. J. Layton]

Long Bone Injuries

Long bone injuries are 'greenstick' bendings and subperiosteal thickenings or frank fractures healing with the usual local swelling and deformity—especially when ignored by the parent in the early stages. These seldom escape x-ray search, but the 'pulled epiphyses' are very easily overlooked by any but the skilled radiologist. His attention to the possibility must be positively requested rather than

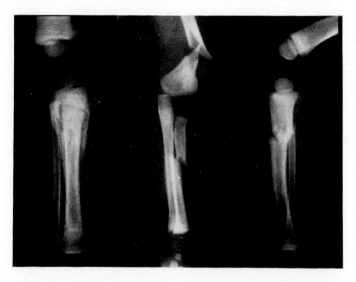

Figure 13. Fractures at three different ages in the same infant—very fresh (two days) in the arm, and some ten days (right) and two or three months (left) leg injuries

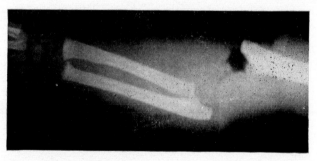

Figure 14. Arm 'pulled right out' through the skin by 'snatching' at the child. The bone end 'came through the skin'

expected, for the films may be several in a long morning's diagnostic work, and the tilted diaphysial disc-end or chipped corner is easy to overlook.

No part of the limb is particularly more frequently involved than any other. An infant may be grabbed by the arms or slung about by the legs, and it is this sudden pull that may cause the epiphysis to separate.

A warning to pathologists about the possibility of a breech-extraction causing a separation of the epiphysis of a long bone is worth scrutiny. The injuries of child abuse seldom start until some weeks have elapsed.

Scurvy, rickets and osteogenesis imperfecta may also require exclusion.

Visceral Injuries

Visceral injuries are quite common, and are commonly discovered only at autopsy. Split liver, usually on the under surface, between the major left and right lobes, probably by crushing against the spine, and bruised or crushed mesenteries, are the common lesions.

It is important to collect and measure the amount of blood lost. Most defending counsel will ask how long it would take 'to lose x ml', and the pathologist must have considered this difficult question before going to court. It is probably best answered by saying, bearing in mind that if it is the only serious injury it is probably the cause of death, that it is likely that an hour or two will have passed to account for any substantial volume to be lost—and to cause death. Such questions can never be answered with mathematical exactness.

Sex Injuries

These are rare. Parents and guardians who batter infants are not in this class. The word 'abuse' has no sex inflection when used to describe the callous beating of children.

Burns

Burns are by no means uncommon, although the revolting cigarette stubbing is fortunately not often seen. It is more common to sit the 'wetting' infant on a hot stove 'to teach it' and thus cause it contact burns of the buttocks. Pressing the body against the bars of an electric fire, pushing the hand or foot into a fire or 'branding' with a poker or steel are also on record. Corrosive fluid burns do not appear in the list of deliberate acts.

Burns are, of course, notoriously difficult to date, even histologically, and the pathologist must be wary of being drawn into this. The usual excuse of 'getting too near the fire' is to be excluded by pointing out that the burns are not diffuse zones as would occur by radiant heat, but strictly localized—indeed sometimes distinctly shaped or patterned areas.

PATHOLOGY

It is as well to remind the hospital morbid anatomist that any infant bearing marks of injury round the face or neck, or showing un-

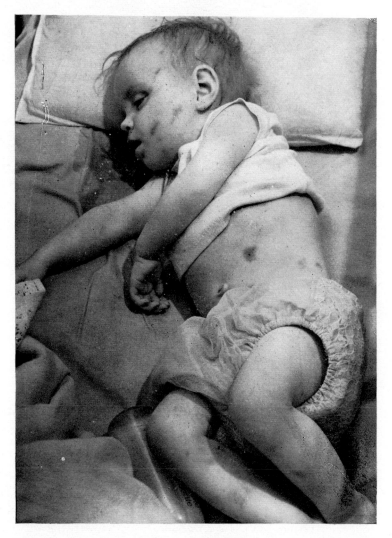

Figure 15. Typical battered baby—'just found dead, like this'—with multiple bruises indicating rough handling. Death was due to a ruptured liver

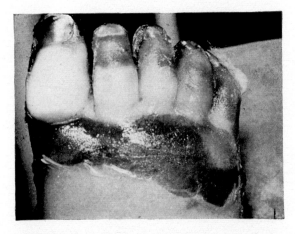

Figure 16. Burns of the toes and foot allegedly the result of an infant aged 2½ years rolling off of a sofa towards an unguarded fireplace. No other (e.g. radiation) burns were present

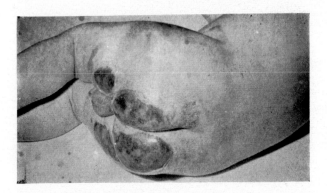

Figure 17. Contact burns of the buttocks from seating an infant of 15 months on an electric stove (metal temperature 112°F) 'to teach it not to wet its nappies'

suspected subdural bleeding (especially multicentric)—with or without skull fracture—or rib or long bone injuries especially of varying date, liver or mesenteric trauma or abdominal bleeding not adequately explained, is likely to become a medico-legal problem that might be handled with more experience by a forensic pathologist. The time to call for one is at the outset, not when the post-mortem is finished and it becomes evident that a criminal case of some substance has arisen. Hospital pathologists who are perfectly competent to handle the routine work of ward and surgical practice do not always emerge well from a testing cross-examination in the Assize Court—often at the hands of counsel who have been well informed by their own forensic medical experts.

The experiences of the forensic pathologist in fatal cases adds to that of the clinician in revealing certain classical injuries in addition to those commonly recognized in clinical practice:

(1) Bruises may not be apparent—becoming revealed only as the tissues, notably the scalp and the back of the body generally, are explored by the numerous incisions and reflections of skin that are necessary to a searching post-mortem. Under the scalp, over the shoulder blades, spine, hip crests, and buttocks and in the orifices of the anus or vagina, a more searching examination commonly reveals further injury. Bruises in the skin of coloured infants commonly escape notice.

(2) The retina may show the traumatic haemorrhage responsible for the partial blindness that can so easily be overlooked in infancy.

(3) The presence of multicentric subdural and subarachnoid haemorrhage—not explained by arterial defect or disease, and of 'commotio cerebri', often without external or scalp injury.

(4) The reverse aspect of the lips may show splits in the mucous membrane or a torn fraenum.

(5) Careful dissection of the neck tissues by the pathologist, not the mortuary attendant (even though no surface skin marks were present), may reveal scattered deep bruises.

(6) Removal of the thoracic cage is an ideal way of obtaining really good x-rays of ribs—often fractured behind, near their angles, by kicking or stamping, punching or throwing the infant against furniture.

(7) Deep loin, deep abdominal (especially mesenteric and liver splitting) injuries may only become apparent upon autopsy. The liver injury is classically set on the under-surface between right and left lobes, and may not be seen unless suspected or sought.

Injured tissues must be removed and preserved for histological dating. Histochemical methods are shortening the time interval after which dating can be effectively made. This and the radiologist's dating of fractures, pulled epiphyses and cortical periosteal thickenings matters much to the lawyer who is trying to relate events to post-mortem findings.

Lastly, the possibility of a dispute over parenthood must be envisaged. Blood should always be retained for an expert forensic serologist grouping. The average haematologist will not be likely to venture far into the rarer family groups, the protein mosaic (other than haptoglobin), the special haemoglobins or enzyme groupings.

The common injuries have been detailed in many articles on the pathology of child abuse, notably Silverman in skeletal injury (1968), Weston in visceral trauma and burns (1968), Adelson (1961), and Camps and Cameron (1964).

MANAGEMENT

Punitive measures are not the aim of any humanitarian. The purpose of early diagnosis in battered baby problems is the safety of the child at risk. Most family doctors are well aware that prevention or cure are the real objectives. To collect all the available information whilst safeguarding the child—if necessary by hospitalization, and then, at interview where the cards are laid out *en plain air*, explanations are given to parents or guardians and plans are produced for protection of the child at risk—often prove enough. Penalties can be kept in reserve: it is often enough to warn both parents of the risk they run of prosecution and utter disintegration of the family. The Children's Officer of the Local Authority becomes the plain clothes policeman with a duty to ensure the peace, help the parents, and protect the child that is 'in need of care or protection'. It must be made clear to the parents that the officer can bring the child before the Court and may obtain an order for its removal from the home. The alternative may well be prosecution for neglect, ill-treatment, or 'actual bodily harm'—or causing death, all of them criminal offences.

The NSPCC, always ready to help where the child is being neglected or is frankly at risk, undertakes an alternative rôle. Much depends on the personal liaison between a particular practitioner and the Society's local officers. Some doctors prefer the unofficial air that attends visits by Society representatives, but some work more understandingly with the Children's Department. There is a gap in the after-care of hospitals, yet the psychiatric care the patient needs is easier to obtain by hospital contact. Co-operative effort from all is needed, and it cannot be over-stressed that the child's interests must come uppermost, even if it is the mother who needs most help and advice.

Under the Children and Young Persons Act of 1933, the penalties in the magistrates court for cruelty were ridiculously ineffectual. A £25 fine (the maximum) for causing permanent brain damage to a child, cutting its plaintive tongue, burning its wet bottom or breaking its limbs were wholly inadequate, and the 1963 Act has increased the maximum to £100. It is not an effective imposition. Even in the event of death a sentence of two years or deferred sentences—which mean that the convicted walk out of Court free, on probation—are no effective way of teaching self-discipline. In the occasional case, such as that reported by Simpson in 1964 of conviction and life sentences for murder (for two successive child killings by a father (R. vs Dean), some kind of protection for other children in the family, if not some lesson to parents and guardians, may seem to have been effected. Such cases form but a small fraction of the whole.

The disinclination of the Crown to press a prosecution where the only basis is the medical evidence is no doubt partly responsible for this. In 1971, two successive baby battering deaths in London in which only medical evidence was available were abandoned before trial—though each passed the scrutiny of medical advisors for the defence and had been committed for trial by the magistrates. The chagrin of pathologists, of police, of coroners' juries who had carefully sifted the evidence and of the magistrates who had committed the case for trial, may well be understood. The difficulty in convincing the lay judiciary of the fact that these are criminal killings wholly comparable with beating up and robbing old ladies, or of the sex murders of children sent to shop, over which no pains to secure a public conviction are spared, is apparent to all who are so concerned with the welfare of the child. The law has need to raise its sights in the prosecution of battering parents and guardians and in the overriding interest of protecting children 'at risk'.

The rôle of the defending solicitor and barrister is more understandable for they have a traditional part to play. It has always been their duty to put their client's case in the best possible light, and whether they believe the explanations or not, to put them forward in court and test the prosecution in every possible respect in the hope of saving a client, even from what would be a proper penalty. Some—though very few—counsel refuse to raise such a defence, though it is open to them to do so, preferring, in fatal cases, to advise accused to plead guilty to cruelty or to manslaughter and to ask for mental treatment. It is a fault of the accusatorial system that counsel can build a repute for himself by successful defence that enables even a guilty client to escape any proper penalty. Doctors and children's departments have indeed many obstacles to overcome in their concern to protect the 'battered baby'.

REFERENCES

Adelson, L. (1961). *New Engl. J. Med.*, **264**, 1345.
Barabas, A. P. (1967). *Br. med. J.*, **1**, 612.
Bodian, M. (1964). *N. Y. St. J. Med.*, **64**, 916.
British Paediatric Association (1966). *Br. med. J.*, **1**, 601.
Caffey, J. (1946). *Am. J. Roentgenol.*, **56**, 163.
Cameron, J. M. (1970). *Br. J. hosp. Med.*, **4**, 769.
— Johnson, H. R. and Camps, F. E. (1966). *Med. Sci. Law*, **6**, 2.
de Francis, V. (1963). *Child Abuse*. Denver; American Humane Association, Children's Division.
Gibbens, T. C. and Walker, N. (1956). *Cruel Parents*. Institute for Study and Treatment of Delinquency.
Gilkes, M. J. and Mann, T. P. (1967). *Lancet*, **2**, 468.
Gill, D. G. (1968). *The Battered Child*, Ed. by R. E. Helfer and C. H. Kempe. University of Chicago Press.
Griffith, J. F. and Dodge, P. R. (1968). *New Engl. J. Med.*, **278**, 648.
Griffiths, D. L. and Moynahan, F. J. (1963). *Br. med. J.*, **2**, 1558.
Harcourt, B. and Hopkins, D. (1971). *Br. med. J.*, **3**, 398.
Helfer, R. E. and Kempe C. H. (Eds.) (1968). *The Battered Child*. University of Chicago Press.
Holzel, A. and Tobin, J. O'H. (1967). *Lancet*, **2**, 723.
— Silverman, F. N., Steele, B. F., Droegemueller, W. and Silver, H. K. (1962). *J. Am. med. Ass.*, **181**, 17.
Kempe, C. H. (1971). *Archs. Dis. Childh.*, **46**, 28.
— (1962). *J. Am. Med. Ass.*, **181**, 17.
Mushin, A. S. (1971). *Br. med. J.*, **3**, 402.
National Opinion Research Centre Survey (1965). University of Chicago.
Schloesser, P. T. (1964). *Bull. Menninger Clin.* No. 28.
Silverman, F. M. (1953). *Am. J. Roentgenol. therm. nucl. Med.*, **69**, 413.
— (1968). In *The Battered Child*, Ed. by R. E. Helfer and C. H. Kempe. University of Chicago Press.
Simons, B. (1966). *Child Abuse Survey*. Denver; American Humane Association, Children's Division.
Simpson, K. (1965). *Br. med. J.*, **1**, 393.
Skinner, A. E. and Castle, R. L. (1969). National Society for the Prevention of Cruelty to Children.
Steele, B. F. and Pollock, C. (1968). In *The Battered Child*, Ed. by R. E. Helfer and C. H. Kempe. University of Chicago Press.
Tate, R. J. (1971). *Br. J. Oral Surg.*, **9**, 41.
Turner, E. (1964). *Br. med. J.*, **1**, 308.
Turner, J. W. A. (1943). *Brain*, **68**, 140.
Weston, J. T. (1968). In *The Battered Child*, Ed. by R. E. Helfer and C. H. Kempe. University of Chicago Press.
Wooley, P. V. and Evans, W. A. (1955). *J. Am. med. Ass.*, **158**, 529.

3 Newer Techniques in Paternity Blood Grouping

ALAN GRANT and IAN D. BRADBROOK

INTRODUCTION

When Lord Merthyr's Bastardy (Blood Tests) Bill was debated by the House of Lords in 1938–39 ABO and MN grouping of the red corpuscles were the only useful tests available. Such tests would exonerate about one-third of wrongly accused men. By 1961, when Lord Amulree's Affiliation Proceedings (Blood Tests) Bill was introduced, grouping tests of the same nature had been extended, especially through discovery of the rhesus system, to a stage that would have permitted exclusion of about 60 per cent of non-fathers. Progress on these lines in the last decade did not significantly increase the proportion excluded but advance in paternity testing accelerated, employing quite different methods. In addition to agglutination tests to group the red corpuscles in the classical manner by identification of inherited factors on the surface, it is now possible to group a considerable range of enzymes within the corpuscles and numerous inherited factors in the blood plasma. These newer techniques employ electrophoresis in hydrolysed starch-gel and other media, double diffusion tests in which antigen and antibody are allowed to diffuse towards each other in clear gels with formation of precipitate lines where antigen meets its specific antibody, and a combination of these two techniques, immuno-electrophoresis. The earliest application of electrophoresis to analysis of this type was in separation of inherited variants in the haemoglobin pigment of the blood. This was of no great value in paternity testing at the time since such variants are rare in the ordinary English population, but haemoglobin grouping has become increasingly useful now that paternity problems involving African and Asian descended infants have to be investigated. However, it was with the discovery of the haptoglobin groups, inherited variants in the plasma globulin, that paternity grouping lost identity with blood transfusion serology. This was not just because of the usefulness of the haptoglobin groups in paternity testing but because Oliver Smithies' discovery of the technique of electrophoresis in gels made from partly hydrolysed potato starch provided the instrument for much of the subsequent advance, and impetus for most of the rest.

Paternity grouping began to swing away from the techniques of the blood bank and is becoming a separate science with methods shared only with departments of human genetics. There is some irony in the situation that, having delayed enactment so long, legislation has at the last hurdle outpaced scientific preparedness and it will be some time before most laboratories will be able to provide the full range of investigation now easily practicable.

The Family Law Reform Act 1969 and the legal aid provisions already available probably constitute the most socially advanced provision for paternity tests in any country. Legal aid apart, the one fundamental difference from Lord Merthyr's original proposals is that the court will not order blood tests on its own initiative; application for a direction must come from one of the parties. The court may place such interpretation as seems right on refusal of blood tests requested by the other party. There is no suggestion that significance could attach to failure to ask for blood tests but it seems likely that the putative father will be advised by his solicitor to apply for blood tests if he wishes to defend the application by denial of paternity. Increased provision for paternity testing may be required because of background pressure from the Act's provisions more than from the actual number of directions made, since it must be more pleasant to have tests by agreement between solicitors than to submit to a court order that can so easily be avoided. We suspect that court direction may come to be a matter of last resort and that a considerable proportion of cases will continue to be investigated before court hearing is commenced. Lord Merthyr suggested that a small number of special laboratories should be set up to carry out paternity testing but the Act relies on a panel of recognized serologists any of whom may be asked to make the tests. Probably more progress would be expected with special laboratories and in this respect the present arrangement has the built-in disadvantage of a standard fee based on the minimum acceptable range of tests. The serologist who wishes to provide more must give both his time and the cost of the equipment and reagents required.

LIKELIHOOD OF PATERNITY

With the present range of blood tests evidence pointing to paternity as well as excluding paternity may emerge. Such evidence has to be treated with caution, not merely from risk of coincidence but because of possibility of a blood relative of the putative father being involved. This risk is greatest in small communities and apart from actual relatives there may be inbreeding in the community as a result of which a gene which is uncommon in the population of the country as a whole may be much more frequent in the inhabitants of a village. If the baby has received one uncommon gene from its father and the named man has this gene, the calculated percentage of possible fathers will be low though all the other factors the child is shown to have received could have been given by quite a large proportion of men. Statistical calculations that give accurate enough answers when applied to the population as a whole may be misleading when applied to the single case.

It is obvious that the mere fact of common possession of blood groups by baby and man does not make him its likely father. This man may never have been within a hundred miles of the mother and for most children it would not involve a long search to find a man whose groups by gene frequency calculations make him a more likely father than the actual father. What we have to attempt to estimate is something rather less tangible: the likelihood that the mother has named by chance a man who is not excluded and whose groups fit this or that well with paternity. If calculation shows that the named man and say 10 per cent of men in the community have groups that are compatible with paternity there are plenty of potential fathers but the mother stood a 90 per cent chance of being shown to be wrong if the man she was naming was not the actual father.

Part I of the report that the tester must supply under the Family Law Reform Act requires 'Comments on value, if any, in determining whether any person tested is the father of the person whose paternity is in dispute'. There can be no easy answer to this question. With the full range of tests now available the mere fact that the man is not excluded must be of some positive evidential value; trial of the blood has not shown the mother to be in error. It will be appreciated that where the proportion of possible fathers is shown to be large this in no way detracts from the case of the applicant mother. This means only that the child received common groups from its father and there is no rare marker such as would give positive support for the mother's contention.

Two methods of calculation are available. The first, which may be called the percentage method, does not attempt to measure the degree of probability of paternity by a particular man. It measures the usefulness of the tests employed in relation to the particular case being investigated. It shows the percentage of men in the community

45

that cannot be shown not to possess all the blood group genes shown by the tests to have been received by the child from its father. Where the range of possible fathers is small and includes the named man, this supports the mother's case. The Law Commission suggested in 1968 that where the percentage of possible fathers was as small as 1 or 2 per cent the tests might be taken as indicating likelihood of paternity. The proposition would be that it is unlikely that the mother has named by chance one of so limited a proportion of men who could possibly be the father if he were not the actual father. It will be noted that the figures considered suggestive of paternity are the ordinarily accepted figures for statistical significance.

The alternative approach seeks to determine the proportion of possible children of the named man that would receive the gene combination that the child has been shown to have inherited from its father and compare this with the proportion of children of all men that would inherit these genes. All the genes that the child received from its father must have been carried in one spermatozoon so it is necessary to calculate the proportion of spermatozoa that would have the required combination. Take one group only: if the child received M from its father a man who is MN is only half as likely as an MM man to pass M to his children since half his spermatozoa will carry N. In practice, the apparent accuracy of this approach turns out to be illusory. Thus, we do not know whether the group B man is BO or BB so 'to be fair' we assume only half his spermatozoa carry B. Usually the calculation starts by assuming that the man possesses factors that the child has been shown to have received from its father when all that the tests have actually shown is that he may have them. Shed of such assumptions there are few cases in which a significant answer can be obtained and this usually depends on child and man having one uncommon factor. With the reservations we have mentioned it is possible by simple multiplication to show that $1/x$ spermatozoa of the named man will carry the gene combination the child received from its father and to calculate from gene frequency tables the incidence $1/y$ of such spermatozoa in men in general. The latter figure is somewhat confusingly referred to as the frequency in a random male. As before, a difference of 50 to 1 might be accepted as significant. The proposition would then be expressed as follows: the man who is claimed to be the baby's father would produce a child with these groups 50 times as frequently as would men in general and it is unlikely that a difference of this magnitude occurred by chance; it is a significant difference. It follows that any less difference is not significant. As we have already indicated absence of significance usually means only that no uncommon gene is involved. In the majority of cases there are no such markers. We feel it better not, on such a chance basis, arbitrarily to divide cases of otherwise equal merit between a small number in which the blood groups point to paternity and the rest in which all we have to say is that we have been unable to exclude paternity.

Before any type of calculation is attempted it is necessary to know the race of the parties involved since there is considerable variation in group frequencies in different parts of the world. There are reliable statistics for the basic populations of western Europe but it would be obviously unrealistic to apply such figures to the baby of, say, a West Indian mother simply because these are the frequencies for most males in the country in which she happens to be living. For most populations there are insufficient data to permit calculations of the type we have been discussing and in anthropologically new communities there is too much variation resulting from comparatively recent admixture of African, European and Asian genes.

We prefer to employ the simple and easily understood calculation of the percentage of men the tests would have excluded and limit this to western European problems. The main value of such calculation is not to point to paternity in occasional cases but to indicate the need for additional non-routine tests when the calculation shows that most men would not have been excluded by the range normally applied.

SECOND ORDER EXCLUSIONS

Classical paternity tests based on identification of red cell antigens were discussed in *Modern Trends in Forensic Medicine—2*. Exclusions of the first order, where the child is shown to possess a blood group gene not present in either the mother or alleged father, present no difficulty. From time to time apparent mutations are reported but later a more likely explanation of the observed anomaly emerges. It is now clear that mutation of the ordinary blood group genes is excessively rare. Unsupported second order exclusions present a more difficult problem. Very occasionally persons have been found who appear to lack any representation at one or other of the blood group loci, the 'minus minus' phenotypes of Allen (1961). As the blood group antigens are so regularly present it may be assumed that they have a purpose, and absence would be likely to be genetically disadvantageous and keep the frequency of such chromosomes low. Apparently no person has been found who lacks both M and N, although an M^gM^g person who might once have been classed as such has been identified. By contrast absence of both the known Duffy alleles Fy^a and Fy^b is quite common in Africans; if there is a third alternative allele in that race it could be an antigenically do-nothing gene rather like O in the ABO system. In Africans the fact that a child is $Fy(a+ b-)$ and the alleged father $Fy(a- b+)$, or vice versa, is not even suggestive of non-paternity. In Africans also S^u or something similar in effect is sufficiently frequent to invalidate apparent second order indications of non-paternity by anti-S, anti-s reactions. By contrast the minus chromosomes of Europeans seem to be so unusual as to justify classification as rare mutants, although it must be remembered that such anomalies will usually be revealed only through instances of seeming non-maternity by tests with both antithetical antisera and that in many of the systems we have to consider such examination has been comparatively limited.

Exclusion is not a word that can normally be qualified but the Family Law Reform Act recognizes the need to disregard minute possibility of error through the unpredictable occurrence of mutation. The definition 'excluded means excluded subject to mutation' should probably be taken as meaning a change in the genetic material in the single reproductive event that resulted in birth of the disputed child but the same difficulty can face the tester from mutation that occurred in a previous generation and might have caused an undetectable anomaly. The significance of an indicated second order exclusion must have regard to the sheer volume of testing that has been carried out with the alternative antisera. Thus, with MN, with Cc and probably Ee there has been a great volume of testing and the risk of error after known safeguarding tests is small. In some systems mother–child tests employing at least two examples of the uncommon alternative antiserum have been too few to establish the genetic system beyond doubt.

With regard to the Fy^aFy^b and Ss groups of Europeans, consideration has to be given to possible occurrence of African genes in the English population. At this time no race is an island serologically and, although in England the immigrant peoples live side by side with the white population so that their paternity problems can usually be considered as if they arose in the country of origin, there is certain to be gradual penetrance of African genes. Adequate enquiry into possibility of African ancestry is necessary before accepting a second order indication of non-paternity that would not be valid for African subjects.

African subjects apart, we have not encountered an apparent second order indication of non-maternity other than in problems of accidentally interchanged babies and one instance of fraudulent exchange. An unexpected hazard was encountered in respect of a white London girl who would have been excluded from maternity of her S +ve, s −ve baby by tests with saline agglutinating anti-S sera all of several examples of which gave negative reactions with her cells. Coombs' reacting antisera gave positive results as did albumen reacting examples. On one occasion we were able to confirm a second order Duffy exclusion by showing that both parents of the alleged father were Fy(a+ b+).

DISSIMILAR TWINS

Some remote possibilities in twin pregnancy that blood group studies have revealed were discussed in the previous volume and we return to the subject to mention an aspect we previously thought of

TABLE 1

Mother	Boy twin	Girl twin	Husband	Co-respondent
O	O	B	A_1 B	O
Ms.Ms	Ms.Ms	MS.Ms	MS.NS	Ms.Ns
Le (a− b−)	Le (a+ b−)	Le (a− b+)	Le (a− b+)	Le (a+ b−)
Gm^a −ve	Gm^a +ve	Gm^a −ve	Gm^a −ve	Gm^a +ve

as a rare possibility but now suspect may not be uncommon. On two occasions in which paternity of unlike twins was disputed blood tests excluded the alleged father from paternity of one twin but not of the other and we thought of this simply as failure to prove non-paternity of the second. In the only case we have examined in which the problem was which of two men was father of the dissimilar twins the informative groups were as set out in Table 1.

It will be seen that the boy twin inherited O, Ms, Le(a) and Gm(a) from his father, none of which the husband could have given. The girl received B, MS and Le(b) from her father, none of which the co-respondent could have given. Quite clearly, one man was father of one twin and the other of the second. The result did not surprise the mother who had noticed the similarity of the girl to her older children and the lack of similarity in the other.

Although twins may be born on the same day conception could be more widely separated. We do not know how long spermatozoa

49

may remain fertile in the female genital tract nor how frequently coitus determines ovulation, but if two sperm populations are present in the appropriate period there would seem to be no reason why a representative of each should not succeed.

It is now clear that exclusion of paternity of one of dizygotic twins is not sound evidence of non-paternity of the other.

VARIANT HAEMOGLOBINS

In the previous volume some account was given of red corpuscle antigens peculiar to African and African-descended subjects and their

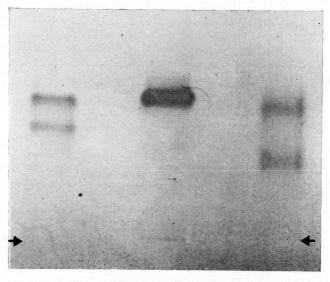

Figure 1. Cellulose acetate electrophoresis of red-cell haemolysates showing three haemoglobin types—left: Hb AS, centre: Hb A, right: Hb AE

value in paternity tests. These tests cannot be applied at random because the most useful antisera are in short supply. By contrast, screening for abnormal haemoglobins by cellulose acetate electrophoresis is rapid and inexpensive.

Haemoglobin variants in Europeans are rare but they are frequently encountered in Africans and their investigation compensates for the lowered chance of exclusion consequent on the sameness of the rhesus groups. In Asians Hb E and Hb D Punjab are encountered from time to time. The former is not easily distinguished from Hb C of West Africans by routine electrophoresis but precise classification matters little when either variant is present in the child and absent in both mother and putative father. Sickle cell haemoglobin provides the most useful marker, being present in over one-fifth of Africans in some regions. This haemoglobin is remarkable in being the one mutant the purpose of which is understood. When inherited from one parent only, the heterozygote state gives protection against malignant tertian malaria. The balance of the polymorphism results from the fact that the child cannot survive long without ordinary Hb A and will die in infancy if Hb S is received from both parents. It is not known whether all Hb S stems from a single mutation in the remote past. Possibly the mutation recurs from time to time but not with a frequency that would detract from the value of Hb S in paternity testing. Where there is no malignant tertian malaria the heterozygote has no advantage over the normal and the homozygote being lethal Hb S will tend to disappear. It is rarely encountered in England where once it may have been more common.

An Irish woman living in England claimed that her baby's father was an Italian born in the south of Italy and unusually blond for a person from that region. The child had negroid physical characters completely lacking in the mother and alleged father. The man was found to have the red corpuscle antigen V, so some element of African ancestry was likely and the question of possible throw-back would clearly arise, although this seemed very unlikely on account of the number of genes likely to be involved in producing the child's negroid physical characters. The child had not received V, the relevant groups being:

Mother   cDE/cde or cDE/cDe, V − ve

Child   cDE/cde or cDE/cDe, V − ve

Man   CDe/cde or CDe/cDe, V + ve

Since V travels with cDe or cde and not with CDe, the child would have been expected to receive V as well as cde or cDe if this man were the father, so V in the man did not point to paternity but virtually excluded the possibility. Haemoglobin typing confirmed this, showing Hb S present in the child and absent in mother and alleged father.

The characteristic of these abnormal haemoglobins is that they travel more slowly than ordinary Hb A on electrophoresis so that a second band is formed nearer the origin. This has to be kept in mind when haptoglobin typing haemolysed blood. When haemoglobin is added to the serum in accordance with the usual practice, a band corresponding with the subject's Hb A component lies in front of a second band formed by his abnormal haemoglobin. This may be confused with Hp 1 in a subject who is really Hp O-O.

Gm BLOOD SERUM POLYMORPHISM

The serum, like the red cells, shows a wealth of inherited group factors. Grubb (1956) showed that red cells incubated with some incomplete anti-D sera are agglutinated by the sera of certain persons with rheumatoid arthritis, and this agglutination is prevented and reversed by a factor which is present in the blood serum of some persons and absent in others. Grubb and Laurell (1956) showed that this ability to inhibit agglutination is inherited as a dominant Mendelian character.

In a simple technique devised by Lawler, group O, D homozygous rhesus positive erythrocytes are prepared as for Coombs' testing using a suitably selected incomplete anti-D serum, and the washed cells agglutinated with the anti-Gm serum in a series of test beds on an opaque tile. Dilutions of the sera to be tested are then mixed with the agglutinated cells, breaking down the agglutinates which re-form if the inhibiting factor is absent.

Grubb's original factor Gm(a), now called Gm 1, is present in some 60 per cent of Europeans. Numerous other Gm factors have since been discovered as well as a shorter related series called Inv. As yet there is no certain information as to which factors are allelic. Some are usually inherited together and all Africans appear to be Gm(1, 5).

The gamma globulin present in the newborn is not its own but has been formed by the mother and transmitted across the placenta, so Gm and Inv studies may be of use where there has been possible mix-up of babies in maternity wards. From about three months onwards the child's own gamma globulin begins to appear coincident with fading of the Gm received from the mother.

So far only first order paternity exclusions are possible. Since there is wide variation of the frequencies of the various Gm factors in different populations, the usefulness of tests for a factor depends on the race of the persons concerned. Grubb (1970) has suggested that in Western Europe the investigation of Gm(1, 2, 4 or 5) and Inv(1 or 2) might be accepted as a good standard in forensic medicine, there being abundant family data. Antisera are numerous but only a minor proportion are sufficiently powerful for medico-legal investigations.

In problems involving race a Gm(−1) child would certainly not have an African father but there could be no such confidence about a West Indian who could have European genes.

SERUM HAPTOGLOBINS

In 1955 Oliver Smithies devised an improved method of separating plasma proteins by electrophoresis in gels formed of partly hydrolysed potato starch. The gel at once provides a supporting medium and forms a continuous sieve with pores of varying size. The smaller the protein molecule the faster it travels since it encounters more pores through which it can pass. Smithies noticed variation in the α_2 globulin bands derived from the plasma of different individuals and, later, Smithies and Walker showed that the differences are inherited; they proposed a simple Mendelian system of inheritance by two allelic genes Hp^1 and Hp^2 resulting in three genotypes Hp 1–1, Hp 2–2 and Hp 2–1. Extensive family and twin studies, particularly by Galatius-Jensen in Denmark and Fleischer and Lundevall in Norway, preceded the application of haptoglobin typing to tests of paternity. As indicated by Smithies and Walker, the pattern of inheritance is identical to that of the MN groups; Hp 1 or Hp 2 cannot be present in a child and absent in both its parents and an Hp 1–1 father cannot have an Hp 2–2 child, and vice versa. In the first months of life it may not be possible to determine the Hp type, possibly because elimination of the excess haemoglobin with which the child is born depletes the serum haptoglobin. This occurs with other conditions that result in intravascular haemolysis, but a puzzling feature is the absence or virtual absence of a haptoglobin pattern in quite numerous healthy individuals. Production of haptoglobin is probably dependent on genetic factors other than those responsible for haptoglobin polymorphism.

On starch-gel electrophoresis sera from Hp 1–1 persons give a single band a little behind that formed by free haemoglobin. The Hp 2–2 person shows no band in this position but a series of slower moving bands that diminish in intensity towards the origin. The heterozygous Hp 2–1 pattern is a series of bands of slightly greater mobility than those of Hp 2–2 with a band in the Hp 1–1 position. An Hp 2–1 (modified) pattern which is not uncommon in Africans shows a pattern in which the slower bands of ordinary Hp 2–1 are absent with increased density of the fastest bands. The multiple band formation is consequent on a tendency of the Hp^2 gene to form polymers, incorporating the product of the Hp^1 gene where this is present.

Atypical patterns are encountered which are easily recognized as atypical but the significance of which cannot be explained with certainty. Provided the haptoglobin patterns are well developed so as to permit unambiguous differentiation as the common phenotypes, haptoglobin grouping is a reliable method of paternity testing.

Table 2, based on the gene frequencies of 1,000 unrelated adults who attended consecutively for paternity tests, indicates the degree of usefulness of haptoglobin testing.

TABLE 2

Haptoglobin System

Gene frequencies in United Kingdom
$Hp^1 = 0.3854$
$Hp^2 = 0.6146$

Phenotype frequencies
Hp 1–1 = 0.1485
Hp 2–1 = 0.4738
Hp 2–2 = 0.3777

Possible matings		Excluded child	Probability of exclusion
Mother	Alleged father		
1–1	1–1	2–1	0.0136
2–2	2–2	2–1	0.0550
1–1	2–2	1–1	0.0216
2–2	1–1	2–2	0.0345
2–1	1–1	2–2	0.0216
2–1	2–2	1–1	0.0345
		Total exclusion probability	0.1808

THE Gc GROUPS

When the protein components of a blood serum are spread out by electrophoresis in a clear agar gel and then allowed to diffuse towards the serum of an animal immunized against human serum a large number of precipitate arcs are formed, each corresponding to an antibody the animal has produced.

In a study of these complex patterns J. Hirschfeld noticed a hitherto unknown component in the α_2 globulin region that showed individual variation. Recognizable only by its group specific variations, the factor was termed group specific component and the polymorphism subsequently recognized was called the Gc system.

Inheritance is controlled by two alleles Gc^1 and Gc^2 giving the three phenotypes Gc 1–1, Gc 2–2 and Gc 2–1. There is no polymer formation such as complicates the haptoglobins; an equal mixture of Gc 1–1 with Gc 2–2 serum gives a typical Gc 2–1 pattern, which permits group confirmation by hybridization experiments. Gc typing has been made easy by commercial laboratory production of adsorbed antisera in which only anti-Gc and suitable markers to assist identification remain. The fast moving homozygote Gc 1–1, the slow

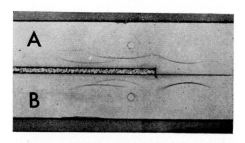

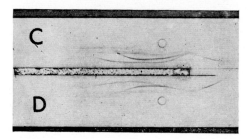

Figure 2. Immunoelectrophoretic patterns of the three common Gc types—A: Gc 1–1, B: Gc 2–2, C: Gc 2–1, D: Gc 1–1

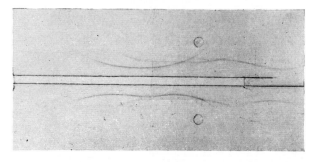

Figure 3. Immunoelectrophoretic pattern of Gc 2–1^{fast} (bottom part of slide) compared with normal Gc 1–1 (top)

C

moving Gc 2–2 and the heterozygote double-arc pattern resembling the spread wings of a seagull are all easily identified. In a small proportion of African subjects and certain other racial groups unlikely to confuse paternity problems in England Gc 1 fast genes occur, resulting in Gc 1–1 fast and Gc 2–1 fast patterns that can hardly avoid recognition or be confused with the trailing prolongation of the Gc arc that may appear with deteriorated serum samples. The exclusion possibilities are shown in Table 3.

TABLE 3

Gc System

Gene frequencies in United Kingdom
$Gc^1 = 0.7274$
$Gc^2 = 0.2726$

Phenotype frequencies
Gc 1–1 = 0.5291
Gc 2–1 = 0.3966
Gc 2–2 = 0.0743

Possible matings		Excluded child	Probability of exclusion
Mother	Alleged father		
1–1	1–1	2–1	0.0763
2–2	2–2	2–1	0.0040
1–1	2–2	1–1	0.0286
2–2	1–1	2–2	0.0106
2–1	1–1	2–2	0.0285
2–1	2–2	1–1	0.0106

Total exclusion probability 0.1586

THE Ag GROUPS

Thalassaemic children whose lives have been prolonged by many blood transfusions occasionally form isoprecipitins to lipoprotein factors in the incidentally transfused donor sera. The Ag system of serum antigens is complex but two genes, Ag(x) and Ag(y), appear certainly to be allelic. Antisera are for obvious reasons in short supply but anti-Ag(x) and anti-Ag(y) when available and free from other Ag antibodies are useful paternity grouping reagents, excluding about 14 per cent of non-fathers, or 8 per cent if only anti-Ag(x) can be used. Grouping is by a simple double diffusion technique in agar gel spread evenly on glass slides. The sera to be grouped are placed in peripheral wells punched in the agar and arranged so as to be equidistant from the central well for the antiserum. After about 12 hours in a humid chamber clearly marked precipitate lines are seen where antigen–antibody reaction has occurred.

The Ag factors are on the beta-lipoprotein molecules, are present at birth and are not transmitted across the placenta. We are fortunate in having been able to apply Ag(x) and Ag(y) tests to paternity problems in the last three years and Table 4 shows the grouping

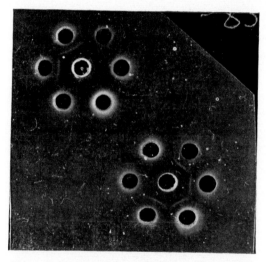

Figure 4. Agar-gel double diffusion of various normal human sera (in the peripheral wells) against anti-Ag(x) in the top centre well and anti-Ag(y) in the bottom centre well. Positive results are indicated by the presence of a line of precipitation between the centre well and the peripheral well

results in 649 cases in which 692 possible fathers were involved. The table is based on the hypothesis of Ag^x and Ag^y being allelic and the agreement between expected and observed exclusions would seem to permit no doubt regarding the correctness of this hypothesis. No blood sample was found to be Ag(x− y−). Fresh sera stored at −40°C for 12 to 18 months showed no obvious deterioration in reaction strength but a fairly rapid fall-off occurred at 4°C. A point to be remembered is that heparin at certain concentrations will precipitate the beta-lipoprotein molecules and therefore the Ag factors. Clotted blood samples are suitable but it is best to employ

TABLE 4

Ag System: Tests with Anti-Ag(x) and Anti-Ag(y)

	Number of cases	Number of alleged fathers	Number of exclusions by genetic markers listed in Table 7	Number of expected exclusions from Table 7	Number of exclusions by the Ag system	
					Observed	Expected
1 man cases	606	606	159	191·8	25	27
2 man cases	43	86	33	40·2	8	5·57
Total	649	692	192	232	33	32·57

dipotassium EDTA as an anticoagulant as this preserves the lipo-proteins to some extent.

Table 5 shows the theoretical usefulness of the system in paternity testing.

TABLE 5

Ag System

Gene frequencies in United Kingdom
$Ag^x = 0.2060$
$Ag^y = 0.7940$

Phenotype frequencies
Ag $(x + y-) = 0.0424$
Ag $(x + y+) = 0.3270$
Ag $(x - y+) = 0.6306$

Possible matings		Excluded child	Probability of exclusion
Mother	Alleged father		
Ag(x+ y−)	Ag(x+ y−)	Ag(x+ y+)	0·0001
Ag(x− y+)	Ag(x− y+)	Ag(x+ y+)	0·0887
Ag(x+ y−)	Ag(x− y+)	Ag(x+ y−)	0·0055
Ag(x− y+)	Ag(x+ y−)	Ag(x− y+)	0·0212
Ag(x+ y+)	Ag(x+ y−)	Ag(x− y+)	0·0055
Ag(x+ y+)	Ag(x− y+)	Ag(x+ y−)	0·0212
	Total exclusion probability		0·1422

RED CELL ENZYME GROUPS

A large number of enzymes are present in the red cells and have been investigated for possible inherited variation between individuals. Numerous polymorphisms have been demonstrated, especially by Harris and his co-workers, using the technique of prolonged starch-gel electrophoresis at 4°C. Cooling of the gel is necessary to prevent loss of enzyme activity and to prevent splitting of the gel. Phospho-glucomutase (PGM) and adenylate kinase (AK) are of established value in paternity testing and adenosine deaminase (ADA) and red cell acid phosphatase (AP) may also be employed. After separation by electrophoresis the group pattern is visualized by application of a reaction mixture containing substances necessary for the particular enzyme-catalysed reaction to proceed. The products of this reaction are then coupled with a dye resulting in the regions of enzyme activity appearing as coloured spots in the gel. The results have to be read at their optimum as diffusion of the spots may occur leading to difficulties in interpretation.

PGM grouping is now routinely employed and excludes paternity of about 15 per cent of non-fathers. AK has less exclusion potential but is of particular value in cases in which Asian subjects are involved, the frequency of the uncommon allele AK^2 being greater. This enzyme is of unusual stability and results may be obtained from blood no longer suitable for classical paternity grouping.

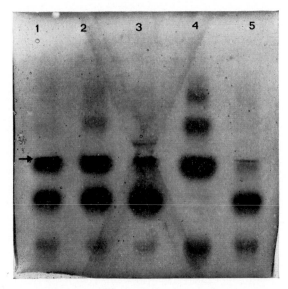

Figure 5. Exclusion by AK groups—left to right: control AK 2–1, mother AK 2–1, child AK 2–2, alleged father AK 1–1, control AK 2–2

Electrophoresis of these enzymes is performed on haemolysates prepared by freezing and rapidly thawing washed red cells. A number of enzyme tests can be made on the same haemolysate and if only a small volume of red cells is available there are micro-methods that may be employed. In our experience acid phosphatase has the drawback of requiring a comparatively large amount of haemolysate to produce convincing results. Also AP activity deteriorates rather rapidly, so the tests are best made at an early stage in the paternity investigation. When the sample from the child is small these factors combine to make AP investigation impracticable. This is unfortunate as the theoretical exclusion possibility is high.

Table 6 illustrates the usefulness of the PGM system in paternity grouping.

TABLE 6

Phosphoglucomutase (PGM)

Gene frequencies in United Kingdom
$PGM^1 = 0.7470$
$PGM^2 = 0.2530$

Phenotype frequencies
PGM 1–1 = 0.5580
PGM 2–1 = 0.3780
PGM 2–2 = 0.0640

Possible matings		Excluded child	Probability of exclusion
Mother	Alleged father		
1–1	1–1	2–1	0.0788
2–2	2–2	2–1	0.0031
1–1	2–2	1–1	0.0267
2–2	1–1	2–2	0.0090
2–1	1–1	2–2	0.0267
2–1	2–2	1–1	0.0090
	Total exclusion probability		0.1533

CHANCE OF EXCLUSION

Table 7 shows the calculated average chance of the non-father being excluded by the routine tests at present employed and Table 8 the actual exclusions obtained by tests in the various systems over a two year period. The exclusion chance will be increased by further extension of the range of tests employed but the law of diminishing returns means smaller and smaller additions to the average exclusion chance. The next step forward is likely to be through use of additional Gm and Inv factors.

At first glance an average exclusion chance of 84 per cent suggests that a non-father is very unlucky if the present tests do not exonerate him but one has only to remember the not infrequent cases in which we are still not able to exclude either of two possible fathers to realize that this view is deceptive. The figure is an average only; the actual chance may be much higher or much lower. If the groups of the

TABLE 7

Non-fathers: Exclusion Chance

System	Exclusion by each system	Total after correction for coincidental exclusions
ABO	0·1760	0·1760
MN.Ss	0·3205	0·4401
Rhesus	0·2800	0·5968
Kell	0·0334	0·6108
Duffy	0·0481	0·6295
Lutheran	0·0333	0·6418
Kidd	0·0286	0·6520
Haptoglobins	0·1807	0·7149
Gc	0·1586	0·7601
Gm(1)	0·0647	0·7756
Ag	0·1422	0·8075
PGM	0·1532	0·8370
AK	0·0420	0·8438

TABLE 8

Exclusion by Routine Tests, 1970 and 1971

Number of cases	Number of men excluded	Calculated number of falsely alleged fathers
649	192	232

System	Observed number of exclusions	Expected number of exclusions
ABO	39	40·8
MN.Ss	88	74·5
Rhesus	74	65·0
Kell	4	7·7
Fy^a	13	11·2
Lu^a	5	7·7
Hp	43	41·9
Gc	39	37·0
Gm^1	26	15·1
Ag	33	32·6
PGM	36	35·6

mother and child happen to be very common and if there is frequent heterozygosity in the numerous systems in which the antithetical factors are now investigated the chance of showing non-paternity may be quite low. In such a situation employment of an additional system may have a much greater chance of showing exclusion than in cases where the tests routinely applied have already given a high exclusion chance.

With the full range of tests now available the fact that such tests have been applied and not shown exclusion is significant but the significance is different from case to case. A report that merely records the groups is no longer adequate; there needs to be some indication of the chance that the investigation gave of showing non-paternity. Where the parties are European the simple calculation of the percentage of men that the tests would not have excluded provides this measure. For other races mathematical calculation is not possible but the serologist is usually able to assess the position and give expert guidance to the court.

REFERENCES

Allen, F. H. (1961). *Transfusion*, **1**, 209.
Grubb, R. (1956). *Acta path. microbiol. scand.*, **39**, 195.
— (1970). *The Genetic Markers of Human Immunoglobulins*, p. 67. London; Chapman and Hall.
— and Laurell, A. B. (1956). *Acta path. microbiol. scand.*, **39**, 390.
Law Commission (1968). Blood Tests and the Proof of Paternity in Civil Proceedings, p. 22 (No. 16). London; Her Majesty's Stationery Office.

C*

4   The Histopathology of Wounds

PETER PULLAR

INTRODUCTION

The microscopic examination of wounds has an ever-increasing rôle in forensic practice. This trend results from the extension of laboratory facilities to which the majority of forensic pathologists now have access. In these laboratories the apparatus and technical skill can apply the classical techniques of standard histological methods to forensic problems. The three most common problems are: Can microscopy confirm the presence of injury? Can the duration of injuries be estimated and did they occur before death? Can the presence of significant natural disease be excluded?

The classical methods have recently been supplemented by the development of relatively simple histochemical techniques and the almost universal use of the cold microtome with the production of enzymatic preparations. Other significant trends are the increasing use in the laboratory of the techniques of electron microscopy and immunofluorescence.

In this chapter the classical methods are reviewed and the development and utilization of the newer techniques, which have some forensic application, are described. These methods can be readily developed and standardized in a routine laboratory. A diagnostic scheme based on their use in a comprehensive forensic practice is also described.

The classical methods of investigating the histopathology of wounds are based on the morphology of the various stages of inflammation, which lead eventually to the process of repair. These processes are well described in the standard textbooks of general pathology and still form the basis of the majority of introductory courses in pathology.

An extensive literature of the various morphological sequences of healing have been summarized, notably by Arey (1936) and Allgower (1956). Another excellent summary of the earlier literature is that of Needham (1952, 1964), in which he considers the healing of human wounds in relation to the spectrum of biological activities of various other species. It emerges that it is not easy to compare regeneration in lower animals with the related process of wound healing in mammals. In general, the regenerative powers are inversely related with a degree of histological differentiation. This can be manifest by a progressive decrease in the power of regeneration in individual animals of many species during their lifetime. He describes wound healing as an epimorphic process, namely a form of regeneration in which there is development *in situ* of the portion lost. This is comparable to the replacement of limbs of the crustacea and the amphibia. In general terms this epimorphic regeneration shows two main phases: (1) regressive, which is subdivided in order of occurrence as wound closure, the demolition of damaged cells and the dedifferentiation of cells to provide new tissue for the process of repair; and (2) progressive, which in its simplest form is divided into three phases, the formation of repair tissue, its growth and differentiation. These three phases are manifest morphologically by migration, mitosis and morphogenesis. There is an overlap of all these various stages, and the whole time scale varies in different organisms and even in different parts of the same organism. This generalization has obvious forensic implications.

The series of events in response to the initial injury generally follow in a definite order and the two main phases described above are generally subdivided, in descriptions of wounds in human tissues, into four periods (Douglas, 1963): (1) the phase of traumatic inflammation which lasts from one to three days after wounding and in which the main histological features are those of the appearance of fibrin and dilated capillaries; (2) a destructive phase, from four to six days, which is characterized with numerous leucocytes and macrophages; (3) a proliferative phase, four to fourteen days, characterized by the presence of fibroblasts around capillaries and some metachromasia of tissue ground substance; and (4) a phase of maturation which is gradually reached over many months and in which collagen formation is accompanied by a decrease in the number of fibroblasts and a progressive increase in tensile strength of the wound. Phases (1) and (2) are described as lag phase or a period with no proper repair. This lag phase was noted earlier by Howes, Sooy and Harvey (1929) who, in the study of the tensile strength of wounds, divided the process into three phases: (1) the lag phase with decreasing tensile strength up to the fourth or sixth day; (2) a period of fibroplasia up to the tenth to fourteenth day, in which the tensile strength rapidly increased and fibroblasts were seen simultaneously; and (3) maturation of varying duration in which the scar assumed its definitive structure.

The earlier morphological changes have been described in great detail by many authorities. Perhaps the earliest sign was noted by Walcher (1930) who described margination of leucocytes on the vascular wall within half an hour of wounding. This in practice is difficult to detect with any certainty in human material from the usual cases of medico-legal interest. There is a note of a definite leucocyte reaction in the tissues some three to five hours after wounding. Our own studies have frequently confirmed the presence of polymorphs within ten hours of wounding, although there are authenticated cases in which this form of exudate has taken still longer to become apparent.

The early studies have been well summarized by Raekallio (1961) and in view of his later studies it is useful to note that in experimental wounds in guinea-pigs he has found polymorphs within eight hours, and at sixteen hours he divides the wounds into two zones, namely, a central zone of up to 500 μ in depth and a peripheral zone. In the central zone there are early degenerative changes with necrosis at some 32 hours; and in the peripheral zone at the same time there is an accumulation of mononuclear cells. At 64 hours there is advanced necrosis in the central zone and mitotic activity in the connective tissue and epidermis of the peripheral zone.

Dann, Glucksmann and Tansley (1941) noted in experimental wounds in rats that while there was a five-day lag period in the repair of connective tissue, epithelial regeneration began at once, as manifest by mitotic activity, and was complete by nine days. The wound was filled with fibrin during the first 24 hours and a cellular infiltrate of polymorphs. These were replaced by histiocytes and fibroblasts at about the fourth day. The fibrin was not completely resolved until about the fifth day when collagen formation began.

The rôle of epithelium in wound healing has received less attention than the mesenchymal components.

Viziam, Matoltsy and Mescon (1965) have studied the sequence of events in epithelialization in small shallow wounds of rabbits. They note three stages: a lag period, a phase of migration of cells and remodelling. The leucocyte invasion, with what they describe as a poly-band, is the first response to wounding and is fully formed after 18–22 hours. It sharply delineates the wounded area from the intact tissues. After about 24 hours the basal epithelial cells from a wedge-shaped mass which moves between the poly-band and the intact dermis. They suggest, therefore, that the epithelialization is not merely a migration but a more complex process involving migration, mitosis and differentiation.

Interest in the regeneration of epithelium in material from human volunteers has been shown by Gillman *et al.* (1955), who note that the epithelium was the first tissue to regenerate and only after several days did a subepithelial exudate appear. As the epithelial tissue grows deeply in a wound they suggest it stimulates a growth response in the young collagen, and that the subsequent invasiveness of the epithelium is brought under control by the connective tissue response. These findings were mainly in superficial, clean cut wounds. They do note, however, that in deep wounds in which there is loss of the dermis and epidermis—these injuries being of the type more closely related to those encountered in forensic practice—there is a totally different course in the form of true granulations building up from the depth of the wounds. These studies on the epithelial component suggest that the process of regeneration is accompanied by an apparent dedifferentiation of this tissue with the assumption of the morphology and histochemical features associated with this process. Thus, the features of epithelium at the edge of a healing wound shows a remarkable similarity to tissues which developed in a form of tissue culture (Pullar, 1964) when various types of epithelium, including human foetal skin, could develop in a chemically defined medium from a primitive two-layered structure with the assumption of squamous morphology and later the formation of keratin. This process was generally complete within four days, and in common with earlier studies of healing wounds no interpapillary processes were noted.

HISTOCHEMISTRY

The standard histochemical methods are well described by Pearse (1968). Montagna (1962) provides a comprehensive account of the application of these techniques to the study of the structure and function of skin. The use of these histochemical techniques for forensic problems with a comprehensive summary of the earlier literature has been given by Gerin *et al.* (1965).

The distribution of histochemically identifiable substances in the two main components of skin will be described in this section and those substances which are found to have particular medico-legal interest will be considered in greater detail.

In the epidermis RNA is moderately intense in the basal cells and becomes less so in the squamous cells, showing an inverse relationship to the degree of keratinization. As demonstrated by the pyronin methyl green/ribonuclease method there is poor cytological detail and the staining is confined to the cytoplasm, apart from moderate intensity in the nucleoli. In skin wounds a great increase in the concentration of this substance is noted when there is active regeneration at the edges of a healing wound. It generally reaches its peak of activity when the cells have bridged the central gap.

DNA is normally confined to the nucleus and by the Feulgen method it is shown in the lower squamous and basal cells to comprise faint purple granules of uniform size. As the squamous cells approach the stratum granulosum there is a rapid but uniform condensation of the nuclei.

The distribution of glycogen (periodic acid Schiff/diastase method) also shows an inverse relationship to the degree of maturity of the epidermal cells, being greatest in the basal cell layer and virtually absent in keratinized epithelium.

The distribution of sulphydryl and disulphide groups show an inverse relationship to each other, the presence of the S–S groups being noted when keratinization is almost complete (dihydroxy-dinapthyl-disulphide method of Barrnett and Seligman, 1952).

The study of the distribution of these components has not proved to be of any practical assistance in an evaluation of wounds for forensic purposes. An increased reaction for RNA, glycogen and sulphydryl groups is noted in actively regenerating epithelium and merely parallels the usual histological stigmata associated with rapid cell growth and some dedifferentiation.

The histochemistry of the connective tissues has been admirably reviewed by Fullmer (1965). He notes that the connective tissues throughout the body constitute the principal means by which repair occurs. These tissues are divided into the cells and intercellular substance, which includes ground substance, elastic tissue and collagen. The fibroblasts, in common with actively growing cells elsewhere, show an increased RNA content in the cytoplasm. Glycogen and metachromatic material are also prominent and most have some alkaline phosphatase activity. There is intense acid phosphatase activity in macrophages and inflamed fibroblasts. A portion of the ground substance is composed of acid mucopolysaccharide. Large quantities of acid mucopolysaccharides are observed in the rapidly growing connective tissues of healing wounds. The elastic fibres are described as being produced by connective tissue cells. They have a remarkable affinity for phenols, naphthols and ferric salts. The basis of the staining methods for these substances is aldehyde fuchsin. Reticulin is characteristically identified by blackening with a number of silver stains. The reactions are well known to be capricious. The collagen stains by Van Gieson and Mallory's methods and their numerous modifications have not resulted in any superior delineations of these components.

Dunphy and Udupa (1955) have summarized the earlier views on collagen formation. It depends on two factors: a protein component, probably produced by fibroblasts, which passes through several stages before becoming collagen, and a carbohydrate component, a complex mucopolysaccharide, which produces homogeneous matrix that is necessary for the ultimate deposition of adult collagen from the soluble non-fibrous protein material. This is produced by the connective tissue cells and the carbohydrate component by either mast cells or connective tissue cells. It is noted that in healing wounds in rats the metachromasia of the connective tissues reaches a peak at about the fifth or sixth day and at this time the first chemical and histological evidence of collagen fibres emerges. As the collagen forms there is a prompt decline in metachromasia.

MUCOPOLYSACCHARIDES

The rôle of mucopolysaccharides in healing wounds has been mentioned. There are now various refinements and combinations of the three basic staining methods, metachromasia with toluidine blue, colloidal iron technique and periodic acid Schiff (PAS). Their use in human wounds at various stages in this laboratory only permits an estimation of their duration in the most general terms. Various other factors including age and nutritional state of the injured person are probably of at least equal importance. This view is shared by Raekallio (1961), who noted that in experimental wounds there was a slight loss of activity in the central zone of injury with an intensification in the peripheral zone after some 32 hours. They have also been used to determine whether wounds were sustained before or after death. Our own experience is that they only place injuries in the peri-mortem period.

Nevelos and Gee (1970) have studied the vital reaction in human material by the alcian blue and dialysed iron techniques with the PAS technique. By the use of extensive controls it was considered that the techniques were specific for the acid mucopolysaccharides of the connective tissue ground substance. They mention earlier investigations when acid mucopolysaccharides disappeared from vital wounds and reappeared during the healing process. They show that acid mucopolysaccharides also disappeared from vital bruises, abrasions and electric marks, while they remained present in the ante-mortem strangulation and hanging marks. They suggest that the alteration in vital wounds and bruises are mainly the consequence of haemorrhage into the connective tissue.

FIBRIN

The studies on fibrin in human wounds have generally either attempted to assess the duration of the injury or, again, whether it occurred before or after death. On the grounds that the blood loses its coagulability after death a clotted haemorrhage was earlier considered to be a sign of vital reaction. Likewise, the presence of fibrin in a tissue haemorrhage was considered to indicate vital injury.

Krauland (1938) studied tissue injuries in persons suffering a violent death. He used haematoxylin and eosin, Weigert's fibrin stain and his own Victoria blue method. He noted that the results had to be based mainly on the haematoxylin and eosin methods. He could detect fibrin in about 75 per cent of the haemorrhages. In many cases it was scanty and located chiefly in the marginal areas; in most the fibrin formed delicate networks. Only occasionally were there thicker bands and, compared with the thicker fibres, the delicate ones usually stained weakly or not at all.

The changes which occur in the morphology of fibrin of varying age have been well described by Cook (1964). With Mallory's phosphotungstic acid haematoxylin and Lendrum's acid picro-Mallory method, haemorrhages in human tissues 4–12 hours old showed a network of fine fibrils with phosphotungstic acid haematoxylin, which after 24 hours gave way to coarser fibrils in layers and a gradually concentrating network. After four days small concentrated areas appeared and after two weeks the solid areas predominated. After one month granular areas appeared amongst the solid areas and at four months only the granular appearance was noted. The picro-Mallory method did not stain the recent haemorrhages and in those older ones staining was less precise. These changes which occurred in the fibrin with age he attributed to proteolytic enzyme action, phagocytosis by leucocytes and compression of tissues into layers.

The alterations in staining reaction have been studied by Lendrum et al. (1962). They note that there are few satisfactory staining methods and describe the method of Martius scarlet blue, which we have found to be an elegant and most useful stain for the examination of wounds. Their material was mainly of the so-called fibrinoid type of lesions of varying age. They note that the staining reactions are dependent on the fine structure of the material rather than on a simple chemical reaction. They suggest that this fine structure probably undergoes changes with age and thus the entanglement of a suitable dye depends on finding the dyes of the right molecular size to match the succeeding structural changes in the ageing fibrin. The newest fibrin stains yellow with Martius scarlet blue, whereas older fibrin—say 16 hours—stains bright red, the corresponding colours with Masson (Lendrum's modification) being red and blue. With picro-Mallory both are red. What they regard as still older fibrin stains with 44/41 Masson, but all the other methods stain it as collagen. This they regard as confirmation of studies with older methods of a gradual change in the fibrils from a positive reaction for fibrin to a reaction for collagen without any other visible alterations.

Although we have found the Martius scarlet blue stain to be a most useful single method for the demonstration of fibrin, the number of positive results are considerably increased when more methods are used, notably Weigert, picro-Mallory and phosphotungstic acid haematoxylin. On occasions the use of all these methods has failed to demonstrate fibrin at a time when it should be present and when other morphological and histochemical changes are in agreement. Thus, a negative reaction may be without validity using these methods. On the other hand they have, on occasions, given positive reactions in injuries which occurred very shortly before death. The presence of fibrin, as demonstrated by these staining methods, can again only be described as occurring at or about the time of death.

PLATELETS

Although thrombosis has been long recognized as an essential reaction to injury and regarded by the earlier writers as an unequivocal sign of ante-mortem infliction, platelets have received scant attention. Sevitt (1970a, b), in reviewing their rôle in thrombosis and embolism after injury, distinguishes four stages: platelet adherence, platelet aggregation, platelet degranulation and platelet disruption. The first two are probably reversible, while the latter are associated with formation of fibrin and the transformation of the platelet plug to a mixed fibrin–red cell–leucocyte mass and the extension of the thrombus.

The rôle of platelets in superficial, human skin-puncture wounds has been studied by Zucker (1949) on both patients with normal haemostasis and those with idiopathic thrombocytopenic purpura. He found that agglutinated platelets arrest haemorrhage in normal skin by rapidly sealing the mouths of all cut vessels larger than capillaries. He has never seen platelet plugs in capillaries which are sealed by a red cell fibrin clot. Platelet thrombosis did not occur in the purpuric patients. He notes that occasionally well preserved platelets are made out within the masses but the bulk of them are already involved in the process of fusion (viscus metamorphosis). The resultant coarsely granular masses stain blue-grey in phosphotungstic acid haematoxylin preparations. A thin, darkly stained band resembling fibrin is present on the margin of the fused platelets. The platelet mass becomes surrounded by secondary clot, composed principally of red cells and fibrin. He believes that there is no evidence that fibrin plays a significant rôle in platelet thrombus formation, although he does concede the possibility that minute quantities of fibrin, not identifiable by routine histological methods, are formed on the platelet interfaces during thrombosis.

ELASTIC TISSUE

A relatively neglected tissue in wound healing is elastic tissue. A classic early study is that of Bunting (1939), who described the formation of elastic tissue in adhesions between serous membranes of the myocardium and pleurae. He notes that elastic tissue is not laid down among the collagen bundles. There may be some new tissue of elastic type laid down in association with the new vessels—parallel to them —and suggests that the development of elastic fibres might be related to protracted alteration of tension in the developing connective tissue.

Gillman et al. (1954) studied the reaction of elastic tissues in skin with various stains. They describe differences in the reaction of normal elastic fibres to what they describe as elastotic degeneration, namely, dermal accumulations of morphologically unusual fibril material. This has been referred to by other authors as an increase in the elastic fibres. They suggest that these accumulations seem to be derived primarily from alterations in the composition of pre-formed collagen or a disturbance during the formation of normal reticular collagen elastic fibres. These fibres stain with Weigert's orcein and Gomori's aldehyde fuchsin. Stains which can differentiate these two substances are haematoxylin and eosin, in which the normal elastic fibres appear pink and the others are blue-grey with pink granules. Toluidine blue is colourless with normal elastic and deep blue-green with the coarsely stained fibres. With Mallory's stain the normal is generally purple and the others pale orange.

Fatteh (1971) quotes earlier studies which suggest that from a microscopic examination of the elastic fibres in skin it was possible to judge whether the wound was ante- or post-mortem, in that in vital wounds there is a remarkable contraction of these fibres and they become wave-like, whereas post-mortem they are straight. The material, which was obtained from operation specimens, was stained by Hart's modification of Weigert's elastic tissue stain. No difference in the nature and distribution of the elastic fibres in the dermis of these wounds was demonstrable.

The study of elastic fibres is, however, of considerable importance in relation to bruises and other skin injuries. It is particularly important in the battered baby syndrome to exclude some familial defect as a suggested explanation for multiple bruises. For this reason normal skin adjacent to injuries is processed and examined routinely.

PIGMENTS

The observation of blood pigments in tissues was described over 100 years ago by Virchow. This and later classic papers are summarized by Muir and Niven (1935), who give interesting observations of these pigments under the headings of: (*a*) phagocytosis of red corpuscles, which in animal experiments is well marked after 48 hours; (*b*) the formation of haemosiderin, and evidence of this may be found after 24 hours; and (*c*) the formation of haematoidin, which is formed within cells at some eight days. They note that in the animals at any rate haematoidin and haemosiderin crystals are present in inverse proportion to each other.

Walcher (1936) noted that haemosiderin in vital wounds occurred only on the ninth day after injury. Hallermann and Illchman-Christ (1943) reported its presence some three days after injury.

Extensive studies with a wide variety of forensic material of differing duration in this laboratory has never demonstrated earlier than 48 hours, and then it is extremely scanty, being found only in an occasional mononuclear cell. Large deposits, such as are readily visible with a scanning power of the microscope, are seldom seen in the dermis of other skin injuries before seven or eight days. It has never been demonstrated in a wide range of material removed at various times *post mortem*.

Although there are numerous references on pigments in wounds in the usual range of laboratory animals, more interesting studies are those of Hamdy, Kunkle and Deatherage (1957a, b), who concluded from a study of cattle, hogs, sheep and rabbits, that the sequence of the visible and measurable chemical changes associated with bruise healing were the same, regardless of the animal species or the site of the bruise. They confirm the findings that younger animals healed significantly more rapidly and they suggest that enhanced healing had been observed in animals which had been bruised previously.

ENZYME HISTOCHEMISTRY

The development of histochemical enzyme techniques permits the study of the intracellular distribution of these substances with a closer correlation of morphology and cell function.

The different enzymes are associated with different forms of cellular metabolism. Thus, the Krebs, or tricarboxylic acid, cycle is associated with the succinic and malic dehydrogenase systems.

The pentose cycle or the hexose-monophosphate shunt pathway is associated with glucose-6-phosphate dehydrogenase. This is an alternative pathway for glucose and converts pentose nucleotides into nucleoproteins; thus an increased pentose cycle activity is accompanied by increased nucleic acid synthesis as manifested by the pyronin methyl green methods.

The glycolytic pathway, also known as the Embden–Meyerhof pathway associated with anaerobic oxidation, is linked to DPN and is manifest by alcohol dehydrogenase and lactic dehydrogenase.

The various enzymes are known to be associated with different parts of the subcellular structure. Thus, acid phosphatase is known to be a lysosomal enzyme, while succinic dehydrogenase, glucose-6-phosphate dehydrogenase, lactic dehydrogenase and NAD diaphorase are thought to be associated with the mitochondria. Associated with the membrane and microsomal fractions of the subcellular component are thought to be alkaline phosphatase, the non-specific esterases and possibly the lipases.

Hydrolytic enzymes are known to be present in lysosomes of polymorphs and macrophages, and are considered to have a fundamental rôle in phagocytosis. The granules of the polymorphs are also thought to contain acid phosphatase, alkaline phosphatase, nucleotidase, ribonuclease, desoxyribonuclease and glucuronidase. The lysosomes can also be stained by acridine orange, methylene blue and neutral red (Curran, 1967).

The distribution of the various enzyme systems has been described in adult human and foetal skin by Montagna (1962), Mustakallio (1961) and Pullar and Liadsky (1965a, b). In general there is agreement as to their distribution in normal skin, although differing

74

methods have been used which in detail produce minor variations in the intensity of staining.

Dawson and Filipe (1969) have given a succinct account of the storage, preparation and staining techniques for the histochemical demonstration of the more important enzymes. The methods described produce readily reproducible results with the use of only simple basic equipment and stains which are readily available. They bring the realm of enzyme histochemistry within the reach of almost all routine pathology laboratories.

The distribution of the enzymes which is now described has been obtained by use of these methods.

Acid Phosphatase

The epithelium is generally unreactive with a dense band of activity at the junction of the squamous and keratin layers—the so-called keratogenous zone of Giroud. There is a weak reaction in the hair sheath and sebaceous glands and the only structure which stains faintly in the dermis is the occasional fibroblast.

Alkaline Phosphatase

In normal skin there is no staining in the epithelium and in the dermis the reaction is generally confined to the capillaries.

Esterases

In the epithelium there is a faint reaction in the basal and squamous layers with a definite intensification in the keratogenous zone. In the dermis there is a reaction in the sweat glands and at the base of the pilosebaceous follicles.

Cytochrome Oxidase

In normal skin there is a moderate reaction in the basal and lower squamous layer with no reaction in the granular layer. A slight reaction is present in the fibroblasts of the dermis.

Aminopeptidase

There is moderate activity in the basal and squamous layers of the epidermis with a possible intensification in the granular layer. In the dermis there is moderate activity in the fibroblasts.

Dehydrogenase

In general, in normal epithelium there is a moderate reaction in the basal layer which becomes less intense in the more superficial layers of the epidermis until in the outermost layer there is no detectable reaction at all. In the dermis there is a faint reaction in the region of the dermal papillae and another faint reaction in the dermal fibroblasts.

These enzyme techniques have been applied to a study of skin wounds. The early studies are mainly on animal tissues and more recently some detailed investigations have been made with human material.

When living tissue is subjected to trauma, the more viable cells at the periphery of the injured part seem to react soon afterwards by synthesizing more enzyme—partly as a defence mechanism and in preparation for the subsequent reparative process. Additional enzyme is brought into the damaged area at first by the invading inflammatory cells, and later also by the proliferating epithelial and connective tissue cells.

Fell and Danielli (1943) studied the healing of experimental skin wounds in rats. They noted that the regenerating connective tissue stained more strongly for alkaline phosphatase than the normal dermis. The intensity of the reaction increased as healing advanced and reached a maximum when the formation of collagen fibres began. At this stage the fibroblasts, intercellular fibres and capillaries stain deeply. In addition they note that the scab was deeply stained because of the high polymorph content.

Detailed animal studies using a wide variety of enzymatic techniques were made by Raekallio (1961) in vital skin wounds of the guinea pig. He distinguished a central zone and a peripheral zone. In the central zone a progressive loss of staining occurred and by enzymatic techniques was demonstrable as little as 2–3 hours after injury, as compared with 8–16 hours with conventional techniques. In the peripheral zone the increase in the activity of the hydrolases could be noted in 2–8 hours, while the accumulation of the leucocytes was not apparent until 8–16 hours after wounding.

Further studies on human material from medico-legal autopsies confirmed the presence of two zones around the vital wound (Raekallio, 1966): (a) again a central zone with decreasing enzyme activity, possibly an early sign of imminent necrosis; and (b) a deep peripheral zone which exhibited an increase in enzyme activity and so possibly an adaptive defence mechanism. The activity of esterases and adenosine triphosphatase increased as early as one hour, that of aminopeptidase in two hours, of acid phosphatase in four hours and of alkaline phosphatase in eight hours. These vital histochemical reactions were recognizable for at least five days after death.

The difference in the timing of the cellular and exudative response in animal and human tissues has been noted earlier. A similar state of affairs has been shown to exist in the enzymatic reaction to injury.

Fatteh (1966) made a histochemical study of wounds in guinea pig and human skin, some wounds being inflicted before death and some after death. He noted that the time sequence in guinea pigs was similar to that of the human but occurred in approximately half the time. Thus, he confirms that a leucocyte response appears in four hours in the guinea pig and takes eight hours in the human. The most rapidly appearing reaction in the guinea pig was that of esterases, being positive in ten minutes, but the same reaction taking some 30 minutes in the human subject. Acid phosphatase was the next enzyme to appear; it took one hour in the guinea pig and as long as six in the human. With alkaline phosphatase and leucine amino-peptidase the figures were three and four hours in the animal and human tissues. The reactions last for some 72 hours *post mortem*.

Similarly Berg and Ebel (1969) note that animal experiments show that all reactions occur considerably earlier than they do in human tissues. They studied the changes in traumatic haematoma, and in their series the earliest reaction was an increased ATPase activity in the adjacent tissues after $2\frac{1}{2}$ hours. Aminopeptidase and non-specific esterase appeared within seven hours; polymorphs appeared within four hours; mononuclear cells within nine hours; haemosiderin after 90 hours; and haematoidin after nine days. They make the point that in unhealthy tissues delayed tissue reactions did occur, and that these delays are irregular and difficult to predict.

A detailed study in the healing process of the three enzymes, aminopeptidase, DPN diaphorase and succinic dehydrogenase, was made by Wolff and Schellander (1965), involving the healing process of autografts in pigs. During the first four days there was a decline in enzyme activity which started at the dermo–epidermal junction and progressed to the deeper parts of the graft, and after four days the process was reversed, in that they re-appeared in the deeper portions and later superficially. They note that in the initial regressive phase the deep portions of the graft showed a less pronounced decrease than the upper part and this they ascribe to diffusion of plasma from the wound bed.

These findings have some similarity to those of Hou-Jensen (1969), who studied the histochemical reactions in wounds from guinea pigs and human ante- and post-mortem material. He notes that in 25 human vital injuries less than eight hours old there were no conventional vital reactions or positive enzymatic reactions. In later injuries (8–32 hours) there was an increase in alkaline phosphatase activity. Tests for adenosine triphosphatase and non-specific esterase gave more variable results. Aminopeptidase and acid phosphatase gave no positive vital reactions in this group. In human controlled injuries inflicted *post mortem* no positive vital reaction was found either by enzymatic or conventional methods. He does note, however, that in some cases there was a diffused increase of enzymatic activity localized on the edges of the wounds. He points out that it is characteristic of vital human and animal wounds that an increase in intracellular enzyme activity is only demonstrable if the inflammatory infiltration is present. In both the earliest sign of increased enzyme activity is that of alkaline phosphatase. Again this increased activity is demonstrable earlier in animal wounds, where it can be observed along with leucocyte infiltration one to two hours after the infliction of the wound. The presence of increased enzyme activity, which is diffused throughout the tissue spaces and along the margins of the wound cavity, is of no value in deciding whether the injury is of vital origin or not in that it can also be shown, though less pronounced, in wounds inflicted *post mortem*, i.e. peri-traumatic activity. He divides this peri-traumatic activity into three phases in which: (1) The initial post-traumatic increase is due to the presence of blood and exudation of plasma and crushed tissues, and this can be observed in both ante- and post-mortem wounds. (2) The second phase of increased activity is due to the cells of the inflammatory infiltrate and depends on the type of the infiltrating cells. This in turn depends on the general condition of the injured individual, notable features being the state of the circulation and blood pressure. (3) The third phase of increased enzyme activity is demonstrable in fibroblast-like cells in the infiltrate and in the normal tissues. It appears to correspond to the increased activity which occurs as a stromal reaction in tissues, with increased activity due to other noxae. He concludes that cellular inflammatory infiltration is the earliest sign of a vital reaction but the demonstration of alkaline phosphatase within polymorphs may occasionally make their recognition easier.

Although wounds of medico-legal importance almost always involve the subcutaneous fat and deeper structures, these areas have been the source of relatively little investigation. The histochemical studies of deeper tissue injury by Hirvonen (1968) are, therefore, of considerable interest. He examined experimental traumatic fat necrosis in the intrascapular adipose tissue of adult guinea pigs. The earlier changes in vital trauma include alteration in cellular detail and the damaged cells lose their enzymatic reaction. All of the enzymes examined were affected within minutes but the process was most obvious in NAD diaphorase, lactic and malic dehydrogenase and non-specific esterase. Less obvious were changes in alkaline and acid phosphatase, ATPase, aminopeptidase and lipase. The cellular reactions were rapid in that polymorphs appeared within 30 minutes and macrophages within one hour. Primitive fibroblasts appeared within one hour, and after four hours a homogeneous ground substance was located extracellularly between the fibroblasts, and subsequently reticulin fibres appeared. Hirvonen comments that the traumatic inflammation in adipose tissue seems to occur much more rapidly than in the skin of the guinea pig or the rat. He notes that the leucocytes showed strong reactions for acid and alkaline phosphatase and a weaker one for aminopeptidase, non-specific esterase and oxidative enzymes. The other phagocytes were strongly positive for acid phosphatase, aminopeptidase and oxidative enzymes. The young fibroblasts reacted for acid and alkaline phosphatase, aminopeptidase, adenosine triphosphatase and oxidative enzymes. The lipase reaction was weak or absent in the phagocytes and fibroblasts. In the later stages when foreign body giant cells appeared after three days they gave a moderate to strong reaction for alkaline and acid phosphatase, ATPase, non-specific esterase, aminopeptidase and dehydrogenase. The primitive macrophages showed a strong reaction for aminopeptidase and a weaker one for acid phosphatase, dehydrogenase, alkaline phosphatase and ATPase.

It is of particular interest that these studies show an early increase in acid phosphatase activity, as has been shown in other situations when the balance between the stroma and the epithelium is disturbed, such as chemical carcinogenesis (Biesele and Biesele, 1944) and human squamous carcinoma (Kawakatsu and Mori, 1963).

Relatively little attention has been paid to the distribution of enzyme activity in regenerating epithelium but current studies confirm that the differentiation of the primitive epithelial cells in healing wounds parallels the process described *in vitro* by Pullar and Liadsky (1965a). The assumption of squamous morphology by conventional staining methods is associated with the appearance of a demonstrable reaction for acid phosphatase, non-specific esterase and cysteine desulphurase. These enzymes show a distinct intensification in the zone between the squamous and keratin layers.

The development of dehydrogenase systems also parallels *in vitro* studies with immature human skin (Pullar and Liadsky, 1965b). With the increasing development of squamous morphology there is an intensification of, in the early stages, DPNH diaphorase and lactic dehydrogenase. Later, when the epithelium appears to be mature and keratin formation has commenced, there is a reaction for the dehydrogenase associated with all three of the main metabolic pathways, namely lactic and DPNH diaphorase (glycolytic pathway), succinic, malic and isocitric (Krebs' tricarboxylic acid cycle) and glucose-6-phosphate (hexose monophosphate pathway). In each case the pattern of distribution is similar—a uniform reaction throughout the squamous layer with some intensification in the basal cell layer and no reaction in the keratin layer. The intensity of the staining, however, does vary, the reaction for DPNH diaphorase and lactic dehydrogenase being considerably stronger than those for other enzymes.

In general, the findings have been confirmed in human wounds of the type encountered in a standard forensic practice. They do permit the recognition of tissue reaction to injury at an earlier stage than is possible by the standard techniques of classical morphology. In practice, however, enzyme histochemistry does not completely solve the question as to whether lesions occurred before or after death. Even with the use of these elegant methods, the forensic histopathologist is still obliged to use the time honoured phrase of 'at or about the time of death'. They are most useful supplements to the diagnostic techniques already available. For satisfactory examination the material should be in a better state of preservation than is usually encountered in medico-legal work. Some enzymes are surprisingly resistant to post-mortem change. This depends on the enzyme under investigation, but Goffin (1968) has shown that the three hydrolytic enzymes in skin and their appendages were very resistant and persisted until putrefaction of the body had commenced. These tougher enzymes, acid phosphatase, alkaline phosphatase and non-specific esterase, are probably worthy of investigation in unpromising material.

More efficient methods are being developed and studies such as those of Jarecki et al. (1969) open up further areas of undoubtedly rewarding investigation. They compared the distribution of esterases using disc electrophoresis in the cathode area. Eight single esterase fractions could be determined. Two of these fractions showed up more intensely in ante-mortem skin wounds compared with un-damaged controls. No difference in the esterase pattern was distin-guished in undamaged skin and post-mortem wounds. More investi-gations of this type may reduce the period during which wounds must be classified as peri-mortem.

IMMUNOFLUORESCENCE TECHNIQUES

When conventional histological methods are used, fibrin in tissue sections gives markedly variable results. This variability is seen to occur even when fibrin clots, formed *in vitro*, are sectioned and treated by the usual histological means for the identification of this protein.

Negative reactions for fibrin in sections when these conventional procedures are employed may be entirely without validity and no adequate evaluation of its presence can be made unless a sensitive method based on immunological specificity is utilized (Gitlin and Craig, 1957).

Beck (1971) has given a short lucid introduction to the background and technique of this method. Although his subsequent illustrations are concerned with auto-immune disease the principles are applicable to a study of wounds.

Woolf (1961) studied the distribution of fibrin within the aortic intima, using a fluorescent antibody technique. With the use of conjugated anti-fibrin serum he showed more fibrin to be present within the tissue section than did the conventional staining methods (mainly Mallory's PTAH method).

Gitlin and Craig (1957) made an experimental study with fibrin clots, following work which showed that fibrin in certain tissue lesions did not stain by standard techniques in the generally accepted manner. Sections from these clots were shown to react specifically with fluorescent labelled rabbit anti-human fibrin antibodies. Comparable sections gave a negative reaction with three standard methods—Mallory's PTAH, Biebrich's scarlet-aniline blue and Pearse's periodic acid-leucofuchsin-haematoxylin-orange G. Exceptions were sections which were prepared in the presence of a concentration of albumin which was greater than 1 g per cent.

Riddle and Barnhart (1964) used the fluorescent antibody method to demonstrate fibrin in leucocytes in areas of fibrin accumulation. They studied the acute inflammatory cellular response to fibrin at ultrastructural level by electron microscopy and by fluorescent microscopy using rhodamine anti-fibrinogen in experimental work in dogs. They were looking for the possibility of fibrin dissolution by a proteolytic enzyme derived from polymorphs in the inflammatory exudate. They note that fibrin is either a network of heavy intertwining strands with orange fluorescence or less intensely stained delicate threads. At ultrastructural level the exudative neutrophils clearly participated in both extra- and intra-fibrin dissolution. Granules which were actively involved were found interposed in areas of lysis between areas of leucocytes and typical fibrin. The fibrin structure was progressively altered as dissolution continued. The typical filamentous structure was first altered to a compact granular mass of moderate density and later appeared as a loosely arranged mass of little density. Exudative neutrophils in contact with the fibrin showed a striking loss of cytoplasmic organelles, chiefly specific granules and vesicles of the endoplasmic reticulum. They suggest that fibrin appeared to have a rôle both as a mediator and perpetuator of the inflammatory process.

Hirvonen (1968) mentions the use of the fluorescent technique in a histochemical study of experimental traumatic fat necrosis in guinea pigs. The damaged fat cells showed a moderate green–yellow auto-fluorescence under ultra-violet light. In the intact tissues only the cell borders fluoresced. He suggests that the fluorescence originated in the degraded triglycerides.

Laiho (1967) has given a useful account of the rôle of fibrin in relation to wounds. He compared the fluorescent antibody technique with the conventional histological staining methods. Human autopsy material, including experimental bruises produced *post mortem*, was studied. The methods were Mallory's PTAH, Lendrum's 44/41 Masson, Martius scarlet blue and Glenner's rosindle. He found that the PTAH method was the best of the conventional methods but the fluorescent antibody technique was superior to them all, fibrin being frequently detectable in fluorescent preparations while the other methods were negative. It also gave sharper delineation. He concludes that the standard histological staining methods for fibrin do not give conclusive evidence that a haemorrhage contains fibrin, and that the absence of fibrin from a haemorrhage does not exclude the possibility that injury was of vital origin. The information obtainable about the presence of fibrin in post-mortem subcutaneous haemorrhages depends greatly upon how soon the samples are taken after the production of the post-mortem lesions. Post-mortem fibrin cannot be distinguished with any certainty on morphological grounds from vital fibrin. A large proportion of post-mortem subcutaneous haemorrhages undergo fibrinolysis which destroys the formed fibrin networks within a day of the haemorrhage. Therefore, well preserved fibrin networks found at autopsy performed two to three days after death appear to point to the vital or agonal origin of a subcutaneous haemorrhage and against its post-mortem origin.

ELECTRON MICROSCOPY

The small size of the sample examined by this method, and the absolute necessity for tissues to be fixed quickly after death, limits its application in a study of wounds of forensic interest. The method has, however, elucidated some of the basic responses of tissues to injury.

Several recent investigations of injury and repair by electron microscopy have produced interesting findings on the finer structure of these processes. The main findings have been surveyed by Curran

(1967), whose interests are centred on the electron microscopic features of fibrogenesis. He reviews the findings on the basis of fibrogenesis with an extracellular precursor—tropocollagen—which consists of three polypeptide chains. Using the colloidal iron technique in electron microscopy in an experimental study of mucopolysaccharides and collagen formation, the Golgi apparatus in the fibroblast is the site of synthesis or completion of synthesis of this compound.

Ross (1964), describing the features in experimental skin wounds in guinea pigs, notes that in the early stages when by light microscopy there is fibrin and the cells associated with an acute inflammatory exudate, with the electron microscope the most prominent features are a large number of free granules which morphologically appear to be similar to the granules found in the intact polymorph and are dispersed between bundles of fibrin in the early wound. He notes that a fibroblast can be recognized by the very extensive system of cisternae of the endoplasmic reticulum. Other characteristics which allow one to distinguish the fibroblast and other cell types are somewhat enlarged mitochondria, peripherally located aggregates of filaments and a prominent Golgi complex. Using these criteria to recognize the fibroblast, a few cells answering this description are already present in wounds at 24 hours, while with the light microscope it had been impossible to recognize such cells before the third day. Later collagen fibrils are present in normal animals by the fifth day; their diameter increases and by the ninth day there are two populations of fibrils which differ in size.

Odland and Ross (1968a) studied, by electron microscopy, superficial incised wounds from human volunteers. Samples were taken at intervals between three hours and 21 days. They divided their parallel light microscopic studies into three conventional phases, namely mitosis, migration and differentiation. The small size of the wounds studied may be reflected in that they note that differentiation, as shown by epithelialization, is invariably complete by three days. Electron microscopy shows that the migrating epithelium is associated with a characteristic ruffling of the cell membranes. The epidermal cells are shown to be phagocytic, enclosing fragments of fibrin and melanin, while the advancing epidermis moves initially through a serous exudate containing fibrin and some red blood cells. Inflammatory cells do not regularly lie in proximity to advancing elements of the epidermis.

The same authors (1968b), in examining the dermal components, note that the neutrophils contain thin membrane bounded vacuoles, some fibrin and serum protein from the wound. Most of the granulocytes lyse and release their cytoplasmic content into the extra-cellular space. The mononuclear cells develop rough endoplasmic reticulum and smooth surface membranes prior to active phagocyto-sis. They can be clearly distinguished from the fibroblasts in which the rough endoplasmic reticulum is highly developed. Immature fibroblast type cells are present in the perivascular connective tissue, and by the fourteenth day the wound contains many collagen type fibroblasts. At this stage the cisternae of the rough endoplasmic reticulum are clearly the dominant feature of the fibroblast. Many small non-banded fibrils are often present within the extracellular space close to the surface of the fibroblast. An interesting observation is intimate contact observed between basal cells of the regenerated epidermis and the monocytes of the wound below. Such contacts were only seen on the fourth to the seventh day after wounding. It was concluded that the inflammatory response and fibrogenesis in human skin wounds are strikingly like those in skin wounds of experimental animals, no important differences being observed.

Electron microscopic features of the long-term structural changes in thoracotomy wounds in guinea pigs were studied by Williams (1970). The period extended over some 84 days, when elastic fibres become a component of the healing wound. Epithelialization is generally complete by the seventh day and the early phase (up to 14 days) is dominated by mucopolysaccharides and collagen formation with actively synthesizing fibroblasts. After 28 days collagenization is advanced and the wounds still cellular, while the fibroblasts retain significant ergastoplasm. At 56 days elastic fibres form an additional component of scar tissue and differ from collagen by their fine structural two-phase system of central elastin cores and peripheral microfibrils (microfibrils appear electron dense in both phospho-tungstic acid and uranyl–lead stained sections). The central core components appear electron dense with PTA but react weakly or not at all with uranyl–lead. They then fuse and form a composite mature elastic fibre. These are found initially in close proximity to fibroblasts. Other fibroblasts are only rarely in relation to the elastic fibres.

BURNS

Injuries of this sort are also examined primarily to determine whether the burning occurred before or after death. Vital reactions which can be determined by the naked eye—namely redness of the burnt area, a red line of hyperaemia around the burn, blister formation and the usual reparative processes—occur too late to be of much practical value.

Early morphological studies (Unna, 1896; Jenecic-Jelacic, 1956) describe some of the microscopic features, such as congestion and oedema, in burns sustained shortly after death. The precise microscopic changes of ante-mortem formation, such as cellular infiltration, appear only after a lapse of several hours.

An extensive study of various histochemical methods involving both ante- and post-mortem burns is that of Cotutiu *et al.* (1964), who note particularly that in post-mortem burns there is a loss of epidermis but no reaction for alcian blue or colloidal iron in the superficial zone. Abundant fat globules are present in the dermis but there is no inflammatory reaction or thrombosis. In the vital burns there is thinning of the adjacent epithelium and an increased reaction for SH groups throughout all layers. In the dermis there is loss of papillae with fragmentation of reticulin, elastic fibres and homogenization of collagen. The superficial zone of the burnt area gives a positive reaction for alcian blue and coloidal iron and a metachromatic fluorescent reaction after staining with acridine orange. Later stages (3–30 days) are characterized by the usual inflammatory reaction with thrombus which is PAS positive and gives an intense reaction for SH groups. Later, at the healing stage, there are numerous fibroblasts, with abundant PAS positive material, some of which is within their cytoplasm.

Pioch (1966) was able to demonstrate, by the use of enzyme histochemistry, earlier changes in ante-mortem changes of the skin than was possible with histological methods. He notes particularly that in burns sustained about the time of death the morphological changes in vital and post-mortem lesions could be almost identical, and in particular the local vascular changes, which had been stressed by earlier workers, were not certain criteria. A positive esterase reaction was noted by the edge of the area of coagulative necrosis some 30 minutes after burning. DPN diaphorase shows negative reaction and at the same time there is an increase in the activity of the ATPase and aminopeptidase of the adjacent mesenchymal cells. There is no essential difference between electric burns and ordinary burns and they could not be separated by microscopic methods.

Malik (1970a, b), on the basis of enzymatic studies, divided burns into two zones. In both experimental burns and human material from forensic cases there were a central necrotic area and a peripheral area of heat damage. The peripheral area showed an increase in enzyme reaction. This was interpreted as a definite indication of ante-mortem origin. None of the post-mortem burns displayed an increase in enzyme reaction in this peripheral zone. The rate of appearance of the increased enzyme activity in this zone varies, the earliest increase being that of non-specific esterase, which appeared as early as 45 minutes after burning; leucine aminopeptidase appeared after two hours, acid phosphatase after three hours and alkaline phosphatase after six hours. A similar sequence was found in the experimental guinea pigs. The reactions occurred sooner and paralleled the time difference taken for the production of inflammatory reaction, which was six hours in the human material and four hours in the guinea pigs. It is noted that the enzymes were stable enough to withstand delays of at least 72 hours between death and the autopsy examination.

BONES

The histological examination of bone injuries has assumed greater importance in recent years largely because of the 'battered baby' syndrome. Microscopic examination is necessary in these cases to exclude the possibility that the bony injuries are due to underlying natural disease. As the injuries are usually multiple it is also necessary to assess the duration of fractures and their possible time relationship to soft tissue and other injuries elsewhere in the body. The healing of fractures is essentially similar to wound healing elsewhere in the body. It comprises vascular and cellular elements and the formation of granulation tissue with the power to form bone. In most cases the specialized form of connective tissue known as callus develops and thereafter seals the gap between the broken ends of the bone.

Most of the earlier histological studies have been concerned with experimental animals but a succinct recent account of the process in human material is that of Sevitt (1970a, b). He notes that, as elsewhere, there are two phases: the first is a preparatory stage and the second is marked by union of the fracture gap and remodelling of the callus. It is the first of these which is of greater forensic interest. There are five main features on microscopic examination.

Haemorrhage

Haemorrhage occurs at the time of the injury. The subsequent haematoma is usually around the fracture rather than within it. Within hours a fibrin network is evident.

Necrosis

Fractures are associated with some necrosis of the bone either

86

from mechanical injury or because of the ischaemic change. Usually this necrosis is recognizable with routine stains in 48 hours.

Traumatic Inflammation

Acute inflammatory changes begin within hours of injury and last several days. After the haemorrhage becomes partly organized the fracture gap may be filled with condensed highly eosinophilic fibrin and within one to two days there may be migration of polymorphs into the necrotic tissues and later macrophages.

Osteogenic Granulation Tissue

This is usually evident by four days. Mitotic figures may be present in the periosteum, and repair which extends towards the fracture zone and progressively involves the fracture tissues. As elsewhere, the process is characterized by the presence of newly-formed blood vessels and mononuclear cells and by about seven days abundant well developed fibroblasts. At this stage there is usually a proliferation and infiltration of osteogenic cells, which subsequently mature into osteoblasts and osteoclasts.

Medullary Callus

Vascular and fibroblastic proliferation in the medullary activity may precede osteogenic activity in onset and location. The fibroblasts lay down reticulin and then collagen fibres, generally away from the fracture at first, and then streams of elongated cells advance towards the gap. This is usually well manifest by ten days and by 15–20 days much of the damaged marrow is invaded by vascular fibrocellular tissue. By 30 days the callus gap is usually obliterated and by three months union has occurred, although the bone is still undergoing reconstructive modelling. Callus is also present in the periosteal region. Again the cellular activity involved begins away from the fracture zone and by ten days the cellular collar, which includes osteogenic cells, is formed. Trabeculae of new bone may be formed but there are numerous fusiform cells which resemble fibroblasts. The outer layer of the periosteum is lifted off this proliferating tissue and eventually the so-formed collars will fuse in the middle. Such a callus is usually well formed by 20 days and may be bridged by this time. The periosteal collars are probably completed by 30 days and the callus gaps virtually obliterated.

The histochemistry of the early stage of the healing fractures has been described by Raekallio, Kovacs and Makinen (1970). They studied experimentally-produced wounds in mice using decalcification methods described by Balogh (1962). The enzymes studied

D

included lactic, isocitric, glucose-6-phosphate, succinate and lipo-amide dehydrogenases, glutathione reductase and cytochrome oxidase. As in skin wounds, in a central zone around the fracture line there was a decrease in enzyme activity which was considered to be an early sign of imminent necrosis. This was histochemically demon-strable some ten hours after injury, whereas the necrosis only became visible by morphology about two days post-operatively. In the peri-pheral zone outside the area of necrosis there was an increase in oxidoreductase activity from the tenth hour onwards in both the osteoblasts and the osteogenic cells of the inner periosteal layer. The strongest activity was noted in lactic and lipoamide dehydrogenase, while succinate and glucose-6-phosphate dehydrogenase showed the least. After some 16 hours the proliferation of the periosteal cells produced an increase in oxidoreductase activity. Similar features were noted in the endosteum where cytochrome oxidase gave the most intense reaction.

Diseases which alter the normal healing process in fractures may confuse the interpretation of the duration of injury. They are, therefore, of obvious forensic interest. Such a condition is scurvy, with its effect on bone and skin.

The classical morphological changes (Wolbach and Bessey, 1942) have been supplemented by the application of more recently de-veloped techniques.

The histological characteristics of abundant proliferation of fibro-blasts which remain immature, and the failure of formation of extra-cellular material, is manifest histochemically by a marked reduction in demonstrable alkaline phosphatase (Pirani and Levenson, 1953). They note that in less severe cases the small amount of extracellular material which may be produced does not become organized into collagen fibres and reticulin fibres persist. In guinea pigs reticulin was present in greater amounts than in the controls. The degree of metachromasia was markedly increased and it was felt that this was due to enhanced reactivity to toluidine blue rather than to an in-creased amount of mucopolysaccharide, probably on the basis of depolymerization of the ground substance, which is thought to occur in scurvy. No alkaline phosphatase activity could be detected in the wounds of these animals.

The basic findings with light microscopy have been confirmed and extended by electron microscopy. Ross (1964) has noted that by electron microscopy scorbutic wounds show three major changes: an apparent vacuolation or rounding-up and separation of the cisternal components of the endoplasmic reticulum in the fibroblasts; an accumulation of large amounts of lipid in the fibroblasts; and a striking absence of collagen fibres in the extracellular regions. In the place of collagen there is a large amount of filamentous material with no banding and this cannot be identified on the basis of its morphology. Thus, the major change in the scorbutic state is in that part of the fibroblasts associated with protein synthesis, namely the endoplasmic reticulum.

STANDARD PROCEDURE FOR
LABORATORY EXAMINATION OF WOUNDS

Injured tissues are removed from the body with a wide margin of 'normal skin'. Skin from areas elsewhere in the body is also removed, including parts which are normally covered and parts which are uncovered by clothing. The tissues are identified by a series of nicks made with a sharp scalpel along the margin of the uninjured area. If necessary, the nicks can be arranged in the form of Roman numerals. Areas for examination are then divided, and one part is fixed in 10 per cent buffered neutral formalin for 24 hours, automatically processed and cut in the form of 5 μ paraffin sections. All sections are routinely stained by: haematoxylin and eosin; Prussian blue reaction; phosphotungstic acid haematoxylin; Martius' scarlet blue; and elastic tissue stain.

Using this scheme the microscopic preparations are available within 48 hours of receiving the specimen. This is generally found to be acceptable for most routine matters under investigation. If the matter is more urgent, with the use of an 'Ultratec', the tissues can be ready for examination the day after removal from the body. These five staining methods used routinely readily permit the recognition of those elements which appear in a wound in response to injury. In particular, the Martius' scarlet blue method is very useful as erythrocytes stand out readily from the background, unlike the standard H and E method. It can also provide beautiful preparations for photomicroscopy.

An examination using these methods permits the estimation of the duration of injury with reasonable certainty into hours, days or weeks. It also allows a comprehensive examination into the possibility of antecedent natural disease.

If the matter is more complex, further paraffin sections are stained for:

Mucopolysaccharides—Hale's colloidal iron (followed by PAS)— acid alcian blue (followed by PAS).

Reticulin—Gordon and Sweets.

Collagen—Van Gieson.

The other block provides cryostat sections, generally cut immediately on receipt. If for any reason this is difficult, the material is stored in a deep freeze and sectioned later, generally within 24 hours. These sections are stained for: acid phosphatase; alkaline phosphatase; non-specific esterase; leucine aminopeptidase; malic and succinic dehydrogenase; and NAD and NADP.

Cryostat sections are also stained with anti-human fibrin serum and examined by fluorescent microscopy using ultra-violet light.

When the procedures are standardized and the laboratory organized for a standard diagnostic scheme it involves relatively little increase in workload, and the results obtained can fully justify any such increase.

REFERENCES

Allgower, M. (1956). *The Cellular Basis of Wound Repair*. Springfield, Ill.; Thomas.

Arey, L. B. (1936). *Physiol. Rev.*, **16**, 327.

Balogh, K. Jr. (1962). *J. Histochem. Cytochem.*, **10**, 232.

Barrnett, R. J. and Seligman, A. M. (1952). *Science, N.Y.*, **116**, 323.

Beck, J. S. (1971). Association of Clinical Pathologists Broadsheet No. 69.

Berg, S. and Ebel, R. (1969). *Munch. med. Wschr.*, **21**, 1185.

Biesele, J. J. and Biesele, M. M. (1944). *Cancer Res.*, **4**, 751.

Bunting, C. H. (1939). *Archs. Path.*, **28**, 306.

Cook, E. (1964). *J. R. microsc. Soc.*, **82**, 215.

Cotutiu, C., Belis, V., Streja, D. and Drugescu, N. (1964). *Ann. Med. leg.*, **44**, 549.

Curran, R. C. (1967). In *Modern Trends in Pathology—2*, Ed. by T. Crawford. London; Butterworths.

Dann, L., Glucksmann, A. and Tansley, K. (1941). *Br. J. exp. Path.*, **22**, 1.

Dawson, I. M. P. and Filipe, M. I. (1969). Association of Clinical Pathologists Broadsheet No. 64.

Douglas, D. M. (1963). *Wound Healing and Management*. Edinburgh; Livingstone.

Dunphy, J. E. and Udupa, K. N. (1955). *New Engl. J. Med.*, **253**, 847.

Fatteh, A. (1966). *J. forens. Sci.*, **11**, 17.

— (1971). *J. forens. Sci.*, **16**, 393.

Fell, H. B. and Danielli, J. F. (1943). *Br. J. exp. Path.*, **24**, 196.

Fullmer, H. M. (1965). In *International Review of Connective Tissue Research*, Ed. by D. A. Hall, Vol. 3, p. 1. New York; Academic Press.

Gerin, C., Fucci, P., Merli, S., Marchiori, A. and Durante, F. (1965). Congress of the International Medico-legal Society (Langue Franc). Atlantida, Coimbra, Portugal.

REFERENCES

Gillman, T., Penn, J., Bronks, D. and Roux, M. (1954). *Nature Lond.*, **174,** 789.
—————(1955). *Br. J. Surg.*, **43,** 141.
Gitlin, D. and Craig, J. M. (1957). *Am. J. Path.*, **33,** 267.
Goffin, Y. (1968). *Acta path. microbiol. scand.*, **73,** 351.
Hallermann, W. and Illchman-Christ, A. (1943). *Dt. Z. ges. gerichtl. Med.*, **38,** 97.
Hamdy, M. K., Kunkle, L. E. and Deatherage, F. E. (1957a). *J. animal Sci.*, **16,** 490.
—————(1957b). *J. animal Sci.*, **16,** 496.
Hirvonen, J. (1968). *Ann. Acad. Sci. fenn.*, 136.
Hou-Jensen, K. (1969). *Dan. med. Bull.*, **16,** 305.
Howes, E. L., Sooy, J. W. and Harvey, S. C. (1929). *J. Am. med. Ass.*, **92,** 42.
Janezic-Jelacic, O. (1956). *Ann. Med. leg.*, **36,** 179.
Jarecki, R., Arndt, U., Schultz, C. and Klein, H. (1969). *Dt. Z. ges. gerichtl. Med.*, **66,** 161.
Kawakatsu, K. and Mori, M. (1963). *Cancer Res.*, **23,** 539.
Krauland, W. (1938). *Dt. Z. ges. gerichtl. Med.*, **30,** 267.
Laiho, K. (1967). *Ann. Acad. Sci. fenn.*, **128,** 1.
Lendrum, A. C., Fraser, D. S., Slidders, W. and Henderson, R. (1962). *J. clin. Path.*, **15,** 401.
Malik, M. O. A. (1970a). *Criminologist*, **5,** 63.
— (1970b). *J. forens. Sci.*, **15,** 489.
Montagna, W. (1962). *The Structure and Function of Skin.* New York; Academic Press.
Muir, R. and Niven, J. S. F. (1935). *J. Path. Bact.*, **41,** 183.
Mustakallio, K. K. (1961). *Ann. Histochem.*, **6,** 275.
Needham, A. E. (1952). *Regeneration and Wound Healing.* London; Methuen.
— (1964). In *Advances in Biology of Skin*, Vol. 5, Ed. by W. Montagna and R. E. Billingham. London; Pergamon Press.
Nevelos, A. B. and Gee, D. J. (1970). *Med. Sci. Law*, **10,** 175.
Odland, G. and Ross, R. (1968a). *J. Cell Biol.*, **39,** 135.
——(1968b). *J. Cell Biol.*, **39,** 152.
Pearse, A. G. E. (1968). *Histochemistry*, 3rd ed. London; Churchill.
Pioch, W. (1966). *Acta. Med. leg. Soc. (Liege)*, **19,** 327.
Pirani, C. L. and Levenson, S. M. (1953). *Proc. Soc. exp. Biol. Med.* **82,** 95.
Pullar, P. (1964). *J. Path. Bact.*, **88,** 203.
— and Liadsky, C. (1965a). *J. R. microsc. Soc.*, **84,** 1.
— — (1965b). *Br. J. Derm.*, **77,** 314.
Raekallio, J. (1961). *Ann. Med. exp. Fenn.* (Suppl. 6).
— (1966). *Med. Sci. Law*, **6,** 142.
— Kovacs, M. and Makinen, P. L. (1970). *Acta. path. microbiol. scand.*, **78,** 658.
Riddle, J. M. and Barnhart, M. I. (1964). *Am. J. Path.*, **45,** 805.

Ross, R. (1964). In *Advances in Biology of Skin*, Vol. 5, Ed. by W. Montagna and R. E. Billingham. London; Pergamon Press.

Sevitt, S. (1970a). *J. clin. Path.* (Suppl. 4), **23**, 86.

— (1970b). *Br. J. hosp. Med.*, **3**, 693.

Unna, P. G. (1896). *The Histopathology of the Diseases of the Skin.* Edinburgh; Clay.

Viziam, C. B., Matoltsy, A. G. and Mescon, H. (1965). *J. invest. Derm.*, **43**, 499.

Walcher, K. (1930). *Dt. Z. ges. gerichtl. Med.*, **15**, 16.

— (1936). *Dt. Z. ges. gerichtl. Med.*, **26**, 193.

Williams, G. (1970). *J. Path.*, **102**, 61.

Wolbach, S. B. and Bessey, O. A. (1942). *Physiol. Rev.*, **22**, 233.

Wolff, K. and Schellander, F. G. (1965). *J. invest. Derm.*, **45**, 38.

Woolf, N. (1961). *Am. J. Path.*, **39**, 521.

Zucker, H. D. (1949). *Blood*, **4**, 631.

5 The Pathologist's Role and Modern Scientific Techniques at the Scene of the Crime

A. KEITH MANT

INTRODUCTION

During the last three decades advances in the scientific investigation of crime have proceeded so rapidly that the forensic scientist now plays a major rôle in almost every form of criminal investigation. The scientific investigations carried out at the scene of a crime are often vital in providing irrefutable evidence against the accused. As the laboratory tests become more sophisticated so it becomes even more important that nothing is done at the scene of crime which may interfere with the material which will undergo laboratory examination. Inadvertent damage to, or loss of, evidence at the scene of crime still occurs and much of this damage arises out of ignorance of the methods and techniques now in the hands of forensic scientists.

Every scene of crime is unique in itself and, therefore, the approach to any investigation will vary from case to case. The purpose of this contribution is to enumerate the basic scientific principles and techniques used in criminal investigation and to evaluate the information which may be gained by their application, in order that those persons who are only called occasionally to the scene of crime may carry out their particular rôle in the investigation without interfering with any concurrent or subsequent examination by the scientists.

In 1960 Detective Superintendent Salter, when addressing the British Association in Forensic Medicine upon trace evidence, said that to him the scene of crime was a sacred place and that he knew that it was the same to many of his audience.

LOCARD'S PRINCIPLE

The basis of scientific investigation of crime is Locard's (1928) exchange principle 'that when any two objects come into contact there is always a transference of material from each object onto the other'. Briefly, this theory implies that anyone entering and leaving a scene of crime will not only leave evidence of his presence there but will also carry away on his person evidence of his visit. Much of this evidence is in the form of contact traces, such as fingerprints, hairs, fibres and dust, and it may be the summation of all these contact traces in a particular case which may provide irrefutable evidence against the accused. It follows at once from this that every investigator entering the scene of crime will also leave evidence of his presence. In order to cut down this interference to a minimum only those investigators with specific functions must enter the scene and they must carry out their particular investigations with as little disturbance to the scene as is possible and leave as soon as they have completed their special tasks. With a trained investigation team the order in which experts visit the scene is an accepted part of the procedure. Although this chapter is orientated towards the pathologist and the police surgeon, it is impossible for them to provide the maximum assistance to the investigation unless they are not only fully aware of their own responsibilities but also of the functions of all other officers who make up the team.

GENERAL PROCEDURES

The most important officer in an investigation is the CID officer who is in charge of the case. This officer not only directs the investigation but co-ordinates the contributions made by all other members of the team. He will be summoned as soon as a major crime is suspected and will establish an Incident Room, which may be a specially equipped mobile unit which can be moved to the scene at the start of an investigation, after which a more permanent room will be set up, often in the local police station, where special telephone lines will be opened to facilitate communications. Information will be fed into this room and from it all directions regarding the investigation will be issued. Although in many homicide cases the solution is soon arrived at, in a proportion the enquiries may go on for weeks or months. A successful outcome of the initial enquiries may not be known for several hours and each case is treated at the outset as one which may require tedious and lengthy investigation. Even in the apparently most straightforward case of homicide all the

set procedures have to be observed with the same meticulous attention as would be given to a case which may demand weeks or months
of investigation. Unsolved cases are never closed and fresh information coming to light some years after a crime may entail a completely
fresh team of investigating officers. It is essential, therefore, that
when a new team takes up an old investigation all the information
gathered at the original enquiry is as clearly presentable to them as if
they had formed part of the original team.

A vital part of any investigation is a complete and accurate
recording of the scene as it was found. This recording in the first
instance is accomplished by accurate diagrams, notes and photography. The photographer is, therefore, one of the first persons to
visit the scene and will, wherever possible, make his photographic
records before anything has been moved or disturbed. He will not
usually, however, be the first person to attend the scene. When a crime
involving homicide has been committed a police surgeon, or possibly
a pathologist, is called at once, and it is of paramount importance
that he is fully aware of his duties at this particular stage of the investigation. The doctor's first duty, whether he be police surgeon or
pathologist, is to ensure that death has occurred. This may usually
be done without disturbing the body in any way. On arrival at the
scene the senior police officer present will normally acquaint him
with the bare facts, tell him whether anything has been disturbed and
possibly instruct him, especially if the body is out of doors, how he
should approach it and what areas he should be careful to avoid.
Certain rules or procedures, such as wearing protective clothing,
would appear obvious, especially if the doctor understands the theory
of interchange before entering the scene. Unfortunately, mistakes are
still made unintentionally, usually because the doctor becomes too
absorbed in the general problems and forgets his specific duties and
functions. He should avoid touching anything, and as an additional
safeguard he should wear a pair of disposable plastic gloves. Disposable anti-static overshoes are also desirable as their use will go far
to eliminate the exchange of trace evidence between the doctor's
shoes and the scene.

TEMPERATURE RECORDING

In many cases it is essential that temperature recordings be taken
of the deceased in order to allow a more accurate estimation of the
time of death to be made. The desirability for such recordings will
have been assessed by the CID officer in charge, who will be aware
of the disturbance to the scene and body which must occur if the

D*

temperature is taken and will have weighed up the advantages against the disadvantages of having the body disturbed before the photographs. If photographs have already been taken the problems are less.

A single recording of the body temperature of the deceased will be of very limited value when estimating the time of death. A minimum requirement is two temperature readings at least two hours apart. The times of the recordings must be carefully noted and the environmental temperature must be taken with each reading of the body temperature. The author has experience of the environmental temperature rising 10°F within an hour in a small room where several police officers were working at the scene.

The body temperature falls evenly until it has cooled some 85 per cent of the initial temperature difference between body temperature and the environment, following a regular cooling curve which flattens out as the temperature approaches that of the surrounding medium. During the last 15 per cent of temperature difference, however, the rate of cooling becomes erratic and, therefore, temperature recordings in this area are of no value (Fiddes and Patten, 1958). If the doctor who first examines the deceased discovers that the body temperature has dropped below that level where useful readings can be taken he should inform the officer of this fact. In many cases this will not be discovered until a temperature recording has been taken.

In most countries the rectal temperature is recorded, and although there are accurate sophisticated electrical temperature recording instruments available which can be used on any part of the body, the laboratory thermometer reading from 0° to 120°F is still the most popular instrument. The range 0° to 120°F ensures that the relevant part of the scale will be well clear of the body. The anus can usually be approached with the minimum of disturbance of the position of the body or the clothing. If necessary a small hole may be made in the clothing to allow the insertion of the thermometer into the rectum, provided that an accurate note is made of the position of the cut and that there is no suspicion of buggery. The thermometer should be left *in situ* for at least two minutes, or until it ceases to rise, before a reading is made. It may, of course, be left *in situ* and recordings taken at regular intervals.

Although the temperature recordings will provide the most accurate data upon which to base an estimation of the post-mortem interval during the first few hours after death, other early postmortem changes such as the distribution of the livid stains and the presence and distribution of rigor mortis should be noted, as these may assist in the subsequent reconstruction of the events.

The value of an accurate estimation of the post-mortem interval cannot be over-emphasized in the investigation of a criminal death. The closer the estimation arrived at, the narrower the time limits in which the police enquiry will be directed, and hence the automatic elimination of many persons from the enquiry. The importance of taking successive temperature recordings of the body at the scene, provided the body temperature has not cooled through 85 per cent of the temperature difference between it and the scene, cannot be over-stressed. In many cases the police surgeon may arrive several hours before the pathologist, and it is his responsibility to make these observations of the early post-mortem changes.

The final estimation of the time of death from the fall in temperature of the body and other early post-mortem changes, however, is the responsibility of the pathologist. His assessment cannot be given until after the post-mortem examination, as certain modes of dying, e.g. asphyxia or certain types of head injury, may cause a significant terminal rise in body temperature. The methods available for the interpretation of the temperature recordings have been well documented (Marshall, 1965), but each pathologist usually develops his own technique. It is important that the less experienced pathologist should appreciate that he is only going to give an estimated time of death, often within fairly wide limits, and that when estimating the time of death of a victim of a homicidal assault there are often many unassessable factors which are absent from the carefully controlled temperature recordings of dead bodies taken in mortuaries or under similar constant conditions. Methods and the interpretation of post-mortem temperature recordings have been reviewed by Mant (1967).

PATHOLOGIST'S EXAMINATION AT THE SCENE

When the photographers have finished there is usually no objection to the body being moved to enable an examination to be made *in situ*. This examination is not normally made until the pathologist who will undertake the autopsy has arrived. By this time the police may already have carried out a preliminary examination of the scene and have several things to show the pathologist, such as possible weapons, the distribution of blood stains and the presence of medicine bottles or, in the case of a suspected abortion, instruments which may have been used. It must be remembered, however, that in most cases only a preliminary examination of the scene by police officers will have been made before the arrival of the pathologist and, although photographs have been taken the collection of scientific evidence will only have just begun. The pathologist, therefore, should inform the senior investigating officer present of anything he proposes to do during his examination of the deceased which may alter the scene.

He should take virtually the same precautions as he would if he were first on the scene. The temptation to smoke at the scene must be resisted, as saliva on cigarette ends may be grouped, thus leading to the possible inclusion or exclusion of suspects. In one case a police surgeon used the last match in a booklet which had originated from a night club to light his cigarette. He then threw the booklet into the fireplace on top of some rubbish already there. It took the police six weeks of enquiries before they traced the matches back to the police surgeon!

The purpose of the pathologist's examination of the body *in situ* and of the scene is to elicit all the information which will assist him in the completion of his report. He will certainly be asked by the investigating officer his opinion with regard to possible weapons and the order in which the injuries have been inflicted. The scene may reveal evidence of a struggle and vital trace evidence may be present on the body. The examination *in situ* should be limited to a search for any such evidence which might be dislodged or possibly lost during the deceased's removal to the mortuary. Wherever possible a correlation should be made between injuries present and possible weapons, or other objects, which might have caused them. The distribution of blood stains and their shape, which may pinpoint the site of the assault, should also be noted.

The distribution of the livid stains must be recorded before the body is moved. An abnormal distribution will indicate that the body has been moved some hours after death. Hypostasis commences with the cessation of circulation, and the longer the body lies in one position the greater will be the permanence of the stains, which will become virtually fixed after several hours, thus providing positive information regarding the position of the body after death. A photographic record of abnormally distributed stains is invaluable to any subsequent reconstruction of events. In one case the body of a strangulated youth was found lying face downwards in a field. Death had clearly occurred several days before. The distribution of the livid stains made it clear that the deceased had been doubled up on his right side for several days, possibly in the boot of a car, before being deposited in the field where he was found.

No attempt should be made to carry out any part of the examination which could be better carried out in the mortuary. Not only is the lighting at the scene of crime usually indifferent but the longer the doctor stays at the scene the more likely he is to disturb something which may interfere with the scientific examination which will be carried out after the body has been moved.

The entire body should be carefully examined before anything is moved. The lie of the clothing should be noted and a preliminary examination made of any injuries. A photographer will always be at the scene during the examination by the pathologist, who may consider it desirable to have further photographs taken for the specific purpose of recording some wound or clothing arrangement *in situ*— anything which he considers important from the medical aspect of the investigation.

It is standard practice in the UK for police photographs prepared as Court exhibits to be in black and white. However, colour photographs or transparencies have such a tremendous advantage over black and white prints as rapidly-interpreted records of the scene or injuries that it is becoming a universal practice for forensic pathologists to make their own colour records of the body *in situ*, of visible injuries and even of the scene in general. The equipment favoured is light and compact, usually basically a 35 mm camera with an electronic flash attachment. The separation of bruises or blood stains from shadows or other marks or smears is thus simplified when refreshing one's evidence before going to Court.

Free hairs, fibres or other small matter which may become dislodged when the body is moved should be carefully searched for, removed and handed to the exhibits officer, who may remove fibres and hairs adherent to the body with adhesive tape. If there is a ligature mark and no ligature *in situ*, the impression should be taped at this stage as it may pick up some fibres left by the ligature, and thus enable the material of which the ligature was made to be identified. It must be remembered that any movement of the body may cause trace evidence to become dislodged or to change its position. If there are any visible bite marks these should be swabbed with a cotton wool swab moistened with saline. In a recent case in which a murdered girl was found with a rather indistinct bite mark, two of the three suspects were immediately excluded following the serological examination of the swab taken from over the bitten area. Such areas must not be touched until swabs have been taken. In cases of rape and murder areas of apparent seminal staining should also be swabbed, and the advantages and disadvantages of combing the pubic hair *in situ* considered.

Saliva swabs may be taken with advantage at this stage, and the precaution of wearing gloves during the taking of swabs must be observed in order to prevent any possibility of the swab becoming soiled with sweat from the pathologist.

Although it is desirable in almost every case to turn the body at the scene in order to examine the back before it is moved, the implications of this procedure must first be considered, and where necessary precautions should be taken to minimize some of the possible complications of such a manoeuvre. Sometimes the turning should be abandoned altogether at this stage, as for instance when the deceased is lying on his or her back, having been stabbed through the front of the chest. In this position the external blood loss is often minimal, or may be virtually absent. When the body is turned, however, a large volume of blood may escape through the stabbed wounds, not only saturating the clothing but also flooding the scene. In this case it is preferable to remove the body to the mortuary and delay the examination of the back until the clothing has been removed.

In cases of suspected criminal abortion where the vulva is exposed, and in cases of rape, vaginal swabs should be taken; and in cases of suspected abortion the strapping of an absorbent pad over the vulva to collect any fluid which may run out during transport should be considered.

The preparation of the body for removal and its actual removal should in every case be supervised by the pathologist. It is important to ensure that no contact traces are lost during removal and, to effect this, certain simple precautions are taken. The hands and feet should be placed in loosely secured plastic bags, and a larger bag should be placed over the head and neck. The legs or ankles must not be tied together. The body should be lifted on to a clean plastic sheet and transported in this sheet to the mortuary. After the body has been lifted the pathologist should examine the place where it has been lying.

Whether certain parts of the external examination should be conducted at the scene or in the mortuary must be governed by the circumstances of each case. The over-riding consideration is always the optimum place for examination and collection of trace evidence, with the minimum opportunity for loss or contamination.

The initial examination of the body in the mortuary will now be described in detail.

EXTERNAL EXAMINATION IN THE MORTUARY

The body will be placed in its plastic covering on the mortuary table and will normally be photographed full length after the sheet has been opened and the plastic bags around the feet, hands and head removed. Saliva swabs, if not already taken, should be taken at this stage. Before the clothing is removed scrapings should be taken from under the finger nails. This operation is normally carried out with the aid of the scientific officer. As a preliminary the hands are examined and the fingers opened. Any visible fibres or other matter in the hand, or adherent to it, should be removed and placed in envelopes, the site of the specimen first having been carefully noted. Before material is actually removed from beneath the nails, ten small envelopes are labelled, one for each finger. There are two means commonly employed for removing material from beneath the finger nails. The first entails the use of the ordinary matchstick, which is cut obliquely and run under the nail; the second is to use instead the apex of a twice-folded Whatman filter paper No. 1, size 4·5 cm. Whichever form of scraper is used, the finger is held over the envelope marked with its number as the material is dislodged, and then the scraper is dropped into the envelope, which is sealed. It is important to avoid contaminating the specimen as far as possible with epithelium or blood from the deceased. If a metallic object, such as a nail file, were used or if the matchstick were to be sharp, there would be a greater danger of abrading or even lacerating the skin and causing blood to ooze. If the nails are long enough they may be cut off with any adherent material. There are other minor modifications of this technique, but any method used has as its primary object the collection of the maximum amount of material with the minimum amount of trauma.

The increasing association of drugs with crime calls for collection of samples even at this early stage. Cannabis resins are fat soluble and will, therefore, stay in the subcutaneous fat of the fingers even after the hands have been washed. A swab soaked in chloroform or petroleum ether is rubbed over the fingers and palms. Samples should be placed in glass containers as plastic is soluble in chloroform. Firearm residues may also be detected on swabs taken from the firer's hand. Multiple swabs should be taken separately and labelled from the fingers, palm and back of the hand.

Heroin is sometimes taken in the form of snuff. It has a marked irritant action on the nasal mucosa, which will appear acutely inflamed. Saline-moistened swabs of the nasal mucosa after heroin-sniffing will yield heroin itself on examination.

The head hair should next be examined. Any apparent foreign matter should be removed with forceps, and then the hair may be combed through for trace evidence. Samples of both cut and pulled hair from at least six different areas of the scalp should be taken and labelled as to their origin.

It is only after these procedures have been completed that the body should be undressed, still on the plastic sheet, which later should be carefully folded for laboratory examination. Each article should be examined as it is removed and placed in its own container and labelled. Tears in the clothing and holes made by knives or other weapons must be noted as these will have to be matched with wounds.

Radiographs are essential before the post-mortem is undertaken in all cases of homicidal firearm wounds and all cases which fall into the suspected battered baby category.

Vaginal and anal swabs are taken at this stage and, if not already collected, swabs from areas of apparent seminal staining. Pubic hair should be combed through in all cases where there is a possibility of a sexual assault. Matted pubic hairs should be cut out with scissors and samples of pubic hair taken.

PROCEDURE WITH DECOMPOSING
AND DECOMPOSED BODIES

When a dead body has commenced to decompose, whether out in the open or under cover, identification, the post-mortem interval and the cause of death will all become difficult to establish. These difficulties increase with decomposition and are usually far greater when the body has lain exposed in the open, especially in the summer. The rate of decomposition is greatly accelerated in warm weather, not only because heat accelerates the onset of putrefaction but because numerous insects attack the body. *Figure 1* shows fly ova deposited beneath the ligature around the neck of a man who was found suspended from a tree within two hours of last having been seen alive. This occurred in a temperate climate. These are ova of the common bluebottle and are laid within hours of death in any accessible natural orifice, for example nostrils, eyes or any wounds. They are only deposited during daylight and will take 8–14 hours to hatch in the summer in a temperate climate. The adult fly will emerge from its pupa after 21–24 days. Between the hatching of the ova and pupation three instars occur. The dead body is attacked by eight separate waves of insects in the open air (Easton and Smith, 1970). The timing of the attacks is dependent upon the state of decomposition. As only one wave of insects attacks at one time a study of the fauna of the decomposing body may provide an accurate estimation of the date of death to within a day or two, provided the samples are correctly collected, and especially if the post-mortem interval is less than three weeks. Each species has its own life span and therefore it is essential that each one is identified and that its state of maturation at the time the body was found is known. Larvae of diptera, which attack the body immediately after death, are extremely difficult to identify unless fully grown. Ideally the larvae are reared to pupae, and eventually to the adult fly, by the entomologist.

In all cases where the timing of death is important samples of ova and maggots, both alive and dead, should be obtained. A few samples of each species should be placed in alcohol, and live maggots should be put in corked tubes with some muscle from the corpse

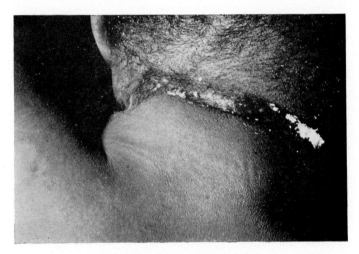

Figure 1. Fly ova deposited beneath the ligature within a very short time of death in a case of suicidal hanging

to feed on. Care must be taken not to put too much food or too many maggots in one tube or the maggots may drown in the excess moisture. In the laboratory, however, they may be reared in large numbers in special cages. Maggots should also be gathered from around and beneath the body and from the clothing, and pupae and any empty pupa cases collected, so that the entomologist can estimate the numbers of generations which have lived on the body. It is important that the specimens be handed to the entomologist as soon as possible after their collection. It is from the state of development of the larvae that the post-mortem interval is estimated and, in the author's experience, the fauna of the cadaver provides invaluable information concerning the time of death which could not be obtained in any other way. Bodies which become fly-blown decompose very rapidly, not only because the larvae feed on the flesh but also because the activities of the maggots raise the temperature of the body, often as high as 100°F, thus greatly accelerating the putrefactive process.

The handling and examination of a decomposing body will be influenced by the state of decomposition when first seen. If decomposition is relatively early and the body is intact it may be moved in the normal way to the local mortuary for autopsy. A rapid autopsy is desirable and if the body is fly-blown an immediate autopsy is essential. Maggots survive refrigeration, and even a deep freeze, for some time and an exceptionally heavily fly-blown body, if merely put in a refrigerator overnight, may consist of little more than skeletal remains the following morning. If the body is commencing to disintegrate it may be necessary to carry out a detailed examination at the scene.

A major consideration in the examination of a decomposing body is the establishment of identity. In a proportion of cases this may be achieved without difficulty merely from the pocket contents, the clothing and general description of the deceased. Where this information is absent, identification may rest upon fingerprints or dental data.

If any skin remains upon the fingers from which a fingerprint impression may be obtained, the finger, or even the whole hand, should be removed at once, provided its removal will not interfere with the general examination. In the United States, where there are very large files of civilian fingerprints, identification may be rapidly established in a high percentage of cases. In the United Kingdom, unless the decedent has a criminal record, no such facilities are available. In cases where the police believe they know the identity of the decedent a search of his house and examination of his personal effects will normally result in several good fingerprint impressions for comparison, even weeks or months after his disappearance. This method may also be used where attempts have been made to destroy the body by burning (R. vs Hearne, 1972).

Teeth, by their nature, resist decomposition, although when the soft tissues disappear they may become loose and fall out of their sockets. Every effort must be made to recover all such missing teeth, and sifting of the earth below and in the region of the skull through a fine sieve will normally produce them. Identification of an individual by his dental data may be specific. However, no matter how much dental data is available in the form of extractions and fillings, it is rarely of any use unless the identity of the decedent is suspected. No dentist is likely to remember details of an individual patient and certainly he could not be expected to go through some thousands of records to see if the dental data of the decedent matches up with one of his patients.

If the body is in a very advanced state of decomposition it may be necessary to lift each part, after it has been examined, into a plastic bag for transportation to the mortuary or laboratory. Great care must be taken when handling the clothing. Clothing frequently reveals names or laundry marks from which the deceased may be traced, but around decomposing bodies it becomes very friable and may disintegrate with all but the most careful handling. Sodden wallets, documents, diaries, etc., found on the decomposing body should be examined in the laboratory after treatment. Any immediate examination may cause irretrievable damage.

When the body has been lifted, decomposed soft tissues which may have run off the skeleton and the layer of soil beneath the body should be collected. Many of the common poisons may be detected in decomposed flesh or in the earth upon which the poisoned body has been lying. The growth of any roots or plants through clothing must be noted and samples retained for examination by a botanist should the time of death become crucial to the investigation.

EXAMINATION OF BURIED OR
PARTLY-BURIED BODIES

Whereas a body found decomposing in the open may have no criminal features a buried or partly buried body *per se* implies that a crime has been committed. In the majority of cases the crime is one of murder or, more rarely, a death following some illegal act such as criminal abortion (Simpson, 1957). Newly-born children are some-times disposed of in this manner and in these latter cases the question of a separate existence may be impossible to determine.

The procedure to be adopted at the disinterment will be influenced not only by the degree of decomposition of the cadaver but also by the terrain in which it is buried. Whatever approach is adopted it must be that which will cause the least trauma to the body during its lifting. Exhumation injuries may confuse the appearances of injuries occurring before burial. In order to minimize this danger the outline of the body must be clearly delineated by moving soil from the top, and the greatest care must be taken to avoid putting weight on any part of the body. This may be difficult to achieve if the body is in an unnatural position.

Bodies that are illegally inhumed are usually buried in shallow graves, and it is the shallow grave which leads to their discovery. Earth may subside around, or even be blown from, part of the body, leaving it exposed. More commonly the grave is found by dogs or foxes, who may carry away a bone, which is recognized as of human origin.

If the decedent has only been buried for a short time and decomposition is early or absent, there are no specific problems associated with exhumation, provided that every precaution is taken to avoid inflicting damage to the cadaver.

Shallow graves, that is to say those with less than 18 in of soil over the body, will allow the access of many insects, and the rate of decomposition will be influenced by seasonal variations in temperature (Mant, 1953). Samples of all insects, their larvae and pupae, must be collected in the same manner as described for bodies decomposing above ground.

Ideally, when any body is found buried without a coffin, a trench should be dug around the body to a depth of about 1 foot deeper than that of the body itself. The body and its covering soil is then upon a raised platform. The trench is essential for several reasons: it allows freedom of access to the cadaver from all sides; it serves as a temporary receptacle for the earth as it is scraped from the body; it allows detailed inspection of roots broken at the original inhumation and their subsequent growth; and finally in wet soils it will act as a drain for water from the actual burial area, although the water itself may have to be continually pumped from the trench. Once the trench has been dug the soil may be gently removed from the top and sides of the cadaver. When the cadaver is reached, the final soil should be removed with the gloved hand, or with brushes should conditions permit. Routine samples of soil should be collected from above, around and beneath the body. Every effort should be made to expose the body and its coverings completely without disturbing any part of it. The body may be then photographed *in situ*. Where skeletal remains only are present, the bones will separate as their earth support is removed and thus should be photographed as they become exposed.

If decomposition is relatively early and no disintegration has occurred, a body sheet may be slipped beneath the cadaver as it lies on the platform and it may thus be transported intact to the mortuary. Where soft tissue decomposition is complete, bones must be removed separately, and the completeness of their eventual reconstruction will depend largely upon the care exercised during the exhumation. In all cases where decomposition of the soft tissues has commenced a very careful search should be made for the components of the larynx as the soft tissues of the neck are some of the earliest to decompose.

Where possible, once the body has arrived at the mortuary, complete body radiographs should be made before there is any examination either of the tissues or coverings. Radiographs may reveal personal effects such as keys or rings which have become embedded in the earth or decomposed soft tissues.

SCIENTIFIC TECHNIQUES

Some of the methods and present-day techniques used by forensic scientists at the scene of crime and in the laboratory, and their importance in the investigation of a case, will now be outlined.

Footmarks

Footmarks, like fingerprints, are an example of transference from an individual to the scene. There, however, except for comparison techniques, the resemblance ends. A recognizable fingerprint is the consequence of the anatomical pattern and physiological properties of the finger. An identifiable footmark pattern, on the other hand, depends both upon the medium, whether soft soil, snow or a hard surface upon which the person has trodden, and also upon the fluid, mud or dust adherent to his sole. A fingerprint is an individual, permanent characteristic peculiar to the person making it, whereas shoes are transferable and wear in time will alter not only the fine details of the sole but also eventually the coarser characteristics.

A footmark, however, may be as specific as a fingerprint, and the increasing awareness of the importance of footmarks in crime detection has led to the development of experts in this field who may find footmarks, or portions of a footmark, which might have been missed a few years ago. A complete footmark is not necessary to establish positive identification. Fawcett (1970), in his paper on the subject, stresses that merely a square inch of a footmark may be quite sufficient to identify positively a shoe or boot (*Figure 2*). A footmark expert may not only be able to identify a shoe with a mark made at the scene of crime but, by his general examination, may ascertain the numbers of persons involved, their actual movements at the scene and their point of entry. Individual impressions, especially in yielding soil, will provide both the shoe size and approximate weight of the individual and also reveal any peculiarity of gait. Just as in ballistics the rifling characteristics may be specific for a particular manufacturer's weapon—although the fine details on the lands and grooves is specific for the actual weapon—so coarse details in a footprint may provide evidence of the make and finer details the specific identification of the shoe.

Footmarks are recorded by photography, casts or lifting, or by a combination of photography with one of the other methods. The technique employed will be governed by the surface and type of mark.

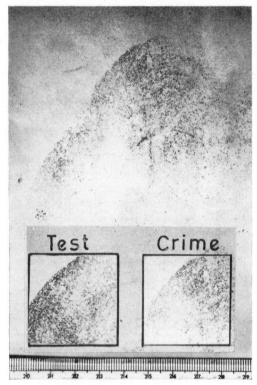

Figure 2. Footmark found on calendar at scene of crime. Below, portion of mark compared with corresponding part of test mark made by suspect's shoe (Fawcett)

Photography

Normally all footmarks are photographed *in situ* before a cast is made or before the print is lifted. On certain surfaces the direct photograph may reveal little or nothing and the mark may then be developed and re-photographed. Characteristic patterns may be developed by the use of oblique lighting, provided note is taken of the angle and direction of the light to exclude optical illusions. In one reported case a house-breaker was identified by a footprint on a soft carpet by the use of lighting techniques (FBI Law Enforcement Bulletin, 1961). Footmarks in snow may be developed by spraying lightly with a dark aerosol paint, and in soil by spraying with a light paint (Fawcett, 1970) (*Figures 3* and *4*). The film of paint is so thin that it will not interfere with the subsequent making of a cast. Footmarks on smooth surfaces have been developed by fingerprint powder. The technique of spraying a footprint is considered superior to the use of oblique lighting as it obviates misleading shadows.

Casts

Casts can only be taken when there is a footmark in depth. The fine detail reproduced on the cast will be dependent entirely upon the medium in which the impression has been made. The finer the grain of the medium, the greater will be the detail. Casts have an advantage in court over photographs as they are three dimensional and thus are easier for the jury to compare with the suspect's shoes.

Lifting

Marks on certain hard surfaces, especially when the colour of the surface is close to that of the footmark, may be suitably lifted with an adhesive fabric.

In view of the great importance of footmarks in crime detection the first officer at the scene will take immediate steps to protect any footmarks already observed and to ensure that all persons entering the scene follow a certain route. When the scene is out of doors any marks will be covered if there is a danger of rain.

Fingerprints

The basic techniques of fingerprint searching at the scene of crime have altered little over the years beyond improvements in the composition of the dusting powder. The practice of lifting prints by means of adhesive tape has become more widespread, and is of particular value when the print is on a coloured surface, unsuitable for developing in the normal manner.

New methods of obtaining prints from decomposing or mummified fingers by means of a rapidly-solidifying silicone-rubber solution have largely replaced the old and lengthy dissection and rehydration procedures.

McKeehan (1970), however, describes a rapid rehydration method for preparing mummified hands for fingerprinting. The fingers are

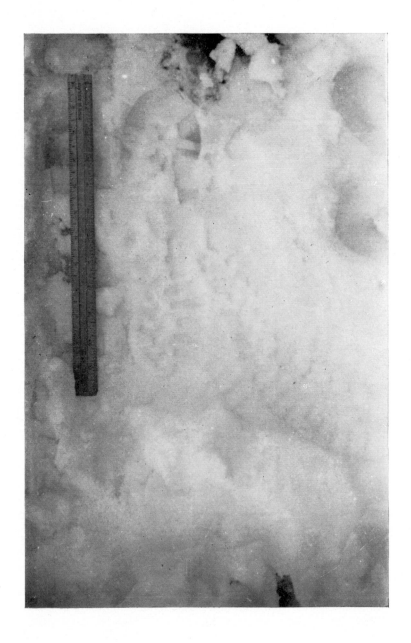

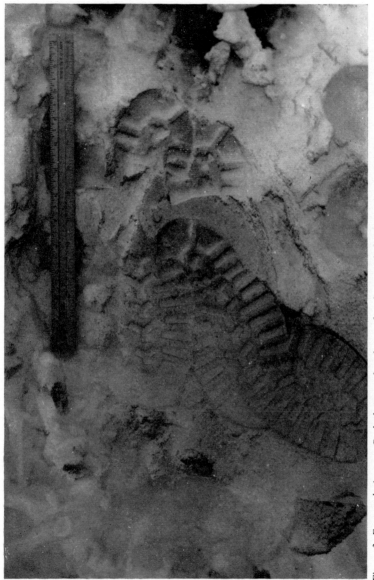

Figure 3. Footmarks in snow. Both photographs taken under the same lighting conditions, the lower one after the impressions had been lightly sprayed with dark brown paint (Fawcett)

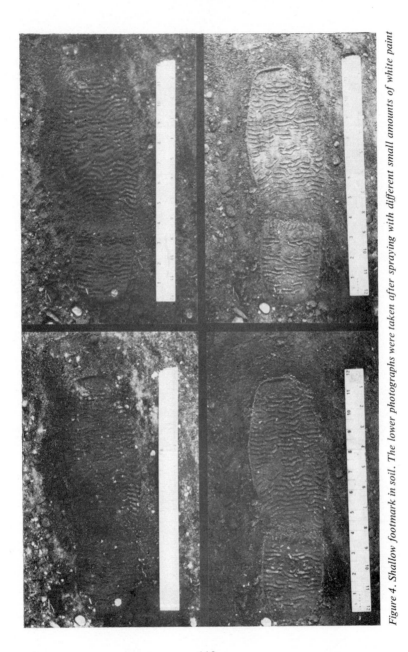

Figure 4. Shallow footmark in soil. The lower photographs were taken after spraying with different small amounts of white paint

removed and soaked in a solution of Eastman Kodak Photo-Flo 200 and the skin becomes soft within 24–48 hours. Owing to the rapidity of rehydration, it is not necessary to add preservatives to the solution.

Research has been conducted in an attempt to develop fingerprints on skin in cases of assault, especially manual strangulation, by the use of radio-active dusting powders and soft x-rays. The optimism engendered by the earlier laboratory experiments has been dampened, however, by the application of the technique in the field.

Research is also being conducted into the migration of chloride from prints in an attempt to establish their age (Sams, 1970).

Blood

Blood has always been the most important forensic body fluid. In certain animal species the blood group systems may virtually allow positive individual identification of the animal. Recent advances in the examination of fresh blood, although not providing proof of identity, have become more and more specific in the field of paternity testing (*see* Chapter 3) and each advance leads to further exclusion or closer identification.

The specificity of the laboratory investigation of a blood stain has always fallen behind that of fresh blood because of the destructive effect of drying and of the action of bacteria and their enzymes upon shed blood. Improved techniques for the examination of dried blood stains are being continuously developed, with the result that the forensic scientist is constantly achieving higher degrees of individuality in the samples he examines.

Species identification has relied for many years upon the precipitin ring test. This test, however, will not distinguish between human blood and that of the higher primates. Many modifications have taken place. Gel diffusion methods, comprehensively reviewed by Crowle (1961), have the advantage that the extracts being examined need not be clear, as is essential in the precipitin ring test. The precipitation-electrophoresis method of Culliford (1964) can also be used with turbid stains, and has the advantage that it is much faster. Double diffusion techniques, which will distinguish the bloods of different primates, are under investigation.

Species identification by the anti-globulin inhibition test was first suggested by Wiener, Hyman and Handman (1949). Since this time the method has been described, developed and modified by numerous workers (Allison and Morton, 1953; Vacher *et al.*, 1955; Mosinger *et al.*, 1960; Periera, 1967; Grobbelaar, Skinner and Gertenbach,

1970a, b). This method is highly sensitive and can be used to distinguish the blood of the higher primates.

Depeids *et al.* (1960) described an electrophoretic method for differentiating adult and foetal haemoglobin.

Blood group determination of dried stains by the absorption-elution method described by Kind (1960a, b) and modified by Nickolls and Pereira (1962), is capable of successfully A, B, O and MN grouping small stains.

The technique has also been used to identify the Rh antigens (Bargagna and Pereira, 1967), although the sensitivity decreases with the ageing of the stains. Lincoln and Dodd (1968a) showed that by careful selection of the anti-sera they could genotype stains up to six weeks old. Blanc, Görtz and Ducos (1971) stress the value of GM typing of stains in determining their racial origin.

A technique has been recently developed for the identification of the Y chromosome in dried blood recovered from both absorbent and non-absorbent surfaces. The cells are stained with quinacrine and examined by fluorescence microscopy, following extraction with a special solution containing magnesium ion (Philips and Gaten, 1971; Phillips and Webster, 1972).

A method for A, B, O and MN grouping of dried blood using cellulose acetate sheets is described by Howard and Martin (1969). Kind and Cleevely (1969) and Chisum (1971) describe a rapid method for the A, B and O grouping of dried stains using ammoniacal extracts. This technique is of especial value in warm climates.

Methods have been developed in recent years for examining other blood group systems, and when these methods have been fully developed the forensic scientist will be able to attain an extremely high degree of specificity. Amongst these newer techniques are those for the identification of haemoglobin variants (Culliford, 1964—haptoglobin types; Culliford, 1966—enzyme systems; Culliford and Wraxall, 1968—adenylate kinase (AK) types).

Hair

The study of human and animal hairs has received continuous attention from forensic scientists. Niyogi reviewed the literature in 1962, and Montanari, Viterbo and Montanari (1967) described their technique for sexing human head hair. Groups of 15 men and 15 women between the ages of 22 and 51 were used in this study. Samples of scalp hair were obtained by pulling; the growing hair follicles were then fixed and, after dehydration and embedding, the root bulbs were cut at 3 μ, stained and examined for Barr bodies.

Each sample was examined five times and a minimum of a hundred nuclei examined on each occasion. Barr bodies were found in the male hair follicles in a proportion of 6 ± 2 per cent and in the female 29 ± 5 per cent.

A mixed agglutination method for the blood group determination of hair was reported by Lincoln and Dodd (1968b). In the series of cases examined the method was 100 per cent successful with shavings, but only just over 40 per cent correct with head hair. Yada, Okane and Sano (1966) have described a method for grouping hair by an elution method.

Wynbracht and Chisum (1971) describe a modified absorption-elution technique for determining the A, B and O groups in a single hair. They took random samples from 50 persons and from different parts of the body. The accuracy was 100 per cent. It was found that the result was not affected by the age of the individual, the length of hair, or the ethnic group, and all the known non-secretors gave positive results, indicating that the antigenic activity is contained within the shaft.

Niyogi (1968) has described certain congenital metabolic abnormalities of the hair shaft, and emphasizes the individuality which these disorders impart to the hair.

Methods of individualizing hair have always been of great interest to the scientist, and the introduction of neutron activation analysis techniques open a new field of investigation. It was even hoped at one time that an examination of head hair might not only provide positive identification of the individual but also provide information of his geographical location.

Activation analysis of trace elements is not only highly sensitive but usually non-destructive. Although the sensitivity of the method varies between elements, some 50 per cent may be detected in amounts of around 10^{-9}g (Hamilton-Smith, 1969). The sensitivity of detection of trace elements, however, is not matched by their quantitative assay, the accuracy of which will vary considerably with the method employed. Hairs, owing to their exposed location on the body, rapidly get contaminants adherent to them, and investigations may lose some of their specificity as all methods of cleaning hairs would appear to cause some damage and alteration in the concentration ratios of the elements (Bernaert, 1968).

As the distribution and concentration of trace elements along the shaft of a hair varies as the hair grows, hair cannot provide a permanent record for identification. However, comparison of a sample head hair by activation analysis with head hair from other persons will reveal significant differences, and analysis of samples may give some indication of occupation and geographical location (Coleman, 1966).

Cornelis and Speeke (1971) carried out a comprehensive study of a unique collection of head hair removed from two brothers over a period of 25 years. They found that zinc and copper levels remained remarkably constant, whereas other elements studied fluctuated considerably, but the concentration range of these elements remained the same whilst the brothers lived together.

Examination of Other Trace Evidence

The forensic scientist now has at his disposal instruments which are capable of quantitating elements which are only present in one part per million in samples as small as a milligram. These instruments will allow full analyses to be carried out on a single fibre, a centimetre length of hair, a tiny flake of paint or a minute fragment of glass.

The modern methods employed include: laser arc emission spectrography, mass spectrometry, atomic absorption, neutron activation, and pyrolysis gas chromatography.

Paint

A paint flake is normally made up of several layers of different composition and often different colours. By use of a 20 micron laser probe and spectrometry, the elements in each paint layer can be quantitated with the minimum destruction to the sample as a whole. Improvement in pyrolysis gas chromatography techniques are permitting identification of the original solvents.

Glass

Glass fragments are common trace evidence. For instance, fragments may be found in wounds as a result of an assault with a broken glass object, in the wounds of road traffic accident victims and in the hair or on the clothing of house-breakers. Although in the United Kingdom the manufacture of glass is largely centralized, there are distinct differences of composition between successive batches and also differences between samples taken from the same batch. These differences enable a surprisingly high degree of exclusion to be achieved.

Measurement of the refractive index of glass fragments has always been a time-consuming operation which may be replaced in the future by an automated system using a microspectrophotometer. The examination of minute fragments of glass by spark source mass spectrophotometry yields a quantitative analysis of the elements present (German and Scaplehorn, 1972). Neutron activation techniques have also been used to determine the origin of minute glass fragments (Schmitt and Smith, 1970).

Glass and paint fragments were shown to be regularly present on suits by Pearson, May and Dabbs (1971), who examined 100 men's suits sent for dry cleaning. Glass fragments were found on 63 of the suits and paint fragments on 97. Although only 18 of the 551 glass fragments collected were over 1 mm the refractive index of 494 fragments was measured. Wide ranges of refractive index were found. Very occasional random matches were found with single layer colour paints and there were no matched samples where more than three paint layers were present.

EQUIPMENT

The equipment needed by a pathologist at the scene of a crime is neither sophisticated nor expensive, except for the photographic apparatus. It is recommended that the following items should be carried by a pathologist visiting a scene.

Protective Clothing

Sensitive duty disposable plastic gloves (Ethicon).
Surgical gloves for any heavy work.
Anti-static overshoes.
Wellington boots for out of doors examination.

Photographic Equipment

35 mm camera, and 50 (+100) mm lenses.
Flash equipment.
Films.
Numbered discs (numbering wounds).
Measuring strips.

Apparatus

Large hand lens.
Dissecting forceps.
Blunt scissors.
Disposable scalpels.
Two thermometers (reading 0–120°F).
Filter papers Whatman No. 1 4·5 cm D.
Throat swabs—in glass tubes.
Ruler.

Tape measure.
Bijou bottles.
Universal containers.
Two small combs.
Pill boxes or small boxes for insects, etc.
Assorted plastic bags.
Assorted envelopes.
Adhesive tape.
Gauze swabs.

Miscellaneous

Normal saline.
Petroleum ether or chloroform.
Clip board.
Paper—body diagrams, etc.
Pencils, etc.
Torch.
Adhesive labels.

ACKNOWLEDGEMENT

The author wishes to thank Dr. A. Fawcett and the Editor of the *Journal of the Forensic Science Society* for permission to publish *Figures 2, 3* and *4*.

REFERENCES

Allison, A. C. and Morton, J. A. (1953). *J. clin. Path.*, **6**, 314.
Bargagna, M. and Pereira, M. (1967). *J. forens. sci. Soc.*, **7**, 123.
Bernaert, F. (1968). Thesis, University of Ghent.
Blanc, M., Görtz, R. and Ducos (1971). *J. forens. Sci.*, **16**, 176.
Chisum, W. J. (1971). *J. forens. sci. Soc.*, **11**, 205.
Coleman, R. F. (1966). *J. forens. sci. Soc.*, **6**, 19.
Cornelis, R. and Speke, A. (1971). *J. forens. sci. Soc.*, **11**, 29.
Crowle (1961). *Immunodiffusion*. New York; Academic Press.
Culliford (1964). *Nature, Lond.*, **201**, 1092.
— (1966). *Nature, Lond.*, **211**, 872.
— and Wraxall, B. G. D. (1968). *J. forens. sci. Soc.*, **8**, 79.
Depeids R., Laurent, G., Cartouzou, G. and Cignoix, D. (1960). *Ann. med. leg.*, **40**, 522.
Easton, A. M. and Smith, K. G. V. (1970). *Med. Sci. Law*, **10**, 208.
F.B.I. Law Enforcement Bulletin (1961), **30**, 18.
Fawcett, A. S. (1970). *J. forens. sci. Soc.*, **10**, 227.
Fiddes, F. S. and Patten, T. D. (1958). *J. forens. Med.*, **5**, 2.

REFERENCES

German, B. and Scaplehorn, A. C. (1972). *J. forens. sci. Soc.*, **12**, 367.

Grobbelaar, B. G., Skinner, D. and Gertenbach, H. N. van de G. (1970a). *J. forens. Med.*, **17**, 103.

— — — (1970b). *J. forens. Med.*, **17**, 112.

Hamilton-Smith, G. (1969). *J. forens. sci. Soc.*, **9**, 205.

Howard, H. D. and Martin, P. D. (1969). *J. forens. sci. Soc.*, **9**, 28.

Kind, S. S. (1960a). *Nature, Lond.*, **185**, 397.

— (1960b). *Nature, Lond.*, **187**, 789.

— and Cleevely, R. N. (1969). *J. forens. sci. Soc.*, **9**, 131.

Lincoln, P. J. and Dodd, B. E. (1968a). *Med. Sci. Law*, **8**, 288.

— — (1968b). *Med. Sci. Law*, **8**, 38.

Locard, E. (1928). *Police J.*, **1**, 176.

McKeehan, H. E. (1970). *J. forens. sci. Soc.*, **10**, 115.

Mant, A. K. (1953). In *Modern Trends in Forensic Medicine*, Ed. by Keith Simpson, p. 84. London; Butterworths.

— (1967). In *Modern Trends in Forensic Medicine—2*, Ed. by Keith Simpson, p. 147. London; Butterworths.

Marshall, T. K. (1965). *Med. Sci. Law*, **5**, 224.

Montanari, G. D., Viterbo, B. and Montanari, G. R. (1967). *Med. Sci. Law*, **7**, 208.

Mosinger, M., Ranque, M., Fiorentini, H. and Bataglini (1960). *Ann. med. leg.*, **40**, 531.

Nickolls, L. C. and Pereira, M. (1962). *Med. Sci. Law*, **3**, 49.

Niyogi, S. K. (1962). *J. forens. Med.*, **9**, 27.

— (1968). *J. forens. Med.*, **15**, 148.

Pearson, E. F., May, R. W. and Dabbs, M. D. G. (1971). *J. forens. Sci.*, **16**, 283.

Pereira, M. (1967). In *Modern Trends in Forensic Medicine—2*, Ed. by Keith Simpson, p. 95. London; Butterworths.

Phillips, A. P. and Gaten, E. (1971). *Lancet*, **2**, 371.

— and Webster, D. F. (1972). *J. forens. sci. Soc.*, **12**, 361.

Salter, G. (1960). *J. forens. Med.*, **7**, 59.

Sams, C. (1970). *J. forens. sci. Soc.*, **10**, 219.

Schmitt, R. A. and Smith, M. S. (1970). *J. forens. Sci.*, **15**, 252.

Simpson, C. K. (1957). *Police J.*, **30**, 26.

Vacher, J., Sutton, E., Derobert, L. and Moullec, J. (1955). *Ann. med. leg.*, **35**, 201.

Wiener, A., Hyman, M. and Handman, L. (1949). *Proc. Soc. exp. Biol. Med.* **71**, 96.

Wraxall, B. G. D. and Culliford, B. J. (1968). *J. forens. sci. Soc.*, **8**, 81.

Wynbracht, F. and Chisum, W. J. (1971). *J. forens. sci. Soc.*, **11**, 201.

Yada, S., Okane, M. and Sano, Y. (1966). *Acta. crim. med. leg. Japonica*, **32**, 173.

E

6 Firearms Injuries

WILLIAM Q. STURNER and CHARLES S. PETTY

INTRODUCTION

During the past several years, there have been significant changes in firearms, ammunition, techniques of demonstrating firing distances, examination of residues and other factors. These have altered the patterns and the interpretations of gunshot injuries which the forensic pathologist encounters in his practice. Not only do some of today's wounds differ from those previously observed, but estimation of range, missile track(s), tissue damage and materials recovered have taken on new dimensions. One can no longer completely rely on standard texts and previous experience in assessing gunshot injuries but must constantly acquire information from manufacturers, governmental agencies and other reliable sources. It is the purpose of this chapter to discuss newer developments regarding the firearm, projectile, examination of the body and clothing, laboratory capabilities, and some experimental studies occurring in present-day activity. Neither a complete historical review nor a comprehensive survey of recent foreign literature will be attempted.

WEAPONS

Changes in firearms which alter an otherwise standard projectile on discharge may pose an identification problem (Petty, 1969). One such innovation is the microgroove system of rifling which consists of 15–20 rounded grooves present on the bore surface of the barrel, rather than the usual 4–8 square lands and grooves. One manufacturer has adopted this system exclusively for rifles, and the missiles fired from such a weapon will have the appropriately increased number of markings (*Figure 1*).

The use of variable or replaceable extensions, called 'chokes', at the end of the muzzle of shotguns has introduced a new factor in the estimation of range. The variable choke, manufactured by one

American firm as 'Polychoke', allows the operator to change quickly the diameter of the barrel (*Figure 2*). Some chokes and even the barrels themselves are replaceable. One must consider these possibilities when asked to estimate the range and to correlate the wound with the probable weapon.

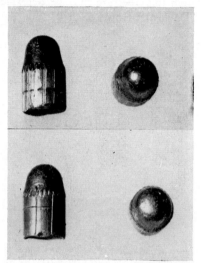

Figure 1. Microgroove markings on 0·22 calibre bullet (above); standard land and groove markings (below)

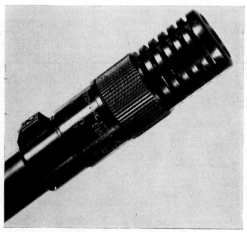

Figure 2. 'Polychoke' attached to muzzle of shotgun

Wounds may be altered by the utilization of 'silencers', which varies the stippling or tattooing seen on the skin or test pattern. Muzzle-brakes and flash-hiders may produce peculiar fouling and tattooing patterns by venting gas in specific directions. A shortened, or 'sawn-off', barrel can result in a narrowing of the muzzle, and bullets fired through this aperture may be deformed or 'squeezed' (*Figure 3*) (Petty, Davis and Howard, 1970).

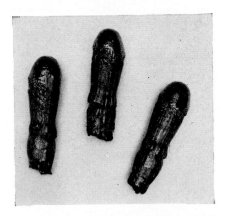

Figure 3. Examples of deformed ('squeezed')
0·22 calibre bullets fired from a revolver with
a crudely shortened barrel

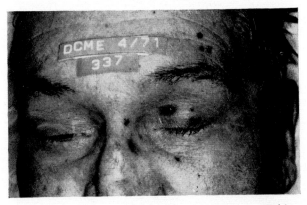

Figure 4. Face of victim with lead fragment injuries caused by a
revolver in which the cylinder did not line up perfectly with the
barrel. One fragment of metal is visible in the left upper eyelid

Tear-gas pen guns are not classified by government agencies in the United States as firearms in their unaltered form, but they may be modified so as to fire ordinary cartridges. The low velocity of the discharged missile is more likely to cause a superficial injury rather than a deeply penetrating wound, unless it is fired from a contact position or very close range (Stahl, 1968). Tear-gas guns do not have rifling, so no such markings are found on the bullet. However, the missile may acquire marks or impressions left by tools used to make alterations. Both 0·22 and 0·38 calibre bullets have been recovered from victims of altered tear-gas guns (Stahl and Davis, 1969). 'Zip guns' and other home-made contrivances have been described and comparison ballistic studies performed (Koffler, 1969, 1970). Air rifles account for a portion of injuries which are rarely fatal (Spitz, 1969).

It should also be remembered that other weapon defects, particularly cylinder misalignment in revolvers, will cause deformities of the missile, with shearing-off of the metal fragments from the bullet occurring when the misalignment is great (*Figure 4*). Lesser defects of this type may cause tumbling (Petty, Davis and Howard, 1970).

AMMUNITION

There has been considerable variation and refinement of ammunition during the past few years, making it mandatory to keep abreast of new developments. Frangible bullets have been employed for some time and are of particular interest and importance because they are designed to fragment upon impact, often to the point of disintegration (Graham *et al.*, 1966). Recovery is difficult due to this shattering characteristic, and does not ensure a match with a test round fired into soft material. Such loads consist of iron rather than lead as the major metallic component of the bullet. The magnetic character may be a useful method of differentiation (*Figure 5*). Such missiles are usually recovered in an eroded state if there is bone penetration, creating further difficulties in comparison tests. It is of historical interest that lead was replaced by iron in bullets used in shooting galleries following reports of plumbism in workers.

Super Vel* ammunition is designed so that the component parts of these bullets tend to separate upon impact. Such bullets are partially jacketed at the base, with the tip remaining as an uncovered lead core. Upon striking, the separated components create their own

* Trade mark registered by Super Vel Cartridge Corporation, Shelbyville, Indiana, U.S.A.

tracks, thus enhancing the capability of damage (Petty, 1969). In addition, they are designed to achieve a greater velocity, primarily by a decrease in the weight of the bullet. Super Vel and other manufacturers' bullets which are partially jacketed, were originally designed for use in revolvers and, more recently, automatic pistols.

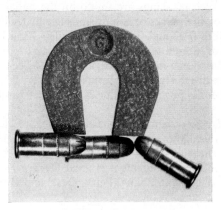

Figure 5. Frangible bullets made of iron. Note magnetic attraction

Other variations include bullets with hollow points and jackets with multiple shallow longitudinal grooves (*Figure 6*). Recovery of a missile and its jacket does not necessarily imply that an automatic pistol was used.

In duplex or tandem cartridges, which are designed to be employed in military rifles, a given round contains two projectiles which enter the target at different points, as much as 30 cm from each other. The forward missile is recessed at its base, allowing the second projectile to fit snugly into its companion (*Figure 7*). The 'follow' bullet has a base not quite perpendicular to its long axis, thereby causing a difference in trajectory.

A bullet designed for increased striking power, commonly called a KTW load, has been recently marketed. It has a tungsten core and the exposed surface is coated with Teflon*. Such ammunition has a greater mass per unit volume than comparable lead missiles. The plastic coating is employed because of the extreme hardness of tungsten, and the bullet, therefore, is not gripped by the rifling. A soft metal combination 'rotating band and gas seal' is also used. This frequently

*Trade mark registered E. I. Dupont De Nemours and Co., Wilmington, Delaware, U.S.A.

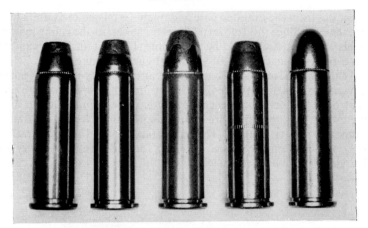

Figure 6. Five available jacketed 0·38 special bullets. From left to right: Super Vel, Smith and Wesson, Remington-Peters, Winchester-Western, and a full jacketed military cartridge

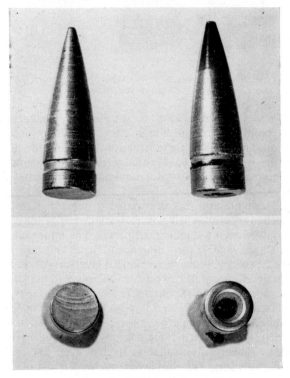

Figure 7. Military duplex load

separates from the tungsten core and might be missed in examination of the body. Since this soft metal band alone carries the rifling marks, ballistic comparison would be impossible. This is a further argument for x-ray examinations in all victims of gunshot wounds.

With the advent of commercial aircraft 'sky-jacking', some governments have installed air marshals on random flights to intercept or deter such occurrences. There have been proposals to arm them with weapons which fire bullets manufactured from a substance similar to plaster of Paris. This projectile, designed for penetration only at close range, provides shocking force sufficient to render an individual momentarily helpless, and thus easy to subdue, with

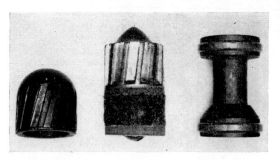

Figure 8. Three types of rifled slugs. From left to right:
Foster, Brenneke and Blondeau

limited danger to other persons and the aircraft. Instances of its use have not been reported, although cases of regular firearms and ammunition employed in these situations both outside and within the plane are well publicized. Plastic bullets have been employed for short range target practice, but wounding in humans has not been described.

Shotgun ammunition has undergone a number of refinements, including changes in the shell closure, constituents of the casing, and the material between the individual pellets. The injury produced by the rifled slug, available for a number of years and now used with increasing frequency, must be recognized (Petty and Hauser, 1968). The initial development of this missile took place in the late 1800s in Germany and was called the Brenneke slug. The Foster type of slug was produced in the 1920s and is now used widely in the United States, while the Blondeau type is a recent French addition to the market (*Figure 8*). At least three other types of slug have recently been made commercially available. In each type, the shell casing contains but one slug. The slug is designed with most of the weight forward so as to increase accuracy. Rifled slugs have been used by law enforcement agencies in riot control and also by assailants in crime. Homicidal shootings employing this type of ammunition are becoming more frequent. Rifled shotgun slugs may display sufficient marking characteristics so that an identification of the offending weapon, as in the case of a 'sawn-off' shotgun, can be made (Townshend, 1970). Wounds involving balled or welded

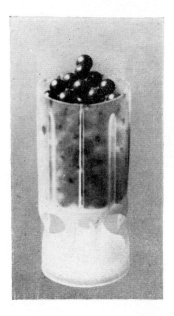

Figure 9. Power-Piston, one form of plastic wad

shot can usually be distinguished (Mant, 1968). The use of rifled slugs (and other appropriate ammunition and firearms) by law enforcement agencies has been suggested (Greenwood, 1966).

Other developments in the changing pattern of shotgun ammunition include plastic wads such as the Power-Piston* variety (*Figure 9*). These are seen more frequently than the older felt or cardboard wads. Western Mark V shotgun shells have a lining of polyethylene or other material, often recovered with pellets and wadding from the wounds (Petty, 1969). Plastic granular substances, some vividly coloured, are used as the interstitial matrix of 'buckshot' ammunition

*Trade mark registered by Remington Arms Co. Inc., and Peters Cartridge Division, Bridgeport, Connecticut, U.S.A.

E*

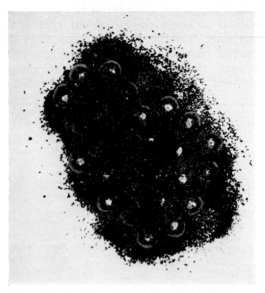

Figure 10. Buckshot, showing interstitial plastic granular matrix

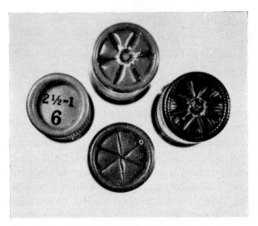

Figure 11. On the left is an old style 'over-the-shot-wad' closure; the other three shotgun shells have variations of the star-crimp closure

and may be seen on and beneath the skin (*Figure 10*). Wad closures have been replaced by what is called the 'star crimp', a stellate-patterned infolding which supplants the 'over-the-shot-wad' used in older ammunition (*Figure 11*). All of the shotgun shell components can leave imprints on the skin, with or without penetration. These wound characteristics should be carefully documented, as they may have relevance in subsequent test firing for estimation of range (Petty, 1970).

WOUNDS

Changes in powder have altered the appearance of firearm wounds. Some of these variations were expected; others were unexpected. The shape of individual punctate defects comprising the stippling pattern in wounds of intermediate range is determined to a degree by the shape of the powder particles. Only recently has ball powder come to be used extensively in other than military cartridges. This powder is formed into small variable sized rounded or flattened spheres. Previously, smokeless powder grains were frequently made into a specific size and shape. The newer ball powder stippling may thus be less characteristic than that caused by other powder grain shapes. There is some evidence indicating that different types of powder have various clothing and skin penetration potentials (Petty, 1970). In addition, the character of the powder grains determine the variations in the appearance of the base of soft metal bullets after discharge (Di Maio, 1971). It has been observed that some stippling can be removed by washing the skin, whereas other stippling remains; the former frequently represents unburned ball powder (Petty, 1969).

The patterns of injury caused by ricocheting bullets and by missiles which have passed through an intermediate target have not significantly changed, but more emphasis on their delineation through experimental studies has taken place. It has been shown that roent-genographic interpretation of the scatter pattern of shotgun pellets within the body may be hazardous and even misleading when used to support an estimation of range. The skin pattern and the location and extent of the injuries to various organs are much more reliable criteria to employ (Breitenecker and Senior, 1967; Breitenecker, 1969). The same conclusion was reached following experimental firing into human tissue, employing 'bird shot' cartridges in a 0·22 calibre double-barrelled pistol (Di Maio and Spitz, 1970).

Missiles associated with ricochets or with intermediate targets may be considerably deformed. Such missiles usually cause asymmetrical or irregular wounds. The discovery of a deformed missile or the finding of an entry wound with unexpected characteristics should arouse suspicion of one of these possibilities. There must then be a search made within the missile track for foreign material arising

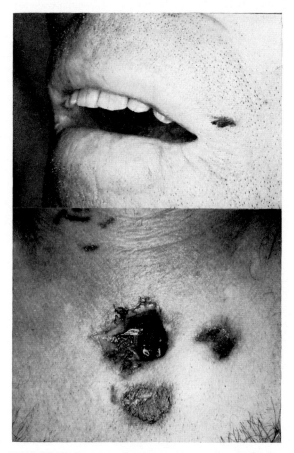

Figure 12. Injury from rifled slug which ricocheted off table. Note asymmetric entry wound, and two abrasions due to wads; note also accompanying smaller abrasions due to wood splinters (lower) and splinter protruding from skin near lip (upper)

from the ricochet site or the intermediate target (*Figure 12*). Other wound peculiarities are seen in industrial injuries such as extensive damage by steel studs used in nailing guns and the rock wool residue from a silencer deposited at the wound margins (Spitz and Wilhelm, 1970). Weapons employed in slaughtering animals and the resulting wounds have been described, and two human fatalities have been noted (Hunt and Kon, 1962).

Foreign material introduced into the bore of a firearm has been noted to alter the appearance of the wound markedly. Such an instance involved firing a rifle after the weapon had been buried in sand; the stippling pattern was thought to be composed entirely of powder residue, but later was shown to consist of ejected silicate particles. A murder charge was dropped following the introduction of this evidence (Birrell, 1970). Similarly, when one encounters tandem bullet wounds with minimal bullet deformity and little or no penetration, it may be suspected that the wrong ammunition was employed in the firearm, or that the proper ammunition, as a result of age, was much less effective (Mason, Rose and Alexander, 1967).

Only in the last decade has emphasis been placed on the histological changes of the skin in gunshot wounds (Adelson, 1961). Combinations of mechanical, thermal, and blast effects are easily demonstrable and the amount and location of powder residue in and about the entrance wounds can be of forensic value. It is of interest that heat injury can occasionally appear to be of equal intensity at both entry and exit sites. Histological studies have not generally been exploited in gunshot wounds, including those of experimental design.

The presence of carbon monoxide in tissues surrounding entrance wounds and, in some shotgun wounds, near both entry and exit sites, has been observed. The associated red to pink discolouration of the involved tissues is often described by the pathologist in his autopsy protocol. Chemical methods for measurement of the carbon monoxide content of homogenates of muscle are available but they generally are not employed in American laboratories. This may be due to insufficient studies to establish the reliability of their interpretation (Sturner and Petty, 1971). It is uncertain whether this compound is present as only carboxyhaemoglobin or a combination of this and carboxymyoglobin. The demonstration of carbon monoxide near the wounds of entrance in decomposed bodies has been noted. Solid matter carried with the bullet into the wound has been demonstrated by a histochemical study of nitrite–nitrate residues (Rolfe, Curle and Simmons, 1971). A preliminary report indicates that such particles can be demonstrated in rifle wounds at a range of 45 metres, even in the presence of body decomposition. This method may be employed to advantage in the investigation of deaths from firearms injuries concealed by burning, and situations where a greater than intermediate range of discharge is suspected. Future applica-

131

tions of this technique will require a larger controlled study employing a number of firearms and ranges.

Reports of wounds from military weapons emphasize the extensive destruction accompanying exit wounds at longer ranges (Dimond and Rich, 1967).

A method with extreme sensitivity for demonstrating elemental substances is that of neutron activation analysis. Using this technique in estimating distances of firing in the intermediate and near contact ranges, it has been shown that, at 15 metres, for example, consistent results are obtained with an error of ± 5 to 10 cm (Krishnan, 1967). The metallic substances determined were copper and antimony; although lead is deposited in greater quantities, it is less easily detected by this technique. Neutron activation analysis has also been used in examining the hands of those suspected of firing weapons (Guinn, 1964). The amount and location of metallic deposits may give an indication of the type of firearm employed. A method of more rapid detection of these residues employing an atomic absorption technique combined with neutron activation analysis has been developed (Krishnan, Gillespie and Anderson, 1971). Despite the fact that neutron activation analysis is costly, time-consuming, and requires much knowledge and skill, it outperforms the perilous 'paraffin test' and its variations which have long been scientifically abandoned (Cowan and Purdon, 1967).

PHYSICAL EVIDENCE

The labelling and preservation of the missile(s) recovered at autopsy is of critical importance. Little further need be said regarding proper markings at the base or, rarely, the nose of the bullet, the use of a sealed envelope or other appropriate container and the 'chain of custody' delivery with receipt from the laboratory—all time-honoured procedures. Lukens and Guinn (1971) have demonstrated by neutron activation analysis of lead alloy, the similar composition of bullets from a common origin, and thus have further narrowed the identity gap of a single unknown missile. One should re-emphasize the importance of recovery of foreign materials from intermediate targets, fabric from clothes, and distinctive casing and wadding components of shotgun shells, all of which need similar evidentiary care (Petty, 1971). Human tissue can be deposited in the offending weapon barrel and even in the revolver chamber due to transfer from victim to firearm.

An equally essential item is the clothing worn by the decedent, optimally removed by the pathologist himself just prior to the autopsy, and retained. Fabrics of different weaves have been shown to admit varying amounts of powder residue during close range firing; one cannot estimate distance from discolouration of, for example, an outer garment without also examining the accompanying underclothes. One should not forget the possibility of a stray or exited bullet intermingled in the clothing. In a recent case of shooting through the hips covered with 'pantyhose', the missile was found

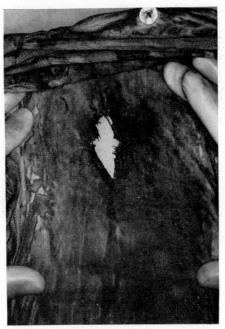

Figure 13. Defect in shirt due to near-contact discharge of 0·38 calibre revolver. Note horizontal multiple punctate defects (between thumbs) due to spray of bullet fragments and powder particles which escaped between cylinder and barrel

within the stocking at the heel. Another example of the necessity for a thorough examination of the clothing was seen in a wound of equivocal range in the flank of a young woman. The inside of her blouse was appreciably fouled, whereas the outer surface was little involved. This supported the theory that a disenchanted lover had held the weapon in a different manner than he first stated. In another instance, escape of metal fragments and powder particles produced a linear pattern of defect some distance from the actual perforation of the clothing (Figure 13). The same principle holds true for the object used for muffling purposes, when a search must be made to resolve inconsistencies concerning weapon, wound and range (*Figure 14*). The use of soft x-ray is another technique for the examination of clothing and body and can be particularly rewarding in a 'back flare' of sheared metal from a misaligned revolver cylinder

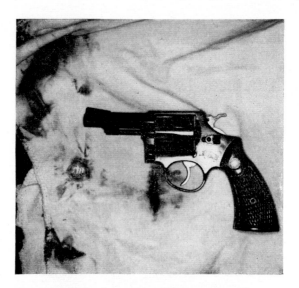

Figure 14. Bullet defect and fouling due to escape of gas between cylinder and barrel on a pillow used as a muffle; barrel length was established by distance between bullet defect and cylinder-barrel fouling

(*Figure 15*). Infra-red photography and the dissecting microscope have yet to be employed to their full advantage in the autopsy room, although they have been used often in clothing examination. Recently, neutron activation analysis together with autoradiography have been used to analyse bullet holes in both biological and inert substances such as cloth and wood (Krishnan and Nichol, 1968). One could conceivably analyse individual powder grains with physico-chemical techniques in order to determine the manufacturer, and possibly even the batch. The newer synthetic fibres of clothing are occasionally fused due to the extreme heat of the bullet or powder gases. There are instances when the outer clothing is torn by the blast because the muzzle was held between the garment and the skin. Careful inspection of the clothing is necessary to avoid interpreting the damage as due to bullet penetration (Petty, Davis and Howard, 1970).

134

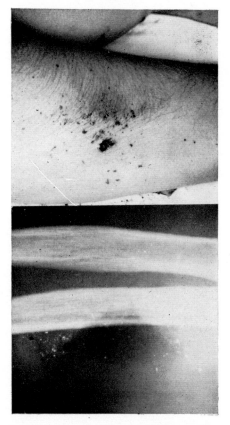

Figure 15. Gunshot wound of entrance from 0·30 calibre rifle with stippling of surrounding skin. The metallic fragments apparent on examination of the x-ray in the absence of injury to bone, must have separated from the bullet and caused at least a part of the stippling pattern

RESEARCH ACTIVITIES

A workshop in ballistics and wounding for 20 experienced forensic pathologists was conducted recently (Petty, 1970). The three-day session consisted of didactic presentations, laboratory and range work, and investigation projects. The didactic subjects included hand loading modifications of cartridges, neutron activation analysis of firearm detonation residues, and information on military cartridges and load innovations. The laboratory activities were concerned with tear-gas projectiles, explosives and bombs, and firearm detonator residues. The investigation projects conducted on the firing range, utilizing experimental animals and carried out by several registrants working together in teams, included: carbon monoxide detection in muscle surrounding close range and contact firearm wounds; breaking-up of partially jacketed high velocity bullets; behaviour of frangible bullets in tissues; potentials for comparison of Teflon-coated tungsten bullets; range of carry of shotgun wads; and stippling pattern variations with ammunition produced by different manufacturers.

The determination of the penetrating potential of different types of ammunition and weapons and the assessment of their striking power is being conducted utilizing high-speed photography (Di Maio, 1971). The results of preliminary studies reveal some unexpected variations with specifications given by the manufacturers and, more important, give further insight into impact, blast effect, and wounding patterns. Other observers have also employed this technique to emphasize the potentials of tissue damage (De Muth, 1966, 1971). There is continuing interest in the use of mathematical probabilities to determine shot dispersion and the penetration of a target with considerations of velocity, energy release and impact area (Mattoo, 1969; Mattoo and Wani, 1969; Mattoo and Nabar, 1969).

REFERENCES

Adelson, L. (1961). 'A microscopic study of dermal gunshot wounds.' *Am. J. clin. Path.*, **35**, 393.
Birrell, J. H. W. (1970). 'Forensic medicine—Cinderella?' *Forens. Sci. Gaz.*, **1**, 5.
Breitenecker, R. (1969). 'Shotgun wound patterns.' *Am. J. clin. Path.*, **52**, 258.
— and Senior, W. (1967). 'Shotgun patterns. An experimental study on the influence of intermediate targets.' *J. forens. Sci.*, **12**, 193.
Cowan, M. E. and Purdon, P. L. (1967). 'A study of the paraffin test.' *J. forens. Sci.*, **12**, 19.
De Muth, W. E. Jr. (1966). 'Bullet velocity and design as determinants of wounding capability. An experimental study.' *J. Trauma*, **6**, 222.
— (1971). 'The mechanisms of gunshot wounds.' *J. Trauma*, **11**, 219.
Di Maio, V. J. (1971). Unpublished observations.
— and Spitz, W. V. (1970). 'Injury by birdshot.' *J. forens. Sci.*, **15**, 396.
Dimond, F. C. Jr. and Rich, N. M. (1967). 'M-16 rifle wounds in Vietnam.' *J. Trauma*, **7**, 619.

REFERENCES

Graham, J. W., Petty, C. S., Flohr, D. M. and Peterson, W. E. (1966). 'Forensic aspects of frangible bullets.' *J. forens. Sci.*, **11**, 507.

Greenwood, C. (1966). 'Police firearms training.' *J. forens. Sci. Soc.*, **6**, 116.

Guinn, V. (1964). In *Methods of Forensic Science*, Vol. 3, p. 47, Ed. by A. Curry. New York; Interscience.

Hunt, A. C. and Kon, V. M. (1962). 'The patterns of injury from humane killers.' *Med. Sci. Law*, **2**, 197.

Koffler, B. B. (1969). 'Zip guns and crude conversions—identifying characteristics and problems.' *J. crim. Law, Criminol. Pol. Sci.*, **60**, 520.

— (1970). 'Zip guns and crude conversions—identifying characteristics and problems.' *J. crim. Law, Criminol. Pol. Sci.*, **61**, 115.

Krishnan, S. S. (1967). 'Determination of gunshot firing distances and identification of bullet holes by neutron activation analysis.' *J. forens. Sci.*, **12**, 112.

— and Nichol, R. C. (1968). 'Identification of bullet holes by neutron activation analysis and autoradiography.' *J. forens. Sci.*, **13**, 519.

— Gillespie, K. A. and Anderson, E. J. (1971). 'Rapid detection of firearm discharge residues by atomic absorption and neutron activation analysis.' *J. forens. Sci.*, **16**, 144.

Lukens, H. R. and Guinn, V. P. (1971). 'Comparison of bullet lead specimens by nondestructive neutron activation analysis.' *J. forens. Sci.*, **16**, 301.

Mant, A. K. (1968). 'An unusual gunshot injury.' *Med. Sci. Law*, **8**, 256.

Mason, M. F., Rose, E. and Alexander, F. (1967). 'Four non-lethal head wounds resulting from improper revolver ammunition.' *J. forens. Sci.*, **12**, 205.

Mattoo, B. N. (1969). 'Shot penetration from ballistic data.' *J. forens. Sci.*, **14**, 521.

— and Nabar, B. S. (1969). 'Evaluations of effective shot dispersion in buckshot patterns.' *J. forens. Sci.*, **14**, 263.

— and Wani, A. K. (1969). 'Casualty criteria for firearm wounds with special reference to shot penetration.' *J. forens. Sci.*, **14**, 120.

Petty, C. S. (1969). 'Firearms injury research. The rôle of the practicing pathologist.' *Am. J. clin. Path.*, **52**, 277.

— (1970). Advanced Ballistics Workshop for Medical Examiners, Southwestern Institute of Forensic Sciences, Dallas, Texas, April 4-6.

— (1971). In *Medical Jurisprudence*, p. 329, Ed. by J. R. Waltz and F. E. Inbau. New York; Macmillan.

— and Hauser, J. (1968). 'Rifled shotgun slugs: wounding and forensic ballistics.' *J. forens. Sci.*, **13**, 114.

— Davis, J. and Howard, L. (1970). 'Factors modifying firearms wounds.' American Society of Clinical Pathology Commission on Continuing Education: Forensic Pathology Seminar, Atlanta, Georgia, September 14.

Price, G. (1965). 'Firearms discharge residues on hands.' *J. forens. Sci. Soc.*, **5**, 199.

Price, G. (1968). 'Recent advances in ballistics laboratory methods.' *J. forens. Sci. Soc.*, **8**, 83.

Rolfe, H. C., Curle, D. and Simmons, D. (1971). 'A histological technique for forensic ballistics.' *J. forens. Med.*, **18**, 47.

Senha, J. K. and Misra, G. J. (1971). 'Detection of powder particles at the crime scene.' *J. forens. Sci.*, **16**, 109.

Spitz, L. (1969). 'Air rifle injuries in children.' *S. Afr. Med. J.*, **43**, 557.

Spitz, W. U. and Wilhelm, R. M. (1970). 'Stud gun injuries.' *J. forens. Med.*, **17**, 5.

Stahl, C. J. (1968). 'Forensic aspects of tear-gas pen guns.' *J. forens. Sci.*, **13**, 442.

— and Davis, J. H. (1969). 'Missile wounds caused by tear-gas pen guns.' *Am. J. clin. Path.*, **52**, 270.

Sturner, W. Q. and Petty, C. S. (1971). 'An analysis of tissue content of carbon monoxide in gunshot wounds of the body.' Paper presented at Twenty-Third Annual Meeting, AAFS, Phoenix, Arizona, February 23.

Thomas, F. J. (1967). 'Comments on the discovery of striation matching and on early contributions to forensic firearms identification.' *J. forens. Sci.*, **12**, 1.

Townshend, D. G. (1970). 'Identification of rifled shotgun slugs.' *J. forens. Sci.*, **15**, 173.

7 The Investigation of Injuries in Road Traffic Accidents

E. GRATTAN, J. G. WALL and J. A. HOBBS

INTRODUCTION

Road traffic accident–injury research has been undertaken in Great Britain, the USA and parts of Europe for the past two decades. It is therefore a comparatively new science but the techniques used are becoming better known and the applications of its findings are beginning to evolve into practical forms. The data obtained are already being applied to the design of motor vehicles and, in addition, a number of countries have embarked on experimental safety vehicle programmes which will make use of many of the results of accident–injury work. In some centres accident causation is investigated as well as injury causation. In this chapter we shall confine ourselves to a consideration of injury investigation.

There is usually a time lag between research and its application. In the case of accident–injury research the information obtained will be from vehicles designed at least three years previously; and the data acquired is likely to be applied to the design of vehicles which may not be in production for a further three years.

THE PURPOSE OF ACCIDENT–INJURY INVESTIGATION

The main purpose of the investigation of road accident injuries using accident collision data is to determine directly, by detailed examination of the results of actual road accidents, the effects of different types and severities of vehicle collision upon the living human body. By this means, together with the experimental determination of loads capable of causing the deformations which result from impact of the human body upon the vehicle interior (or, in the case of pedestrians, the vehicle exterior), it would seem likely that more accurate information relating to mechanisms of injury will be obtained than is possible from simulated impacts using anthropometric dummies, live animal subjects or cadavers.

The following factors are investigated:

(1) The patterns of injury and of death in various groups of road users.

(2) The time interval between accident and death.

(3) The causes of injury in relation to specific parts of the vehicle.

(4) The direction in which force acts on the human body to produce injury.

(5) The levels of human tolerance to dynamic loads applied to different parts of the body.

(6) The effectiveness of various safety design features in terms of reduction in frequency and/or severity of injury. These currently include the following: (a) occupant restraint; (b) energy-absorbing steering columns; (c) high penetration resistant windscreen glass; (d) padding, including deformable sheet metal structures; (e) anti-ejection devices; (f) strengthening of the passenger compartment against intrusion.

THE PROCEDURE OF ACCIDENT–INJURY INVESTIGATION

The general procedure of accident–injury investigation used by the authors at the Road Research Laboratory is the same for all classes of road users whether they be vehicle occupants, pedestrians or motor cyclists. The research team is inter-disciplinary and consists of medical scientists, physicists, engineers and professional photographers; it should be added, however, that it would not be possible to undertake this work without the willing co-operation of hospitals, police, garages and the motoring public.

The standard procedure of investigation consists of a medical interview and medical examination of the injured person(s), with a follow-up study of the vehicle(s) damaged in the accident, including photography of the vehicle(s), interview of the police officer concerned with the accident and, if necessary, other witnesses; and finally writing up the accident in detail. Analysis of results is undertaken when the number of accidents reaches an adequate level.

Medical Investigation of Casualties

The medical investigation of casualties is usually undertaken in hospital, the patient's permission having first been obtained. The interview and the examination include both clinical and radiological findings, and all injuries are classified according to their severity as minor, moderate or severe (Road Research Laboratory Leaflet, 1969). The exact site and nature of the injuries are recorded on diagrams (*Figure 1*), and whenever possible a photographic record in

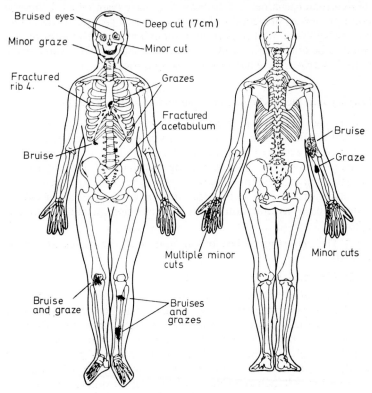

Bruised eyes

Minor graze

Fractured rib 4.

Bruise

Deep cut (7cm)

Minor cut

Grazes

Fractured acetabulum

Bruise

Graze

Multiple minor cuts

Minor cuts

Bruise and graze

Bruises and grazes

Car occupant: Driver of Ford Cortina saloon

Direction of impact on car: Centre head (frontal)
Point of contact : (1) Right knee into facia
          (2) Left knee into heater unit
          (3) Chest into steering wheel
          (4) Head on roof and windscreen.

Figure 1. Injury diagram

colour is made. In the case of fatalities post-mortems are attended and full details of all injuries are recorded, including the time elapsing between injury and death and an assessment of the cause (or causes) of death.

141

There is no selection of cases, except that all the casualties examined were admitted to hospital other than some which, if dead on arrival at the hospital, would not have been admitted. Such results as are obtained refer, therefore, mainly to the more seriously injured road casualties and to those who have been killed. From the point of view of prevention of injury these two groups of road users are probably the most important, although much useful information can also be obtained by studying severe crashes in which some or all of the occupants have not sustained serious injuries.

Enquiry into the Accident and Examination of the Vehicles

It is necessary when attempting to determine injury causation in road traffic accidents to be able to reconstruct with reasonable accuracy the events of the accident in relation both to vehicle and to occupant movement. Whether using 'on-the-spot' techniques, i.e. investigation at the scene of the accident, or retrospective techniques, i.e. investigation at a convenient time interval after the accident, a three-phase investigation of the accident circumstances is undertaken:

(1) The reporting police officer and other witnesses are interviewed.

(2) The accident site is examined.

(3) The vehicle(s) are subjected to careful scrutiny.

When using retrospective techniques it has been found possible to obtain certain basic data from the reporting officer regarding the accident which will include the directions in which the various vehicles involved were travelling, their final positions after the accident, and a rough estimate of pre-accident speeds. Further information will include evidence of ejection, or otherwise, trapping of the occupants and confirmation of the use or non-use of seat belts.

In the retrospective studies currently being undertaken at the Road Research Laboratory the vehicles involved in an accident are investigated at the garages to which they were taken after the accident, provided that they are still in their accident condition and that owners' permission has been obtained. A careful examination is made to determine the precise direction of impact. By direction of impact is meant not necessarily the point at which the vehicle was struck, but the direction from which the impact came that caused the damage. For example, the offside of the vehicle may be struck from an oblique frontal direction or the front from an oblique side direction.

The direction of impact has a bearing upon injury since the occupants of a vehicle in an impact tend to move, relative to the vehicle, in the opposite direction to this force, i.e. in a frontal impact they move forwards relative to the vehicle.

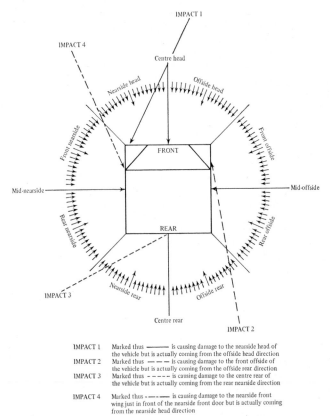

IMPACT 1	Marked thus ———— is causing damage to the nearside head of the vehicle but is actually coming from the offside head direction
IMPACT 2	Marked thus — — — is causing damage to the front offside of the vehicle but is actually coming from the offside rear direction
IMPACT 3	Marked thus - - - - - is causing damage to the centre rear of the vehicle but is actually coming from the rear nearside direction
IMPACT 4	Marked thus -—·-—·— is causing damage to the nearside front wing just in front of the nearside front door but is actually coming from the nearside head direction

Figure 2. Direction of impact

Figure 2 shows the four central directions of impact—namely, centre head (CH), centre rear (CR), mid-offside (MOS) and mid-nearside (MNS), in which forces are applied in a direction at 90 degrees to the front, rear, offside and nearside of the vehicle respectively. These particular directions of impact can only result from forces applied at these respective vehicle surfaces although at any position along the surfaces. The other eight directions are oblique forces varying in the extent of their frontal, rear or side components.

143

For example, direction offside head describes a force with a large frontal component and a smaller side component, front offside a force with a large side component and a smaller frontal component, and similarly for the directions nearside head and front nearside and the oblique rear impacts. The square in the centre of *Figure 2* represents a vehicle, and the four directions of impact given serve to illustrate these points. Overturning accidents are classified separately.

Certain basic measurements are taken in order to record the overall deformation of the vehicle. From these measurements the severity of the damage on a damage index scale is calculated. Damage scales of different kinds are widely used by investigators in this field but most refer only to deformation and are not therefore a measure of collision severity except in respect of the particular model under consideration. In our investigations the damage index is divided by the unladen weight of the vehicle (in cwt) to produce a ratio which has been shown empirically to give an indication of the severity of the impact on the car (Moreland, 1964), enabling the severity of impacts involving different models and makes of cars to be compared.

In addition to investigating damage severity and direction of impact the area of impact is noted, e.g. a full width collision with a wall or a localized collision with a tree or similar object, or by a car under-running the rear overhang of a heavy commercial vehicle.

Examination of the car interior will show whether or not the damage inside the vehicle was caused directly by the vehicle impact or as a result of the secondary collision between the occupant and the vehicle interior. It is usually possible to relate the injuries previously recorded by medical examination of the occupant (or occupants) to deformation caused by occupant contact with the interior of the vehicle. Some parts of the human body, notably the shin or the knee, leave characteristically shaped indentations on certain components of the passenger compartment, usually the parcel tray or facia panel, and there may be other evidence of body to vehicle contact such as blood, hair, skin, etc. A careful note is made of various construction details, e.g. the material used in the construction of the parcel tray or facia panel, the thickness and type of windscreen, the angle of the steering column, and the presence or absence of any safety features incorporated within the car to reduce or to prevent injury.

Photography is used extensively in all accident–injury investigations. A routine set of photographs in black and white and in colour are taken of the exterior and interior of the accident vehicle(s), using where necessary a wide angle lens, and any occupant impact areas of particular interest are also photographed. In this way a permanent pictorial record of each accident is obtained.

The scheme of accident investigation which has been outlined concerns the study of injury causation to vehicle occupants. The same general procedure applies to the investigation of injuries sustained by pedestrians and riders or passengers on two-wheeled vehicles. In pedestrian accidents it is necessary to attempt to ascertain whether the injury was caused as a result of the pedestrian being struck by the vehicle or as a result of contact with the ground. A careful examination of the exterior damage to the vehicle will frequently reveal deformations caused by contact with various parts of the pedestrian's body and some estimate of the subsequent pedestrian trajectory may be possible.

In reconstructing accidents to two-wheeled vehicles much attention has to be paid to the evidence of witnesses. An attempt is made to determine whether the injuries sustained by the rider or passenger were received as a result of contact with their own machine, as a result of contact with the other vehicle or object struck, or as a result of being thrown from the machine and making contact with the ground.

THE RESULTS OF ACCIDENT–INJURY INVESTIGATION

A few of the results of accident–injury investigation are very briefly summarized in Tables 1 and 2 and some results of the related experimental work are considered in the following section (*see* pp. 148–153).

As an example of injury patterns found in road accidents, Table 1 shows the overall pattern of injury amongst 526 seriously injured unrestrained front seat occupants of passenger cars and light vans involved in accidents irrespective of impact direction.

A considerable amount of information has now been collected which delineates the interior components causing injury to vehicle occupants. Table 2 shows the components causing skeletal injury to the lower limb amongst 426 seriously injured vehicle occupants.

The Appendix at the end of the chapter gives a number of examples to show the relationship between specific injuries and specific parts of the vehicle, the effects of different directions of force acting upon the body, an experimental method of determining levels of human tolerance to dynamic loads and the effectiveness of various safety design features.

It will be seen that the evidence of causation of injury in the examples given appears to be conclusive. However, not all accidents

TABLE 1

Percentage Distribution of Injuries Among 526 Unrestrained Front Seat
Occupants of Cars and Light Vans Admitted to Hospital Following Road
Accidents

All Directions of Vehicle Impact

Region of injury	Surface injury only	Skeletal injury with or without surface injury	Deep soft tissue injury with or without skeletal and/or surface injury	Total injuries
Head	66	13	7 (Intra-cranial or Intra-orbital)	86
Neck	5	2	2	9
Upper limbs, including shoulder girdle	46	20	1	67
Back	5	4	—	9
Chest	30	17	7 (Intra-thoracic)	54
Abdomen, including pelvis	13	6	3 (Intra-abdominal)	22
Hip joint	—	13	—	13
Thigh	24	18	—	42
Knee	57	8	4 (Intra-articular)	69
Lower Leg	44	15	—	59
Ankle and foot	14	6	—	20

Note 1—The figures denote the percentage of front seat occupants with a particular injury. Whilst
these figures are additive for a particular part of the body (as shown in column 5) they are *not*
additive for the body as a whole.
Note 2—Skeletal and deep soft tissue injuries were usually accompanied by surface injury. Intra-
thoracic injuries were usually accompanied by fracture of the rib cage, and intra-cranial injury by
fracture of the skull.
Note 3—Intra-cranial injury did not include mild concussion.

Reproduced from Grattan ,Clegg and Hobbs (1970) by courtesy of the Road Research Laboratory.

TABLE 2

The Relation Between Skeletal Injury to the Lower Limb and the Interior
Structure of the Vehicle Among 426 Seriously Injured Vehicle Occupants.
All Directions of Vehicle Impact

Injury	Point of contact	No. of cases
Hip joint: Posterior dislocations and posterior fracture dislocations	Facia	14
	Parcel tray	3
	Bulkhead	1
	Centre support rear seat	1
		19

Fractures of the roof of the aceta-bulum	Facia	4
	Parcel tray	2
	Heater unit	2
	Unknown	2
		10
Central fracture dislocations	Door	5
	Ejected	1
		6
Femur: Single transverse fractures with or without comminution	Facia	8
	Parcel tray	6
	Door	5
	Steering wheel	4
	Gear lever	3
	Bulkhead	2
	Heater unit	1
	Seat back	1
	Ejected	1
		31
Double comminuted fractures	Facia	6
	Door	6
	Parcel tray	2
	Wheel	2
	Rear seat back	1
	Unknown	1
		18
Spiral or oblique fractures	Facia	3
Supracondylar fractures	Facia	4
	Parcel tray	4
	Seat back	1
		9
Patella: Comminuted and non-comminuted fractures	Facia	13
	Parcel tray	9
	Heater unit	5
	Steering column	2
	Segment of fence pierced car through bulkhead	1
		30
Tibia and fibula: Plateau fractures	Parcel tray	15
	Bulkhead	4
	Lower edge facia	1
	Ejected	1
		21

Reproduced from Grattan and Hobbs (1968) by courtesy of the Road Research Laboratory.

147

investigated present such clear-cut proof of the mechanism of injury and there are a few injuries to some parts of the human body for which the precise method of injury in road accident collisions is still open to debate. Example 1 shows one of the ways in which the head can be injured in pedestrian accidents; about one-half of the pedestrian fatalities due to head injury appear to be caused by the head being struck by some part of the front of the vehicle and about one-half by the head striking the ground. Example 2 shows a typical mirror injury to a driver of a car. Example 3 shows a parcel tray injury, in which both driver and passenger sustained plateau fractures of the tibia and fibula; the majority of plateau fractures are caused by the lower leg impacting on the parcel tray (*see* Table 2). Example 4 shows the effects of differences in direction of force applied to the same region of the human body. Posterior dislocations or posterior fracture dislocations of the hip joint are produced by knee impact, usually upon the facia panel, in frontal impact accidents; whereas central fracture dislocations appear usually to be the results of force applied to the great trochanter in side impacts (*see* Table 2). Example 5 shows the relationship, in this instance for the hip joint, between accident–injury data and the experimental work being undertaken to determine the thresholds of injury tolerance for the human body to dynamic loading, described on pp. 150–151. Example 6 illustrates the effectiveness of safety belts, when correctly worn. Two similar cars collided with each other, the severity, direction and site of impact being the same for both vehicles. The restrained driver sustained only minor bruising due to the belt; the unrestrained driver was killed. Example 7 illustrates the intrusion that may occur in collisions between heavy commercial vehicles, which usually result in severe injury; in our present sample of accidents the risk of trapping of the occupant, as a result of intrusion, appears to be about eight times greater among injured occupants of heavy commercial vehicles than among injured car occupants. Example 8 shows that energy-absorbing devices, when fitted to the more horizontal types of column, appear to produce a reduction in severity of chest injury. Example 9 shows that the more vertical types of steering column possess more satisfactory yielding characteristics and cause less injury to the chest than the more horizontal types of steering column.

RELATED EXPERIMENTAL WORK

The investigation of injury occurring in road traffic accidents would be insufficient in itself to provide all the information needed to determine the requirements for the safer design of vehicles and their equipment. A great deal of additional experimental work is required to supplement the accident–injury investigation data and to assist in its interpretation.

Thus the simulation of pedestrian accidents using anthropometric dummies is an important means of assisting in determining the probable trajectories of pedestrians after being struck by a vehicle, and the results of such experiments may be a valuable guide to the accident investigator when attempting to associate injuries received by a pedestrian with a particular part of the car struck or with the road surface.

In the same way a knowledge of the results of controlled impact tests on complete vehicles containing anthropometric dummy occupants has assisted accident–injury investigators in assessing the probable trajectories of human occupants in actual crashes and in associating the injuries received with the part or parts of the vehicle interior struck by the person(s). An impact rig (*Figure 3*) is used at the Road Research Laboratory to simulate various vehicle impacts. In this way information on the movement of occupants during impact can be gained without expending a vehicle for each test.

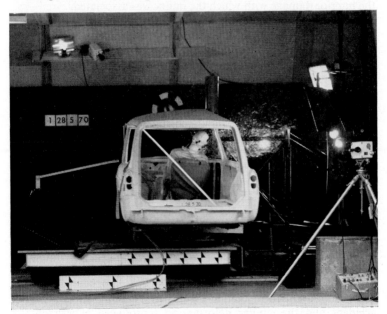

Figure 3. Impact rig. Full scale impact rig being used to project a car body sideways into a rigid vertical pole at 29 km/hour (18 miles/hour)

The information from accident–injury investigations can be used to indicate which parts of a vehicle are likely to cause injury and often to postulate the probable mechanism of the injury. Before a vehicle can be re-designed to optimize the safety of the occupant it is necessary to know the maximum force that the occupant can sustain without receiving serious injury, because in an impact it is desirable that any protective structure or padding should absorb as much energy as possible in the space available. To do this in severe impacts the restraining load exerted on the occupant by the device should rise as quickly as possible to a load which is just below that which would cause serious injury to the occupant and should remain constant at this level until the occupant is brought to rest.

The data obtained from accident–injury investigations can be used to determine human tolerance levels if it is supplemented by experimental simulations of accident damage to the vehicle interior. This is done by reproducing the damage to the interior of a vehicle, which was associated with a particular occupant injury, under controlled laboratory conditions on a similar undamaged vehicle. The force required to reproduce this damage is measured. It is equivalent to the force which acted on the occupant in the accident and produced the interior damage with which the injury was associated.

By investigating a number of accidents, in which damage to a particular part of the car interior caused by a particular part of the body has occurred to varying extents, and in which a range of injury severity to that particular part of the body has been produced, it is possible to construct a table relating force to degree and frequency of injury and so estimate the probable tolerance level for that part of the body.

As an example Table 3 shows the results obtained from a series of tests to determine the tolerance of the hip joint to blows received on the knee when the subject is in a seated position as in a car.

Table 3 correlates the occurrence of skeletal injury to the hip joint of front seat occupants with the dynamic load required to reproduce the associated degrees of facia damage. The peak loads obtained for different types of facia panel or on different parts of the same facia panel are shown in the first column of Table 3 and the number of cases with or without hip injury in the remaining two columns. From the results it appears that the threshold of human injury tolerance for this particular type of impact injury lies between 2 and 4 kN (450–900 lb force). Example 5 (in the Appendix) shows the deformation caused to the facia panel by knee impact in an actual accident and the similar deformation reproduced experimentally. The simple knee form shown has a mass representative of the effective

TABLE 3

Dynamic Load Required to Reproduce Facia Damage Associated with the Occurrence of Posterior Dislocation or Posterior Fracture Dislocation of the Hip Joint in Front Seat Occupants, Produced as a Result of Loads Transmitted along the Femur (Lister and Wall, 1970)

Estimated load (kN)		Cases with skeletal injury	Cases without skeletal injury
Greater than	6	3	2
Less than	6	2	3
Of the order of	5	3	3
Greater than	4	1+1*	2
Less than	4	0	3
Of the order of	2	1*	12

mass of the knee–thigh–hip complex, and is swung under gravity into the car structure being investigated at a speed sufficient to cause the damage found in the accident–injury investigation. The force acting on the knee form during the laboratory impact is recorded.

A further example of levels of human tolerance, obtained in this instance by determining the dynamic loads required to deform steering columns of a similar type, but with different bending strengths, is shown in Table 4.

From Table 4 it will be seen that a 25 per cent reduction in the load (8·5 to 6·2 kN) required to deform the steering wheel and column assembly corresponds to a 70 per cent reduction in the incidence of serious injury to the chest. Thus it is inferred that a steering wheel and column assembly of this type which deforms when subjected to a dynamic load of 6·2 kN (1400 lbf) is nearer to the optimal level of loading for the chest than one which deforms at 8·5 kN (1900 lbf) and that the optimal level may be under 6 kN.

Using experimental methods of this kind the tolerance levels to loading of various parts of the human body can be inferred directly from accident–injury investigations. This information is vital for the optimum design of occupant protection devices. Data obtained in this way have the advantage over inferences drawn from cadaver or animal tests in that they are relevant to living human beings in actual accident situations; and in particular to that group of vehicle occupants who are being injured in accidents and for whom it is desired to give protection. It is to be noted, however, that the injury tolerance

151

TABLE 4

Severity of Chest Injury in Unrestrained Drivers Related to Steering Column and Wheel Assembly Strength
Showing also the Severity of Vehicle Impact

No. of cases	Type of vehicle	Angle of column to horizontal	Distance of wheel from the steering column/facia bracket	Peak force (kN) (when tested to SAE J 944)	Severity of chest injury			Severity of vehicle impact. Damage index/car weight ratio		
					Serious	Minor	None	Low	Moderate	High
15	Morris 1100	45 deg	240 mm	6.2	13%	33%	54%	7%	20%	73%
12	Austin 1100	45 deg	150 mm	8.5	42%	25%	33%	25%	33%	42%

Reproduced from Annual Report of Road Research Laboratory (1970) by courtesy of Her Majesty's Stationery Office.

limits of the body to loading, particularly for the skeletal system, may vary between different persons, depending upon such factors as age, size, presence or absence of disease or disuse, and so on.

THE RECORDING AND ANALYSIS OF DATA

Most accident–injury investigation teams collect a sufficient quantity of data to permit the use of computer analysis of the data. At the Road Research Laboratory each accident investigated is manu-scripted in full for future detailed reference. In addition, the data collected is stored and analysed by means of a computer programme using a general purpose method of producing tabular analysis on a 4/70 computer (Harris, 1971). This general programme enables the data collected on a survey report form of the type used for national accident data to be analysed by staff with little or no computer experience. The accident–injury data from each accident file is transferred to a specially designed survey report form which presents the data exactly as it is punched on to 80-line Hollerith cards. These are read by the computer, the data is stored on magnetic tape and the information is then ready for future analysis.

SUMMARY

Some indication has been given in this chapter of the purpose, procedure and results of accident–injury investigation, including the related experimental studies presently being undertaken at the Road Research Laboratory. The data that is being acquired is part of the necessary background information needed for the safer design of motor vehicles.

Example No. 1—Pedestrian Injury

Case No. P48. This pedestrian was hit by the front of a Ford Thames 15 cwt van. His head struck and dented the offside windscreen pillar of the van, causing a depressed fracture of the right frontal bone.

Windscreen pillar of van

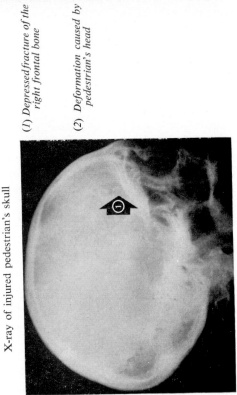

(1) *Depressed fracture of the right frontal bone*

(2) *Deformation caused by pedestrian's head*

X-ray of injured pedestrian's skull

Example No. 2—Mirror Injury

Case No. 822. The injured car driver, who was not wearing a safety belt, was travelling in a 1966 Austin 1800 saloon car which was involved in a frontal collision with an oncoming BMC box van. His head struck the interior mirror, breaking the glass and causing lacerations to the face and scalp.

Interior mirror of car

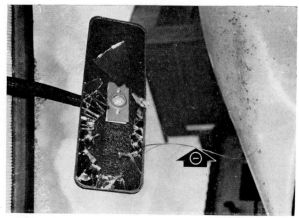

(1) Hair from scalp adhering to mirror

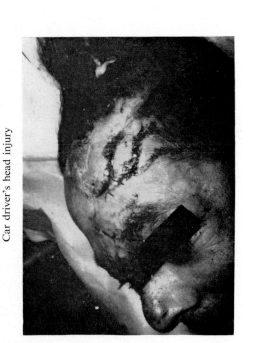

Car driver's head injury

155

Example No. 3—Parcel Tray Injury

Case Nos. 258 and 259. The injured car occupants, who were not wearing safety belts, were travelling in a 1965 Wolseley Hornet saloon car which was involved in a frontal collision with an oncoming Bedford van. Both occupants sustained plateau fractures of the tibia and fibula. The passenger sustained fractures to both legs, and the driver to his right leg, caused by impact of the lower legs on the parcel tray, which shows deformations corresponding to the fracture sites. The mechanism involved in producing a fracture of this type is a shearing force applied to the proximal end of the tibia and fibula.

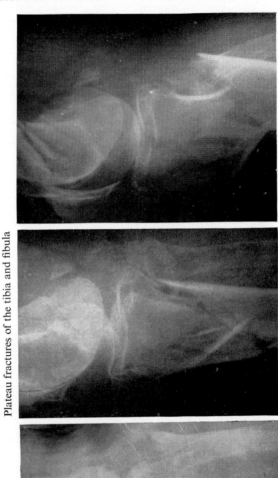

Plateau fractures of the tibia and fibula

Driver's right leg   Passenger's left leg   Passenger's right leg

Interior of Wolseley Hornet saloon

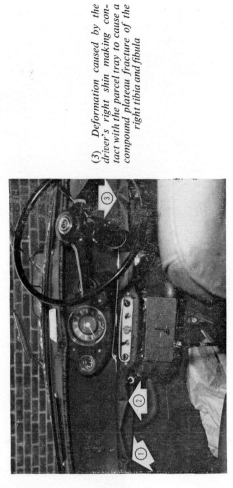

(1) Deformation caused by the front seat passenger's left shin making contact with the parcel tray to cause a plateau fracture of the left tibia and fibula

(2) Deformation caused by the front seat passenger's right shin making contact with the parcel tray to cause a plateau fracture of the right tibia and fibula

(3) Deformation caused by the driver's right shin making contact with the parcel tray to cause a compound plateau fracture of the right tibia and fibula

157

Example No. 4—Direction of Force Applied to the Body

The following two cases illustrate clearly that the direction in which force is applied to a particular part of the human body has an influence on the nature of the resulting injury.

Case No. 177. Posterior fracture dislocation of the hip joint. The injured driver, who was not wearing a safety belt, was travelling in an Austin 1100 saloon car which was involved in a frontal collision with an oncoming Austin A50 saloon car. He sustained a posterior fracture dislocation of the right hip joint, caused by his right knee striking the lower edge of the facia to the right of the steering column. His right knee was grazed and bruised and the patella fractured. The force was transmitted via the shaft of the femur to the hip joint, causing the posterior fracture dislocation.

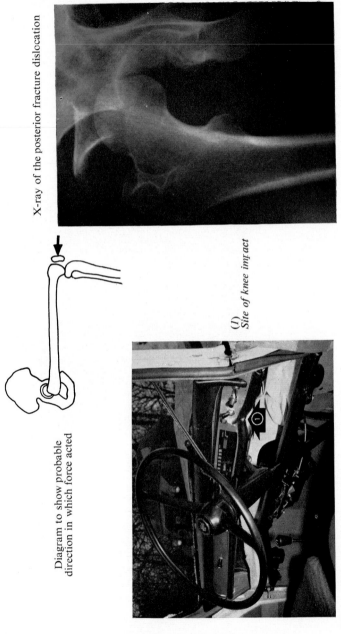

X-ray of the posterior fracture dislocation

Diagram to show probable direction in which force acted

(1)
Site of knee impact

158

Case No. 304. Central fracture dislocation of the hip joint. The injured front seat passenger, who was not wearing a safety belt, was travelling in a Renault Dauphine saloon car which was involved in a side collision with the front of a Morris Minor 1000 saloon car, the point of impact being on the nearside front passenger door. As a result of being struck by the incoming nearside bodywork of the passenger compartment of her car she sustained a central fracture dislocation of the hip joint, the load being applied to the great trochanter.

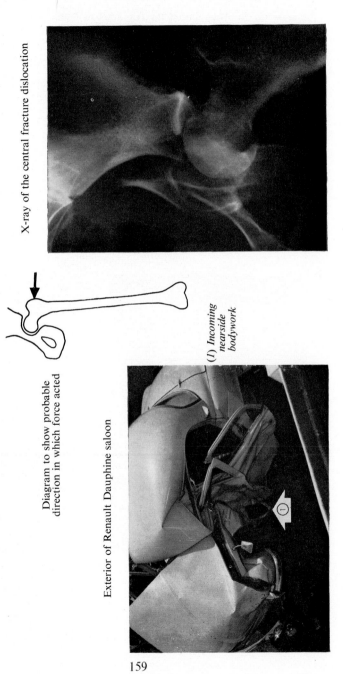

X-ray of the central fracture dislocation

Diagram to show probable
direction in which force acted

(1) Incoming
nearside
bodywork

Exterior of Renault Dauphine saloon

159

F*

Example No. 5—Tolerance of the Hip Joint to Loads Applied through the Knee with the Thigh Flexed at a Right Angle

Case No. 594. The injured front seat passenger, who was not wearing a safety belt, was travelling in a 1963 Morris 1100 saloon car which was involved in a frontal collision with the nearside of a Rover 75 saloon car at a cross roads. She sustained a posterior dislocation of the left hip joint, without fracture of the acetabulum, when her left knee struck the facia and underlying metal beam fixed between the two A-posts. Her left knee was grazed and bruised, the force being transmitted via the shaft of the femur to the hip joint to cause the posterior dislocation.

The damage seen on the facia and underlying metal beam was simulated under controlled laboratory conditions. The dynamic load required to produce this damage was recorded. This was equivalent to the force acting on the occupant's knee during the accident which caused the hip injury.

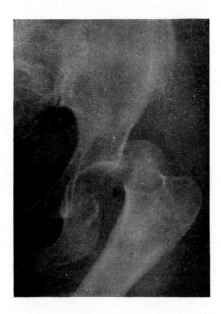

Posterior dislocation of
passenger's left hip joint

Morris 1100 saloon car involved in accident

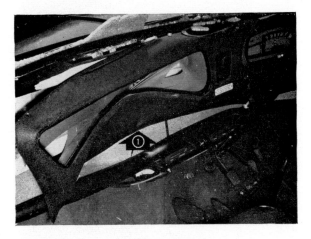

(1) Site of knee impact

Laboratory simulation of accident damage on a body shell of a
Morris 1100

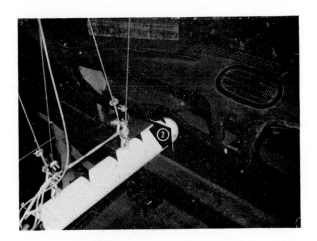

(2) Knee form striking facia

Example No. 6—Safety Belts

Case Nos. 732 and 735. The two occupants were the drivers of Ford Cortina saloon cars which collided with each other. The dynamics of the collisions were similar for both vehicles. In both cases the impact was frontal and the degree of damage to both cars was the same. The driver of the white 1966 Cortina (*Case No. 735*) was wearing a lap and diagonal (static type) safety belt correctly adjusted. He was adequately restrained and sustained superficial injuries only, his chest and lower abdomen being bruised due to pressure from the safety belt. The driver of the dark green 1968 Cortina (*Case No. 732*), who was not wearing a safety belt, sustained fatal chest and abdominal injuries as a result of striking the steering wheel and column. His injuries were: a stove-in chest, a torn pericardium and bruising of the heart, collapse of both lungs, a lacerated liver and a ruptured spleen.

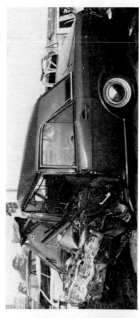

Dark green Ford Cortina Mk II saloon (Case No. 732)

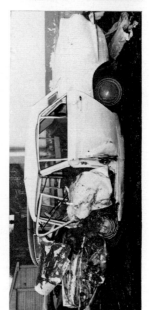

White Ford Cortina Mk I saloon (Case No. 735)

162

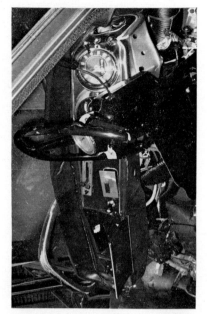

Unrestrained driver—steering wheel and column badly deformed as a result of being struck by the driver's chest and abdomen (Case No. 732)

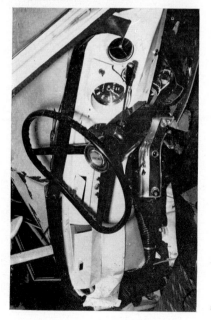

Restrained driver—steering wheel and column almost undamaged (Case No. 735)

Example No. 7—Steering Columns Fitted with Collapsible Energy-absorbing Devices

For the more horizontal steering columns it is now normal practice to incorporate a collapsible energy-absorbing device in the steering wheel or column.

Case No. SC2. The driver, who was not wearing a safety belt, was travelling in a 1970 Vauxhall Viva saloon car which was involved in a severe frontal collision with an oncoming lorry. The driver struck the steering wheel but sustained no chest or abdominal injury. In this example the energy-absorbing device consisted of a column with a collapsible outer tube and a telescopic inner tube; the column being fastened to the underside of the facia by shear plugs designed to break free if the driver's body strikes the steering wheel. It will be noticed that there has been collapse of the mesh and that the shear plugs have separated from the facia.

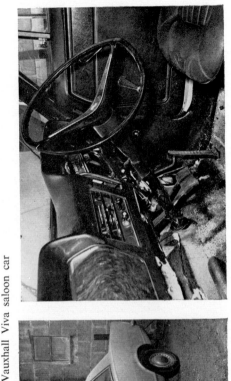

Vauxhall Viva saloon car

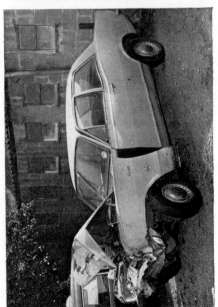

164

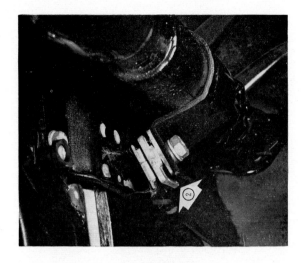

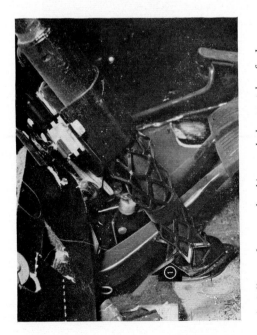

(1) *Collapse of energy-absorbing meshed outer tube of column*
(2) *The fixing point of the column to the underside of the facia has sheared as a result of the impact of the driver on the steering wheel*

Example No. 8—Intrusion

Case No. 489. The injured driver, who was not wearing a safety belt, was travelling in a 1962 Bedford T.K. tipper lorry which was involved in a frontal collision with the rear of a Commer lorry. As a result of this impact the front of the cab of the Bedford, a forward control vehicle, was crushed backwards causing intrusion into the driving compartment. Resulting from the intrusion of the front of his cab the driver sustained bilateral fractures of the pubic rami, a simple transverse fracture of the shaft of the right femur, a compound fracture of the shaft of the left femur, and a compound fracture of the left tibia and a fractured left fibula. The pelvic and femoral fractures were caused by being struck by the incoming steering column and steering wheel respectively, and the fractures of the left lower leg by being crushed between the seat pan and the incoming front of the lorry cab. The driver was trapped by the incoming structures.

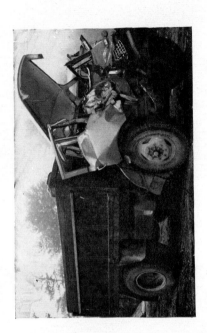

Bedford T.K. tipper lorry

Severe frontal impact with the rear of the load platform of a Commer lorry. Note: windscreen pillars cut in order to release the driver

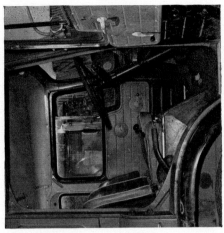

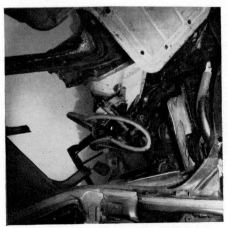

Left: Driver crushed between the incoming front of the cab, the steering wheel and column and his seat

Right: Undamaged vehicle for comparison

Example No. 9—Injury Potential of Steering Columns Related to Steering Column Angle

Two frontal impact accidents are illustrated to show the relation between different steering column angles, i.e. steering columns with a different rake, and the severity of chest injury.

Case No. 1301. The driver, who was not wearing a safety belt, was travelling in a 1965 Austin Mini estate car which was involved in a severe frontal impact. This car has a more vertical type of steering column. He struck the steering wheel and column which bent forwards under the load applied to it by his upper body. He sustained no chest or abdominal injuries.

Case No. 269. The driver, who was not wearing a safety belt, was travelling in a 1965 Vauxhall Velox saloon which was involved in a frontal impact of moderate severity. This car has a more horizontal steering column. He struck the steering wheel and column which did not bend, and sustained severe chest injuries, i.e. a fractured sternum, a fracture of the tenth right rib in the mid-axillary line, a small right haemo-pneumothorax, but no abdominal injury. It will be noticed that in this accident there was also some backward penetration of the steering column towards the drivers' seat as a result of the frontal impact on the car.

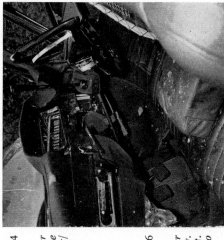

Car with a column angle of 44 degrees to the horizontal

Left: Case No. 1301. Driver sustained no chest injury. Severe frontal impact. Damage index/ car weight ratio ≡84

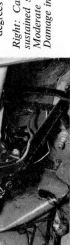

Car with a column angle of 26 degrees to the horizontal

Right: Case No. 269. Driver sustained severe chest injury. Moderate frontal impact. Damage index/car weight ratio ≡51

REFERENCES

Grattan, E. and Hobbs, J. A. (1968). 'Mechanisms of serious lower limb injuries to motor vehicle occupants.' Road Research Laboratory Report No. 201.

— Clegg, Nancy G. and Hobbs, J. A. (1970). 'Chest injuries in unrestrained vehicle occupants who survived a road accident.' Road Research Laboratory Report No. 320.

Harris, P. (1971). 'Road accident tabulation language (RATTLE).' Road Research Laboratory Report No. 377.

Lister, R. D. and Wall, J. G. (1970). 'Determination of injury threshold levels of car occupants involved in road accidents.' International Automobile Safety Conference Compendium SAE 1970.

Moreland, J. D. (1964). 'Damage index. A scale for assessing car damage.' *J. Inst. auto. Assessors*, **15**, No. 3.

Road Research (1970). *Annual Report of the Road Research Laboratory*. London; H.M.S.O.

— (1969). 'The classification of injuries sustained in road accidents.' Road Research Laboratory Leaflet No. 130.

8 Investigation of Mass Disaster

PETER J. STEVENS

An event in which ten or more persons are killed is generally referred to as a mass disaster, although the number ten is purely arbitrary. In certain parts of the world nature is frequently responsible for mass disaster with floods, hurricanes, avalanches or earthquakes killing hundreds, if not thousands, of people. During the five-year period 1965–69 over 113,000 died in 170 or so such catastrophes. About 88,000 of these perished in five massive disasters, four of these being in East Pakistan. In these really enormous disasters, when whole communities are wiped out, there can be very little detailed investigation; the task would be far too great and the most that could be attempted would be the identification of some of the bodies of the dead. When disaster on a smaller scale occurs, the casualties being numbered in tens or at most a few hundreds, and especially when it is connected with man's activities and therefore almost certainly with man's fallibility, a proper investigation is both possible and desirable. There are many of these lesser disasters. Few countries escape in any given year; often a single state will suffer several in the same year. Between 1965 and 1969 there were at least 36 mining accidents which took over 2,200 lives, but one-quarter of these casualties were accounted for by two accidents in 1965, one in Turkey and one in India. Some 80 explosions and fires during these years killed nearly 2,000 persons; 48 railway accidents killed over 1,600; 100 road traffic mass disasters killed 2,400; over 5,200 died in 90 marine accidents; and a further 1,500 or so died in 40 miscellaneous catastrophes such as collapsed buildings, panic and stampede in crowds and so forth. In addition to any technical investigation into the event itself, examination of the bodies of the victims by pathologists is necessary for two main reasons:

(1) To identify each body and to establish the cause of death for legal purposes so that a death certificate can be issued.

(2) To discover evidence relating to the investigation of the disaster itself.

This is perhaps most pertinent in the context of aircraft accidents where, as has been shown in recent years (Mason, 1962; Reals, 1968; Stevens, 1970), the medical evidence following a fatal crash can contribute a great deal to the general reconstruction of the accident and to the discovery of the cause or the exclusion of possible causes of the accident.

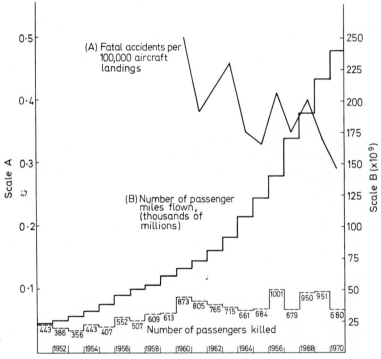

Figure 1. The statistic 'fatal accidents per 100,000 aircraft landings' is probably the most reliable index of flight safety in public transport aviation and like all other measures of flight safety it shows that there has been a steady improvement over many years. Nevertheless, there is a trend towards an increasing annual death toll in this form of aviation explained by the very marked increase in its volume.
The figures for 1971 are: Killed 859, fatal accident rate (A) 0·33

Although aviation in general, and public transport aviation in particular, gets safer year by year, the volume of aviation, showing no decline in its annual rate of increase, is likely to result in an increasing toll of life (*Figure 1*). During the second half of the 1960s, about one-sixth of the 180 or so annual disasters involved aviation and an average of 31 fatal aircraft accidents occurred, killing an average of 28 persons each; during the first half of the 1960s the annual average was 28 accidents, with an average of 27 deaths per accident. It is likely, however, that the 1970s will see a change in this pattern; it is to be hoped that the safety trends will continue and that there will be fewer accidents, but the much larger aircraft now in service make the single aviation disaster with well over 300 deaths merely a matter of time.

The establishment of the identity of the dead to the satisfaction of the local legal authority is generally regarded as the duty of the police. Most, if not all, police forces have personnel trained in this work. However, in many disasters the extent of damage to bodies and their clothing by traumatic forces or by fire is such that specialized examination of the bodily remains is necessary to establish identity. It is therefore considered highly desirable that, from the outset, very close liaison should be established between the police and the pathologist appointed by the local legal authority—H.M. Coroner in England and Wales—to carry out the post-mortem examinations.

There is much to be said in favour of the Scandinavian practice which provides for the appointment by a Prefect of Police of an identification commission including a policeman, a doctor (usually a pathologist) and a dentist, whenever the need arises by reason of mass disaster or crime (Keiser-Nielsen, Frykholm and Strøm, 1964). This commission collects evidence of identity of the bodies recovered, each member working in his own field of competence, and jointly it reviews all the evidence and determines whether or not in each case the evidence warrants a particular identity being assigned to a particular body.

Whether or not the circumstances of the accident are such that a medical and pathological contribution to the accident investigation itself is called for, or whether the pathological assistance is required solely to assist in identification, the co-operation of pathologists and police can be conveniently considered in three phases. The first relates to the procedures to be carried out at the accident site, the second to the tasks in the mortuary and the third to the problems of reviewing the evidence collected, comparison of records and of follow-up investigations of various sorts.

THE FIRST PHASE—AT THE ACCIDENT SITE

Priorities in the initial stages of the post-disaster situation will generally be self-evident. There may be survivors to be rescued and all possible means will be used to save life without unduly endangering rescuers from the various continuing dangers that may exist, fire being an obvious example. As soon as it is clear that no further lives can be saved, those in charge should pause to take stock of the situation. It is important that there should not be hurried retrieval of bodies without thought for the preservation of evidence that may contribute both to their identification and to the investigation of the accident itself in its widest sense. The first tasks involve the location of the bodies, labelling them with a number, photographing them *in situ* and preparing a plan of the disaster site, so far as this is possible, showing the main pieces of wreckage and the position of the bodies. If the terrain is suitable the position of the bodies can be staked. The way these tasks are carried out and whether each step is rigidly observed will very much depend upon the type of disaster and the judgment of the senior police officer in charge. A map of the site showing the main pieces of wreckage and the location of the bodies is clearly more appropriate in the context of an aircraft accident than, say, a hotel fire, for in the latter a written record of which numbered bodies were found in which rooms might be considered to suffice.

The exact location of a body at a disaster site may prove to be very important, however, whatever the disaster. In a hotel fire, the room in which it is found may be one of very few clues to its possible identity; in an aircraft accident, the seat in which a body is found may help to determine its identity, for it may be known to whom a particular seat was allocated; after a railway accident, the identification of one of a group of bodies in a particular railway compartment may provide a clue to the identity of others when a family or friends were known to be travelling together. The location of a body in an aircraft accident may be of considerable importance in the reconstruction of the accident; a passenger's body amid the wreckage of the flight deck and among the bodies of the flight deck crew might be fortuitous, but on the other hand might indicate that an accident had occurred during a failed attempt at air piracy.

The elimination of possible causes of a disaster is as worthy an achievement as the demonstration of the true cause. When a BOAC aircraft broke up in the air over Japan near Mount Fujiyama in 1966, sabotage was immediately suspected. Painstaking mapping of the location of the bodies and their individual identification, with the knowledge that the aircraft had split in two in the region of the bulkhead between the first class and economy class passenger sections of the cabin, permitted certain deductions to be made (Stevens, 1970, p. 46). Bodies retained in the forward section were those of the flight deck crew, the first class cabin steward and certain first class passengers. Those retained in the rear half or thrown out at ground impact were all economy class passengers and were found near to their appropriate seats (a passenger seating list was available). The bodies that were scattered over a wide area and at a considerable distance from the aircraft wreckage were all those of persons who had occupied seats immediately in front of or behind the split in the aircraft. The bodies of a steward and two stewardesses were found near the wreckage of the rear galley. This routine reconstruction of where each person was located at the time of this catastrophe did little more than show that the operating crew were in position on the flight deck, that there was no evidence of an additional person on the flight deck, and that there was no evidence of any 'unauthorized' person in the forward first class cabin; it appeared that all passengers and cabin staff were in their appropriate places, with the cabin staff attending to their routine duties. It is largely on such pieces of evidence that the completed jigsaw puzzle of an aircraft accident reconstruction is composed, none of them having the nature of a 'vital clue', but each essential for the complete picture.

The work of identification of the bodies and accident reconstruction from medical evidence therefore commences at the site of the accident to the extent that bodies are labelled and photographed and a record made of their precise position. I do not believe that further procedures should be carried out on the bodies at the site; detailed examination of the bodies, their clothing and the contents of clothing should be left until the corpses have been transferred to a mortuary where facilities are adequate for these further examinations to be carried out without fear of overlooking or mixing up evidence. The best course is for the rescuers, properly supervised by an experienced police officer, perhaps in co-operation with the pathologist, to recover each body and place it in some sort of a suitable container for transfer to a mortuary. In the process of placing a body in the container, clothing and associated property or even parts of the body that have become detached in the process of handling (as is not unusual when a body has been severely burnt) must be transferred to the same container; but only provided it is certain that they *do* belong to that particular body. Great care must be taken by those engaged in this task to ensure that things belonging to one body are not assigned to another.

Figure 2 shows a partially burnt address book placed in the container with body 31 by the rescuers following a certain aircraft accident. The rescuers had found this book lying on or beside body 31, which was very badly burnt, and the book had apparently dropped from a pocket of the jacket which had been largely destroyed by fire. This documentary evidence was accepted as a clue to the identity of the body since those whose names appeared in the address book were found to know only one man travelling on that aircraft. This tentative identification was proved wrong beyond doubt when confirmation was sought from dental evidence; it transpired that there had been several burnt bodies in a pile (a fact that had not been

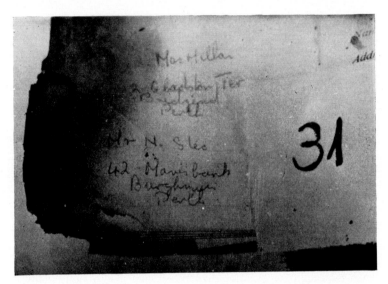

Figure 2. Partially burnt address book associated by rescuers with Body 31. It transpired that this book had, in fact, fallen from the burnt clothing of another body in close proximity to Body 31 and it was therefore a false clue to the identity of Body 31 (reproduced by permission of Professor J. Milçinski)

recorded by the rescuers) and that the address book had in fact come from another body in that pile. Loose property or a separated part of a body assigned by the rescuers to the wrong cadaver can result at best in considerable extra work for those in charge of the identification, or at worst in an incorrect identification.

There are several types of container which can be used to transport bodies from the scene of a disaster to the mortuary. The author has experienced many types of *ad hoc* arrangements made when local authorities have not planned to deal with a disaster situation. Hessian sacks and polythene sheeting can often be produced at short notice. I have known of makeshift wooden coffins being quickly produced, their construction being more influenced by the urgency of the situation than the potential skill of the carpenter. The result has been that defects in the sides or floor have produced a risk of loss of fragmented contents, and even total disintegration of a coffin has resulted during handling and transit. Most impromptu arrangements are less than ideal. Some type of burial sack or pouch, preferably disposable, may be best (*Figure 3*). It should be sufficiently robust that, with a body inside, it can be handled from the accident site to a point where it can be placed on and strapped to a stretcher or directly placed in transport. There are situations—on the side of a

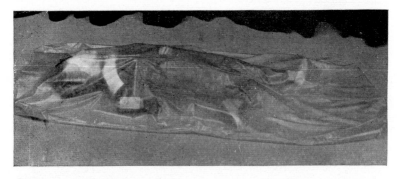

Figure 3. A simple, cheap, but in most circumstances efficient plastic pouch in which corpses may be transported from accident site to mortuary

steep mountain for example—where, though it may be possible to put a body into a burial pouch at the spot where it is found, it may be difficult to get even a light-weight stretcher to the area and then carry that stretcher down the mountain. In such uncommon circumstances the pouch itself has to be manhandled for a distance and needs to be strong enough to remain intact. The pouch shown in *Figure 3* has the advantage of being sufficiently cheap to be disposable, consisting only of a plastic envelope with a plastic single zip. Being semi-transparent it is possible to see the numbered label attached to a body without need for further labelling on the outside. Its disadvantages are that it does not have handles to facilitate carrying and if it is necessary to carry it for a distance a stretcher of some sort is probably essential. A more sophisticated pouch with carrying handles costs much more and the need to clean and re-use more expensive articles would probably arise. Authorities with the foresight to prepare disaster plans would do well to consider having available a stock of containers such as the one illustrated. It weighs approximately 3¾ lb, folds to occupy a volume of approximately $11 \times 8 \times 1\frac{1}{2}$ in and, at the time of writing, these pouches cost about £2 each.

Although it is true that there are few authorities or organizations which can afford to disregard the cost of fulfilling their functions, it is well that the economics of mass disaster investigation should be viewed in perspective. These investigations are expensive. Their value with regard to the legal, sociological and humanitarian aspects of recovery and identification of the bodies of the dead and the consequent speedy issue of death certificates is difficult to quantify. When the disaster is one like an aircraft accident and the investigation is directed also towards the discovery of the cause of the accident so that other similar accidents may be prevented, the economic value of the whole investigation is more easily understood. In October 1971 a BEA Vanguard crashed in Belgium. It was announced within a few weeks that the cause of the accident was corrosion of a rear bulkhead. If this discovery resulted in similar damage being found and repaired in but one other aircraft with a similar accident thus prevented, the saving in financial terms, let alone in terms of human life, make the cost of the whole comprehensive investigation of the accident well worth while. It follows, therefore, that there is a strong case for planning and executing disaster investigation in liberal fashion, with sufficient manpower (but properly supervised) for search and rescue procedures, with the quickest possible transportation to the scene for the specialist investigators, and with the provision of a sufficient quantity of efficient modern equipment. When it is a case of too little and too late, the value of an investigation is seriously jeopardized.

PHASE TWO—IN THE MORTUARY

Mortuary accommodation, and in particular refrigeration, are likely to be problems following any major disaster. Bodies should not be dispersed to numerous small mortuaries if this can be avoided for it makes the task of a co-ordinated investigation very much more difficult. It is preferable that a building of suitable size be designated a temporary mortuary; a village hall or a disused hangar near an airfield or some other building where there is sufficient space and light is required. If the available accommodation is in general terms suitable, but the permanent lighting source inadequate, temporary efficient lighting may be provided by mobile generators. In the absence of more sophisticated facilities it is possible to proceed in such a building with an external examination of the bodies. In certain types of mass disaster, where identification is not difficult and evidence in the bodies cannot contribute in any way to a reconstruction or explanation of the accident, only external examinations may be required.

When, as is the rule in aircraft accidents, a full autopsy is required from the point of view of the accident investigation itself, then better facilities—a properly equipped autopsy room—become essential. It may be necessary to transfer bodies one or two at a time from a temporary mortuary to the main autopsy room some distance away. With careful organization and relatively few bodies, this can be done quite successfully. Following one particular aircraft accident in a tropical country the bodies were transferred two at a time from refrigerated accommodation seven miles away to the small hospital autopsy room that was available for their examination. This was found not to present any serious problems—but there were only 16 victims; it would not have proved so satisfactory if there had been 116.

It is ideal to have in close proximity an autopsy room, refrigerated mortuary accommodation, an area for embalming and casketing, rooms for interviewing relatives and viewing bodies if necessary and a suitable room for use as a communications headquarters. Rarely will this ideal be available, and less desirable arrangements may have to suffice. The ideal is likely to be most closely approached when there has been pre-planning by the appropriate local authorities (in particular the police) before a disaster situation of medium to considerable magnitude occurs, with decisions having been taken in advance about what accommodation could be brought into use in the event of a disaster of a particular size.

It is rare, in particular, for sufficient refrigerated mortuary accommodation to be available in one place. One solution to this problem is for the accommodation most suitable in other regards to be selected and a number of refrigerated trucks hired and parked in the vicinity of the autopsy room. A large number of bodies can be held in such temporary accommodation and this has proved a very useful arrangement following several large aircraft accidents in recent years. An alternative approach to the problems of refrigeration is the installation at certain centres of large, walk-in types of refrigerator which can be adapted rapidly to accommodate several hundreds of bodies if necessary. Such equipment is being provided in certain United States medico-legal departments, but their use in dealing with a mass disaster may well involve transport of large numbers of bodies for a considerable distance; there could be also the attendant disadvantage of temporary divorce of the medical investigators from the other accident investigators while carrying out their respective duties—a real disadvantage in aircraft accident investigation, but not so serious a disadvantage perhaps in many other types of disaster.

The author is firmly of the opinion that the procedures in the mortuary should be a matter for team work involving at least a pathologist and a police officer, usually a forensic odontologist and occasionally other specialists, such as a radiologist when appropriate to the particular circumstances and conditions of the bodies. It is always important to count the number of bodies recovered. This is easy enough when there has been little or no mutilation and fragmentation, but when the traumatic forces of the accident have been severe the total number of items of human remains recovered may far exceed the number of persons killed. It will then be found helpful to introduce in the mortuary a new set of body or cadaver numbers. If, for example, about 130 persons are believed to have been killed and some 250 or so numbered items of remains have been recovered from the accident site, a suitable set of numbers to choose as cadaver numbers would be 401 *et seq.*

If the circumstances are judged to warrant the use of a new series of cadaver numbers, the first body selected for examination will have a label bearing the first new number attached to it. It must then be photographed to show clearly both the labels it now carries, the one with its site location number and the other the cadaver number. As subsequent remains are brought to the table for examination, cadaver numbers will be assigned to those which constitute more than half a body. The whole task is facilitated if the bodies selected for examination in the early stages are those which are likely to be easily identified and are substantially whole, or at least comprise more than half a body.

Figure 4 shows the relative value of various types of evidence used in the identification of a series of aircraft accident victims. A similar histogram was constructed by Mason (1970) from another series of aircraft accidents although he did not use precisely the same grouping of means of identification and included a concept of primary and secondary means of identification. Primary identification is a term that could apply either to the first clue to identity discovered in a given instance, whether it be strong or insubstantial evidence, or to the most valuable clue, judged in retrospect, when all evidence has been adduced. The categorization of pieces of evidence as primary or secondary is probably of little practical consequence; the only practical approach is, in the writer's opinion, to seek routinely from the outset to establish identity by all or several of the different means and not to rest content unless identity has been established and confirmed by at least two different means if at all possible.

179

Visual identification is the standard method used by police to establish the identity of a dead body that falls within a coroner's jurisdiction. While visual identification of facial features can be reliable when a body is intact or but little damaged externally, the effect of burns and traumatic injury reduces its value very considerably in many disaster situations; either visual identification is impossible or—and perhaps more serious—if attempted, incorrect identifica-

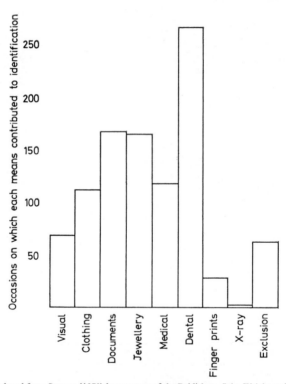

Victims identified	577
Unidentified	28
Total	605

Figure 4. Histogram showing the means of identification of the bodies from 13 fatal public transport accidents and the relative values of the various types of evidence

tions may be made either in a positive or a negative sense; this has been reported on several occasions (Stevens, 1970, p. 142). In these circumstances any statement made by a person attempting a visual identification should be regarded as a clue to, not proof of, that body's identity.

When a body has been selected for examination and brought to the autopsy table, given its cadaver number if necessary and a photographic record made to relate body, site and cadaver numbers, additional photography must be considered as the subsequent steps in the examination are undertaken. Even if facial features are unrecognizable, photographs of distinctive clothing, personal possessions or physical characteristics may be recognizable by friends or relatives and it is desirable that a photographer remain at hand throughout the examination of a corpse.

After the initial photography, clothing and jewellery must be removed from a body, examined and catalogued. This is primarily for identification purposes and would be normally carried out by the police member of the team who might well take samples of material from any clothing that was distinctive, and such manufacturers' labels or laundry marks as might provide valuable clues to the identity of the wearer. But during the removal and examination of this clothing the pathologist must have an opportunity to examine it for evidence that might bear upon his primary task. It might be that evidence of vomit, blood or other stains upon the clothing could prove to be important. Damage to clothing is likely to have arisen during the accident sequence but occasionally evidence in the clothing may relate to the cause of the accident such as the damage that might result from the explosion of a saboteur's bomb.

There follows the careful external examination of the body and, though primarily in the province of the pathologist, experienced police officers may well contribute by their observations. At this stage the examination of the body will be directed at determining its sex, measuring or estimating height and weight, recording such bodily features as hair colour, location and abundance, colouring of skin and, if possible, of eyes, external abnormalities such as birth marks, tattoos, surgical or traumatic scars and any anatomical abnormalities, congenital or acquired. The external examination of the body is also directed to the discovery of injuries which have arisen during the accident and in particular any that could be related to the cause of the accident. Any injuries suggestive of having been due to an explosion would be especially carefully examined for the possibility of there being, in or around the wounds, trace evidence which would need to be preserved for special examination. Specimens of tissue possibly containing metallic fragments or saved for chemical analysis should be deep frozen, while samples intended for histological examination should be preserved as usual in 10 per cent formol saline.

It is then necessary to consider whether, if available, radiographic examination should be used. The ideal would be to take a complete set of skeletal x-rays of each victim, but in many instances the effort and expense may be correctly judged unjustified. If there is any suspicion of sabotage full skeletal radiography should be carried out. When bodies are extremely badly burnt and there is likely to be difficulty in identifying them, radiographs can sometimes be helpful in revealing the presence of articles embedded deeply in charred muscle which would probably be otherwise overlooked. On several occasions such objects revealed by x-ray examination have led to identification of the body. A further advantage of a skeletal survey is that a permanent record of the bone injuries is obtained and reduces the time spent in assessing and recording these during the autopsy.

There follows the full internal autopsy in the course of which again evidence relevant to identification will be collected, such as the surgical absence of internal organs, the presence of post-surgical states such as a gastroenterostomy, evidence of pre-existing disease, of internal injury and the precise cause of death. During the autopsy, specimens of certain organs and tissues will be collected for routine histological and toxicological examination—the former in 10 per cent formol saline, the latter deep frozen if solid, or in 1 per cent sodium fluoride if fluid such as blood and urine. The value of histological examination of the lungs in trauma has been well documented by Mason (1962, 1965); appropriate specimens of other organs may reveal a disease which would be relevant to a consideration of impaired function if the body be that of operating crew or expectation of life should medico-legal problems concerning compensation subsequently ensue. Autopsy evidence and histological confirmation of the presence of Hodgkin's disease was the first clue to the identity of a particular body in an aircraft accident investigated by the author in 1964.

It will be noted from *Figure 4* that finger-prints have been of limited value in the identification of victims of aircraft accidents in the writer's experience. This is, of course, in some measure due to the nationality of most of the passengers in the aircraft being in question. In Britain only criminals and merchant seamen have their finger-prints permanently recorded. In the United States of America a considerable proportion of the civilian population have their finger-prints filed either by the Federal Bureau of Investigation or by one of the government departments of an individual state. It is estimated that in the USA there are of the order of 160 million finger-prints available for comparison with those of unknown persons. Indeed, the column in *Figure 4* results almost entirely from American subjects. On one or two occasions it has been possible to search the home of a British passenger or member of crew for finger-prints to match with those of one or more of the victims; this has been attempted only when the number of unidentified bodies has been reduced to the difficult few. At some stage in the joint examination procedure, therefore, the finger-prints of the victims must be taken. It is probably best that this should be done at the end of the autopsy after all other possible evidence has been collected from the examination of the body including the unstained hands.

Also at a suitable stage in the joint examination procedure, again probably best at the end of the autopsy, a dentist should make an examination of the jaws and teeth. The value of dental evidence in identification has been long established and has become widely recognized in recent years, particularly as a result of the work of Scandinavian forensic odontologists such as Strøm (1954), Keiser-Nielsen (1963) and Gustafson (1966). The general principles of comparison of dental charts of known persons with findings in cadavers are too well known to be laboured at length once again here. It will suffice to re-state that a positive identification can be made when there are a number of points of similarity as between teeth missing and points of matching in restorations by a particular tooth and surface, and when there are no incompatible inconsistencies. The minimum number of points of similarity required for a confident identification to be made cannot be stated dogmatically. Seven or eight are often quoted as a suitable number; but each case must be considered on its merits and a judgment of those merits is part of the expertise required of the forensic odontologist. Clearly a match between one or two acrylic crowned incisors would be relatively of greater significance than a match of three or four molars each having a single occlusal surface amalgam filling. It is well to keep in mind the principle of the compatible and incompatible inconsistency. A tooth missing in a cadaver (not resulting from the trauma of the accident) but recorded as present in the chart of the known person is no bar to identity when there are several matching features, especially when the chart of the known person is not a recent one. Similarly a restoration present in the body not recorded in the known person's chart is not an incompatible inconsistency; the tooth in question could have been extracted or filled, as the case may be, between the last available charting and the accident. But a tooth present in a cadaver recorded as extracted in a known person, or an intact tooth in the body recorded as having been filled in the known person's chart, is an

183

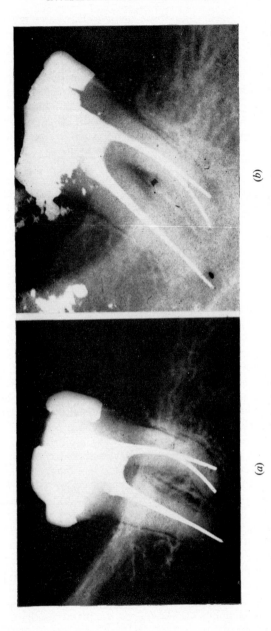

(a)   *(b)*

Figure 5. Comparison of a post-mortem radiograph of a fragment of jaw bearing a single tooth (b) with an ante-mortem film (a). It is difficult to conceive of stronger evidence of identification

[Reproduced from Stevens (1970) by courtesy of the publishers, John Wright and Sons]

incompatible inconsistency; it can only be disregarded in the face of overwhelmingly forceful evidence that the inconsistency is due to mischarting or some other artefact—perhaps in the telegraphed transmission of the dental notes or chart.

In the context of mass disaster in which traumatic forces are severe the value of the dental charts is reduced and the value of radiographs is enhanced. It is quite common for a body to have retained but one or two fragments of jaw—perhaps with but one or two teeth. These teeth may have a restoration or two, but they may be commonly filled teeth and a chart may be quite inadequate in its detail of the size and shape of the restorations for the evidence to be strong enough to form the basis of an identification. If an ante-mortem radiograph of the relevant part of the dentition is available, however, it may prove to be of the greatest possible value for comparison with the post-mortem radiograph of the fragments recovered (as is shown in *Figure 5*).

The above references to dental evidence as a means of identification have been primarily in connection with the comparative approach to this work. The author's experience has been largely in the field of aircraft accidents when the names of all the persons involved in the accident are nearly always known with a considerable degree of certainty and the comparative approach is the most appropriate. When a completely unknown body is found, or when a mass disaster involves quite unknown persons as is usually the case in a department store fire or a railway disaster, the reconstructive value of dental evidence is more often utilized. The teeth may reveal much about their owner: his or her country of origin, perhaps, from characteristic restorative work; his or her occupation, such as the notching of upper incisors that may occur in hairdressers, for example; and the teeth can be a good guide to age. Gustafson (1950), Dalitz (1962) and Miles (1963) have all contributed to the subject of the estimation of age from the examination of the dentition; Johanson (1971) has recently taken the six criteria that Gustafson used in a single regression line giving each criterion equal value, and he has shown that they are of unequal importance in ageing. He advocates the use of multiple regression with a different value given to each criterion; with this statistical evaluation Johanson improves on Gustafson's standard deviation by about two years.

One of the main problems in the field of international forensic odontology has been the lack of a common dental nomenclature. The many systems used by dentists in various countries were reviewed in 1962 by Frykholm and Lysell. The possibilities of confusion after a mass disaster involving people of many nationalities, when dental information is received in telegraphed form was emphasized by these authors, and I can, from personal experience, vouch for the truth of this. A great step forward was made at the International Dental Federation meeting at Bucharest in 1970 when a new two digit system was proposed and adopted for recommendation for international use. It is very simple (*Figure 6*) and it is to be hoped that it will find general favour quickly. The first of the two digits refers to the quadrant; the digits 1–4 are given to the quadrants in a clockwise direction, beginning at the upper right, and they indicate the permanent denti-

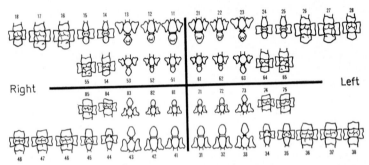

Right   Left

Figure 6. Two-digit system of dental nomenclature recommended by the International Dental Federation. The first digit indicates the quadrant and whether the tooth is of the permanent or deciduous dentition and the second digit indicates the position of the tooth in the quadrant. The digits denoting a tooth are spoken separately, i.e. 'two five' (not 'twenty-five') means the upper left second pre-molar. This illustration shows the two-digit system combined with a pictorial chart of a type recommended for forensic odontological practice

tion; the digits 5–8 are given to the quadrants to indicate deciduous teeth. Within the quadrants teeth are numbered 1–8 from the midline backwards or 1–5 in the case of the deciduous teeth. Thus 34 (spoken as 'three four') refers to the lower left first premolar and 16 ('one six') to the upper right first molar; 51 ('five one') is the upper right deciduous central incisor. This new nomenclature has been incorporated into the new Interpol form and into the other forms referred to below.

Other means of identification, more sophisticated than those referred to in the foregoing, may be required either when mutilation is extensive or when difficulties arise for other reasons. Stewart (1970) has edited a collection of papers on subjects such as multivariate analysis for the identification of race in crania, the identification of the scars of parturition in the skeletal remains of females, and neutron activation analysis of hair. Incidentally, there is some doubt as to whether neutron activation analysis of hair is as valuable a technique for identification as was at first thought (Cornelis, 1972). Such advanced and complicated methods referred to in Stewart's volume would be justified in criminal investigations such as ordinary murder or perhaps wartime atrocities (Mant, 1970), and certainly they would be justified in any accident investigation when the identification of particular bodies appears to be crucial to very important conclusions concerning the accident cause. Whether there is a point beyond which efforts need not be taken to identify the bodies of those suffering an accidental death is perhaps debatable.

The last task to be performed in the mortuary is the examination of any fragments of bodies, with, so far as possible, matching of those fragments with the bodies from which they originated. It will sometimes prove possible to identify a body only after clues have been discovered in a detached part. In one accident in 1964 the author found it possible to identify a body when jaws and part of a face had been found amid the fragmented human debris and these parts had been shown anatomically to have come from a particular cadaver; dental identification of that body was then made. Not only may clues to identity be found in separated fragmented remains but, occasionally, important evidence about the cause of the accident awaits the diligent pathologist carefully pursuing this, perhaps the most unpleasant part of his duty.

THIRD PHASE

Comparison of records and identification

During recent years the need for practical record forms in the context of a mass disaster has come to be appreciated and, as a result of a suggestion put forward by the Australian police, Interpol recently produced a disaster victim identification form (*Figure 7*). This document is most useful, perhaps, when there is a relatively small number of victims and when identification is the main aim rather than a medical investigation of an accident. The Interpol form, however, provides little or no space for autopsy findings—even when these might be appropriate to identification itself. One of its biggest disadvantages is, in my opinion, the fact that the form is designed for use both as a record of findings in a cadaver and as a record of details concerning a missing person. The different parts of the form are annotated: 'For completion only when disaster victim identification form is used to detail description of missing person'; or: 'For completion only when disaster victim identification form is used to detail description of deceased victim of disaster', with

187

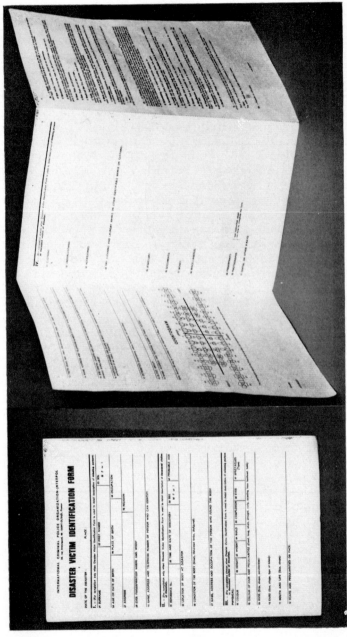

Figure 7. Views of the Interpol Mass Disaster Victim Identification form showing its face and that it is a form comprising three pages; the last page, having only instructions for the use and completion of the form, can be torn off and discarded

PLATE I

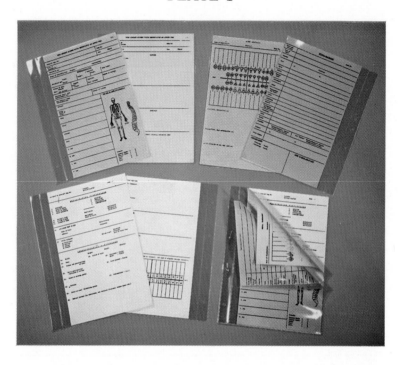

The pink and yellow forms shown face up are for female bodies, and the blue and orange forms shown on their reverse sides are for male bodies. Both face up and on the reverse is the white 'information-about-missing-persons' form, and the simple means of clipping together the plastic envelopes to form a dossier when a body's identity has been established is demonstrated. This dossier remains in a form facilitating easy reference should the need arise. The forms illustrated were developed jointly by the author and J. K. Mason on the basis of their personal experiences, and have been included by the International Civil Aviation Organization in the 4th Edition of the *Manual of Aircraft Accident Investigation*; earlier simpler documents from which the present forms were evolved were described by Stevens (1965a, b)

To face page 189

sections to be completed in both cases. If, therefore, one had a disaster involving 200 persons, there would be 400 identical forms varying only in the sections which had been completed and the task of comparing records, which is the basis of the process of identification, would not be nearly so easy as it could be.

The forms which have evolved from 15 years of practical experience by those pathologists who have worked in the Royal Air Force Aviation Pathology Department at Halton consist of four different coloured forms and a white one. Two of the coloured forms are for males, the other two for females. The white form is for information about missing persons. Each form is a single sheet printed on both sides. One of the coloured forms for each sex is designed to record all the external features of a body relating particularly to identification and also the dental evidence. The other two coloured forms (again one for each sex) are primarily for the autopsy findings; they include a skeletal diagram for use as the simplest means of indicating missing parts or a level of bisection if there has been gross mutilation. These single-sheet forms are inserted each into a transparent envelope upon completion so that they may be handled thereafter with ease and are protected from being soiled. Because they are coloured and are single sheets of paper, the subsequent paper exercise of matching records and 'proving' the identification of the bodies is very much simplified. As identifications are completed the transparent envelopes containing the relative forms can be clipped together to form a single dossier (Plate I).

Reference has been made above to forms used to record information about missing persons. Identification of bodies of course depends upon accurate information about those who are believed to have been involved. When the persons killed are of the country in which the disaster occurs it is probable that the normal police communications system is the best for the collection of the required information. Either it can be obtained from those who telephone the police disaster communications centre to make enquiries about individuals, or the police can actively initiate the collection of information by telephoning or visiting relatives or friends of the deceased, their dentists and doctors. The latter is only possible of course where there is some information about the names of the persons involved; this is usual after aircraft accidents, likely in many hotel fires but will not be available normally after a rail accident. In the case of aircraft accidents and in particular accidents to British aircraft abroad, the airlines themselves or a company of funeral directors representing those airlines have provided an efficient information service as has been described elsewhere (Stevens, 1970, p. 176).

Review of Evidence and Accident Reconstruction

In a disaster such as that at Aberfan in 1966 there is little or nothing that pathological examination of the bodies of the victims can achieve beyond providing evidence leading to identification and confirmation of an obvious cause of death. At the other end of the scale, experience has shown during the last decade that a comprehensive pathological investigation of an aircraft accident can help a very great deal to reconstruct the accident, sometimes to the extent of revealing the cause, though more often perhaps helping to exclude possible causes.

The autopsies on the pilots and the subsequent laboratory investigations on samples of tissue may reveal serious disease as a likely cause of an accident: Stevens (1970, pp. 65, 101, 103) recorded a number of instances of death due to acute coronary artery insufficiency in pilots while at the controls of gliders and light aircraft; Mason, Townsend and Jackson (1963) and Buley (1969) reviewed this disease as a cause of airliner accidents; certainly one major accident killing 83 persons was due to coronary artery disease in the pilot (Civil Aeronautics Board, 1967).

It is important to keep in mind, however, that even if naked eye or histological evidence of even severe disease is discovered it does not follow that it is related to the cause of the accident. Mason (1963), among others, has advocated caution in ascribing an accident to coronary artery disease found in a pilot since quite advanced disease is compatible with normal function and efficiency for long periods and, with the relatively high incidence of this disease in the general population, it may only be an incidental finding in a pilot (or any other vehicle operator) whose machine has crashed due to some entirely dissociated technical fault. This is equally true of other conditions such as isolated focal myocarditis when the unwary might too lightly attach significance to the finding without giving sufficient weight to the incidence of the condition in the normal 'healthy' population (Stevens and Ground, 1970).

At the time of going to press a Public Inquiry is being held on a Trident aircraft which crashed in the summer of 1972 at Staines, Middlesex. This case is especially relevant to the matters referred to above and it remains to be seen whether the Commissioner accepts that the undoubted coronary artery disease present in the pilot with apparently a recent haemorrhage into an atheromatous plaque was, in the light of all the known circumstances and other investigators' evidence, the probable basic cause of the accident.

In 1968 an initially inexplicable disaster, apparently due to a navigational error, was only understood when routine toxicological

190

tests on the tissues of the three pilots showed carbon monoxide intoxication, the source of which was shown to be a malfunctioning cockpit heater exhaust system (Stevens, 1970, p. 31).

As already implied, the bodies of either crew or passengers may reveal evidence to raise or support a suggestion of sabotage as a cause of an accident. At least one major aircraft accident has resulted from the pilot being shot by a passenger (Doyle, 1968), the case of Mason and Tarlton (1969) is a good example of medical evidence supporting engineering evidence of an in-flight explosion due to a bomb.

On more than one occasion a careful analysis of the injuries of the pilots, particularly those in the hands and arms, has led to conclusions about who was piloting the plane at the time of the accident (Civil Aeronautics Board, 1967; Board of Trade, 1967).

An appraisal of passengers' injuries and correlation with damage to seat structures and other solid structures within the aircraft may permit a reconstruction of the precise causes of injury and death. This will show the relative safety of different parts of the aircraft in the circumstances of the particular accident and may suggest means of improving safety and the chance of survival in a similar accident. Where an accident has been partly survived it is especially important that such a reconstruction be undertaken so that an assessment of the factors affecting aircraft evacuation can be made; the training of cabin crew, the adequacy of restraint by seat belts, the number, location and ease of operation of escape exits and devices and the adequacy of gangways should all come under review. This can only be done if the location of bodies at the site has been recorded, their identification effected and the injuries and precise cause of death determined and related to the state of the aircraft wreckage and the history of the accident as given by survivors.

The principles briefly outlined in this chapter are applicable in part or in whole to any mass disaster. Those concerning recovery of bodies and their identification can be adopted with advantage in virtually all types of disaster. Those relating to a reconstruction of the accident from medical evidence clearly have a more restricted application. They are appropriate in particular to aircraft disasters but in a more limited way can be followed in other instances—in particular other transportation accidents.

REFERENCES

Board of Trade (1967). CAP 310, *Report on the Accident to DC46-ASOG at Frankfurt on 21st January 1967*. London; H.M.S.O.

G*

Buley, L. E. (1969). *Aerospace Med.*, **40**, 64.

Civil Aeronautics Board (1967). *Aircraft Accident Report SA* 392 *File No.* 1-0001, *American Flyers Airline Corporation, Lockheed Electra—L188C, N183H, 22nd April* 1966. Washington; CAB.

Cornelis, R. (1972). *Med. Sci. Law*, **12**, 188.

Dalitz, G. D. (1962). *J. forens. Sci. Soc.*, **3**, 11.

Doyle, B. C. (1968). In *Medical Investigation of Aviation Accidents*. Ed. by W. J. Reals, p. 38. Chicago; College of American Pathologists.

Frykholm, K. O. and Lysell, L. (1962). *Int. dent. J., Lond.*, **12**, 194.

Gustafson, G. (1950). *J. Am. dent. Ass.*, **41**, 45.

— (1966). *Forensic Odontology*. London; Staples Press.

Johanson, G. (1971). *Odont. Revy.*, **22**, Suppl. 21.

Keiser-Nielsen, S. (1963). *J. dent. Res.*, **42**, 303.

— Frykholm, K. O. and Strøm, F. (1964). *Int. dent. J., Lond.*, **14**, 317.

Mant, A. K. (1970). In *Personal Identification in Mass Disasters*, p. 11, Ed. by T. D. Stewart. Washington; Smithsonian Institution.

Mason, J. K. (1962). *Aviation Accident Pathology*. London; Butterworths.

— (1963). *Br. med. J.*, **2**, 1234.

— (1965). *Med. Servs. J. Can.*, **21**, 316.

— (1970). *Commun. Hlth.*, **2**, 36.

— and Tarlton, S. W. (1969). *Lancet*, **1**, 431.

—— Townsend, F. M. and Jackson, J. R. (1963). *Aerospace Med.*, **34**, 858.

Miles, A. E. (1963). *Third International Meeting in Forensic Immunology, Medicine, Pathology and Toxicology. Abridged Proceedings*. International Congress Series, No. 80, p. 35. Amsterdam; Excerpta Medica.

Reals, W. J. (1968). *Medical Investigation of Aviation Accidents*. Chicago: College of American Pathologists.

Stevens, P. J. (1965a). *Aerospace Med.*, **35**, 641.

— (1965b). *Milit. Med.*, **130**, 653.

— (1970). *Fatal Civil Aviation Accidents: Their Medical and Pathological Investigation*. Bristol: Wright.

— and Ground, K. E. (1970). *Aerospace Med.*, **41**, 776.

Stewart, T. D. (Ed.) (1970). *Personal Identification in Mass Disasters*. Washington: Smithsonian Institution.

Strøm, F. (1954). *Int. dent. J., Lond.*, **4**, 527.

9 Recent Improvements in Estimating Stature, Sex, Age and Race from Skeletal Remains

T. D. STEWART

INTRODUCTION

Nearly 20 years have elapsed since Boyd and Trevor dealt with the above-listed problems of skeletal reconstruction in the First Series of *Modern Trends in Forensic Medicine*. Their objective was to present, within the limits of a 20-page chapter, what was then known about the subject. Yet naturally they stressed new developments, and of these the one that absorbed them most was Dupertuis and Hadden's (1951) set of regression equations for estimating stature from the long limb bones of males and females in general. Unfortunately, however, by the time the volume appeared (1953) the Dupertuis and Hadden equations had been challenged by more promising, if less general, ones (Trotter and Gleser, 1952). Moreover, the succeeding years saw the experts in bone identification—mainly physical anthropologists—giving far more attention than previously to the forensic aspect of their endeavours. Since this recent trend has included the improvement of numerous other identification techniques besides stature estimation, a progress report, rather than another cumulative account, is in order.

Logical arguments can be advanced for dealing with the subdivisions of the subject in different ways. Boyd and Trevor started with the most general (or phylogenetic) problem—race—then considered sex and age, and ended with the most individual (or ontogenetic) problem—stature. My own order preference in another connection (Stewart, 1954) was sex, age, race and stature, largely because age estimation depends upon sex and because stature estimation depends upon sex, age and race. On the other hand, I have frequently realized that when I look at a skeleton my initial impression is likely to be a general age distinction—adult vs sub-adult—and then the sex (partly indicated by size). In this instance race comes last. However, since my objective here is a progress report on the advancement of knowledge in a limited field, the order of considering the problems is of secondary importance. Having already made reference to stature estimation, I will carry on with it. If more logic is needed, this means starting where Boyd and Trevor left off.

STATURE

Correction of Stature Estimates for Ageing

Trotter and Gleser's initial contribution (1951) to the subject of stature estimation had to do with the effect of ageing on stature. This paper, although given as a reference by Boyd and Trevor, was not mentioned in their text, presumably because the contents had no application to existing equations. Thus it was not until 1952 that Trotter and Gleser pointed out how knowledge of the rate of decrease in stature following maturity gives a degree of accuracy to their equations not possessed by any of the earlier ones. As will appear, however, this is not the only reason why their equations have received wider acceptance than those of Dupertuis and Hadden.

Previously, when regression equations for estimating stature from long limb bones had been derived from cadavers, the statures of these individuals measured in life had been unavailable. Trotter and Gleser got around this problem by using the remains of American white and Negro soldiers killed in the Pacific 'theatre' during World War II. This enabled them to match up the post-mortem measurements of the long bones with the corresponding statures recorded at induction. It was relatively simple then to adjust the statures for whatever growth took place between the dates of induction and death.

Since the military sample was predominantly young—18 to 49 years of age—Trotter and Gleser supplemented it with a civilian sample derived from the Terry collection—the remains of white and Negro dissecting-room cadavers that had been assigned to Washington University School of Medicine in St. Louis over some 22 years. By comparison of the two samples they arrived at a reasonable correction for cadaver stature as measured in that institution. This resulted not only in the inclusion of females, but in an extension of the age range of the total sample to 99 years.

Because the study was cross-sectional in nature (i.e. it dealt with samples of successive age groups measured at the same time), and the age range of the Terry collection is so great, the secular and ageing factors affecting the stature curve could be separated and the rôle of ageing alone evaluated. By secular factor is meant the change in stature attributed to evolutionary trend and environmental influences; by ageing factor is meant the change in stature attributed to degenerative alterations of the joints (mainly those of the trunk). Without going into details, Trotter and Gleser were able to show that, when 30 years is assumed to be the age of beginning stature decrease, the rate of decrease due to ageing alone is 0·06 cm per year, or 1·2 cm in 20 years. French cadavers measured in 1888 by Rollet show the same rate of decrease, which suggests that the figure can be applied generally.

The establishment of the rate of stature decrease due to ageing enabled Trotter and Gleser to formulate regression equations that give estimates of maximum living stature reached in the age period between 18 and 30 years. The same equations can be used for estimating the stature of older individuals simply by subtracting from the results 0·06 (age in years −30) cm.

General vs Specific Equations for Stature Estimation

Like their predecessors, Trotter and Gleser (1952) presented equations based on all six long limb bones, either singly or in combination. In addition, they showed the advantage of using their favourite equation (that involving the femur alone) to estimate the means of the American and/or European samples of Pearson (1899), Breitinger (1937), Telkkä (1950) and Dupertuis and Hadden (1951). Actually, this equation, when applied according to the indications of sex and race, *considerably underestimates* the means of the Dupertuis and Hadden sample, as do the corresponding equations of the other investigators mentioned, whereas the corresponding equations of Dupertuis and Hadden (not one of the general equations) *considerably overestimates* the sample means of Trotter and Gleser, as well as those of the others.

This still leaves unanswered the question as to how well the Dupertuis and Hadden *general* equations estimate stature as compared with the Trotter and Gleser *specific* equations. In this connection it is important to note that Dupertuis and Hadden obtained their general equations by averaging the slopes and origins of the Pearson (1899) equations for whites and their own equations for whites and Negroes, and by giving Pearson's smaller population half of the weight of the other two. In considerable part this procedure was designed to reconcile the above-noted divergencies in estimation of stature by the two sets of equations.

Table 1 gives an answer to the just-posed question through comparison of the results of applying the femur equation from each of the two sets of equations to the series of actual individuals listed in Boyd and Trevor's Table 3. Ignoring the seeming inaccuracies of the basic data, it appears that the differences slightly favour Trotter and Gleser, in spite of (or perhaps because of) my inability to apply their correction for ageing due to the lack of ages in the data

TABLE 1

Comparison of the Stated Statures of 10 Individuals with the Estimated Statures of the Same Individuals as Determined from their Stated Femur Lengths by Means of General and Specific Regression Equations

Known person*	Femur length (cm)*	Actual or presumed stature (cm)*	Dupertuis and Hadden (1951) general equation 'a'†		Trotter and Gleser (1952) specific equation for whites‡	
			Est. stature	Diff.	Est. stature	Diff.
		Male				
Mathelin	50·1	180·0	181·2	+1·2	180·6	+0·6
Sellier	45·2	173·4	170·4	−3·0	169·0	−4·4
Kaps	44·5	171·7	168·7	−3·0	167·3	−4·4
Dr. 'P'	46·8	169·0	173·8	+4·8	172·8	+3·8
Riviere	44·7	168·3	169·1	+0·8	167·8	−0·5
Gamahut	42·7	165·2	164·6	−0·6	163·0	−2·2
Alorto	44·8	160·9	169·4	+8·5	168·0	+7·1
Monsieur 'A.B.'	39·5	156·0	157·5	+1·5	155·4	−0·6
		Female				
Isabella Ruxton	42·4	160·5	159·6	−0·9	158·8	−1·7
Mary Rogerson	39·8	152·4	153·6	+1·2	152·4	0·0
Total difference with regard to sign				+10·5		−2·3
Total difference without regard to sign				25·5		25·3
Range of difference				−3·0 to +8·5		−4·4 to +7·1

* Data from Boyd and Trevor (1953), Table 3, page 149.
† Male: 2·24 Femur + 69·09; female: 2·32 Femur + 61·41.
‡ Male: 2·38 femur + 61·41; female: 2·47 femur + 54·10.

provided. On the other hand, the objection can be raised that Dupertuis and Hadden require the averaging of estimates from all 10 of their equations, whereas only the estimate from one equation has been used here. This is not a valid objection, because the best estimate is obtained from the limb bone having the highest correlation with stature, which is always a lower limb bone. No amount of averaging can improve on the estimate from the best equation (*see also* Keen, 1953, 1955).

What is lacking in Table 1 is a racial comparison. How do the two kinds of equations work out when applied to racial groups other than whites? Allbrook (1961) has come nearest to answering this question. Working out of Kampala, Uganda, he took percutaneous tibial and ulnar lengths, along with stature, on 229 living males of six East African groups of varying ethnic origin and provenience, and on 200 living British soldiers. Ages ranged from 18 to 34. The tallest group (30 Nilohamites—mean stature 177·7 cm) had the longest tibiae and ulnae; the next tallest group (200 British soldiers—mean stature 172·1 cm) had the shortest bone lengths; and the shortest group (185 East African Bantus—mean stature 164·4 cm) had bone lengths significantly longer than those of the British soldiers. Perhaps partly because of these disproportions, and partly because of the different methods of measuring the bones, Allbrook found that Trotter and Gleser's, Dupertuis and Hadden's and Breitinger's tibial equations all gave excessively high estimates of stature for the groups studied. This is further support for the generally accepted principle that for the best stature estimate it is necessary to use an equation with the lowest error derived from the population in question. Such being the case, it is noteworthy that specific equations have been provided during the period under discussion, not only for East Africans (Allbrook, 1961), but for Western Europeans—mainly French (Lorke, Münzner and Walter, 1953) and for Japanese (Fujii, 1958).

In concluding this aspect of the subject it is noteworthy that the Trotter and Gleser equations received their first extensive test following the Korean War when the U.S. Army was again identifying its war dead. In a study of a large sample of these war dead Trotter and Gleser (1958) could find little wrong with their original white and Negro equations and were able to add to them equations for estimating the stature of Mongoloids (North American Indians) and Mexicans living in the United States. The equations from the 1952 and 1958 studies recommended by Trotter (1970) are given in Table 2.

Estimation of Stature from Fragmentary Bones

In 1935 Gertrude Müller, using German skeletal samples without regard to sex, defined certain segments of the humerus, radius and tibia, and gave for each the percentage of whole-bone length. The length of the bone estimated in this way could then be used in one of the available equations for estimating stature. Steele (1970), using documented American white and Negro skeletal samples (again from the Terry collection), has now taken sex into account and altered this method in three ways: (1) by substituting the femur for the radius; (2) by developing regression equations to estimate whole-bone lengths—with standard errors; and (3) by developing regression equations to estimate stature—with standard errors—directly from one or more preserved segments of a specified bone. Unfortunately, space is lacking here to reproduce both the definitions of the segments and the numerous equations to which they relate.

TABLE 2

Selection of Equations for the Estimation of Stature—with Standard Errors—from the Long Limb Bones of Several Racial Groups between the Ages of 18 and 30 years* (Trotter, 1970)

White males		Negro males†	
3·08 Hum + 70·45	±4·05	3·26 Hum + 62·10	±4·43
3·78 Rad + 79·01	±4·32	3·42 Rad + 81·56	±4·30
3·70 Ulna + 74·05	±4·32	3·26 Ulna + 79·29	±4·42
2·38 Fem + 61·41	±3·27	2·11 Fem + 70·35	±3·94
2·52 Tib + 78·62	±3·37	2·19 Tib + 86·02	±3·78
2·68 Fib + 71·78	±3·29	2·19 Fib + 85·65	±4·08
1·30 (Fem + Tib) + 63·29	±2·99	1·15 (Fem + Tib) + 71·04	±3·53

White females		Negro females	
3·36 Hum + 57·97	±4·45	3·08 Hum + 64·67	±4·25
4·74 Rad + 54·93	±4·24	2·75 Rad + 94·51	±5·05
4·27 Ulna + 57·76	±4·30	3·31 Ulna + 75·38	±4·83
2·47 Fem + 54·10	±3·72	2·28 Fem + 59·76	±3·41
2·90 Tib + 61·53	±3·66	2·45 Tib + 72·65	±3·70
2·93 Fib + 59·61	±3·57	2·49 Fib + 70·90	±3·80
1·39 (Fem + Tib) + 53·20	±3·55	1·26 (Fem + Tib) + 59·72	±3·28

Mongoloid males‡		Mexican males§	
2·68 Hum + 83·19	±4·25	2·92 Hum + 73·94	±4·24
3·54 Rad + 82·00	±4·60	3·55 Rad + 80·71	±4·04
3·48 Ulna + 77·45	±4·66	3·56 Ulna + 74·56	±4·05
2·15 Fem + 72·57	±3·80	2·44 Fem + 58·67	±2·99
2·39 Tib + 81·45	±3·27	2·36 Tib + 80·62	±3·73
2·40 Fib + 80·56	±3·24	2·50 Fib + 75·44	±3·52
1·22 (Fem + Tib) + 70·37	±3·24		

* To estimate stature of older individuals subtract 0·06 (age in years −30) cm; to estimate cadaver stature, add 2·5 cm .
† Can be used also for Puerto Ricans.
‡ Primarily for North American Indians.
§ Only for those resident in the United States.

Estimation of Foetal Stature

The reason for dealing with this subject here is the fact that the lengths of the diaphyses of the foetal long limb bones have a high correlation with foetal stature, which in turn is a good indicator of foetal age (*see* page 207). Actually, crown-rump length or sitting height can be used for this purpose just as well as total height (stature) and is said to be measurable with greater accuracy. In 1954 I published a graph showing the plot of femur lengths of 65 foetuses (the two sexes combined) against their crown-rump lengths subdivided by months of pregnancy. The slope of the added regression line provides a means for quickly ascertaining the approximate age. In the meantime Olivier and Pineau in France (1960) and Fazekas and Kósa in Hungary (1966) have investigated series of foetuses numbering 40 and 138, respectively. Their findings differ slightly, but on the whole are very similar to mine, although reported in terms of stature rather than crown-rump length (*see Figure 4* and Table 5). However, they also give the following regression equations for estimating foetal stature (in cm) from each of the long limb bones:

Olivier and Pineau:	*Fazekas and Kósa:*
7·92 Humerus − 0·32 ± k 1·80	7·52 Humerus + 2·47
13·80 Radius − 2·85 ± k 1·82	10·61 Radius − 2·11
8·73 Ulna − 1·07 ± k 1·59	8·20 Ulna + 2·38
6·29 Femur + 4·42 ± k 1·82	6·44 Femur + 4·51
7·39 Tibia + 3·55 ± k 1·92	7·24 Tibia + 4·90
7·85 Fibula + 2·78 ± k 1·65	7·59 Fibula + 4·68

Note that only Olivier and Pineau give an error of estimate and that it is preceded by the factor 'k'. This gives me the opportunity to explain a rule that is usually unstated but applies to all regression equations. It is simply this: if 'k' is given the value of 1, the error encompasses 68 per cent of cases; if given the value of 2, it encompasses 95 per cent of cases.

SEX

The newest advance two decades ago in the area of skeletal sexing to which Boyd and Trevor gave attention was Washburn's (1948) ischium–pubis index. It is clear now that Washburn's finding of only a small overlap between the ranges of this index for the two sexes stimulated a number of investigators to search for other skeletal characters and statistical procedures capable of yielding even more accurate estimates of sex. Since an index, such as the one used by Washburn, shows the relationship between two measurements only, a more sophisticated statistical procedure is needed to express the relationship between a greater number of measurements. Multivariate analysis or discriminant function serves this purpose in a way not very different from that used in estimating stature from more than one long limb bone.

Giles (1970) has explained how the sex of a specimen is arrived at by means of a discriminant function by applying the procedure to an actual forensic case (an unknown Caucasoid skull). The data in this instance consist of eight cranial measurements compatible with an existing discriminant function (*Figure 1* and Table 3). By weighting the measurements and totalling the results according to sign, as shown in Table 3, a discriminant function score is obtained. This can be interpreted by reference to the sectioning point in *Figure 1*.

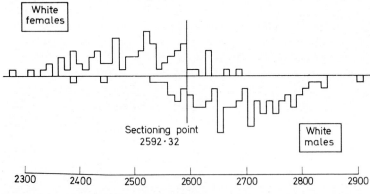

Figure 1. Distribution of Giles' discriminant function No. 2 scores for 108 male and 79 female skulls

Reproduced from Giles (1970) by courtesy of the National Museum of Natural History, Washington

TABLE 3

Application in a Test Case of a Discriminant Function for Estimating the Sex of a Caucasian Skull*

Names of measurements comprising function 2	Discriminant function weights		Measurements (in mm) of test specimen		Products
Glabella-occipital length	3·400	×	168	=	571·200
Maximum width	−3·833	×	140	=	−536·620
Basion-bregma height	5·433	×	128	=	695·424
Basion-nasion diameter	−0·167	×	94	=	−15·698
Maximum bizygomatic diameter	12·200	×	125	=	1525·000
Basion-prosthion diameter	−0·100	×	93	=	−9·300
Prosthion-nasion height	2·200	×	72	=	158·400
Mastoid length	5·367	×	29	=	155·643
				Score	2544·409

* Assembled from Giles, 1970, pages 101 and 103.

200

In Giles' words, 'A score for this specimen of 2544 puts it on the female side of the sectioning point of 2592 but . . . not far from the demarcation line. In fact, this skull, though small, had a number of unmeasurable indicia of maleness, which presumably are reflected in the position of its discriminant function score relative to the majority of females' (page 101). Giles reports also that the discriminant function used in this case gives 86·4 per cent correct results.

We are indebted to Giles for summarizing all of the discriminant functions for sexing (with definitions of measurements) developed up to 1970. These apply to three racial groups and involve 49 measurements of skeletal parts. For Caucasians and American Negroes there are six functions based on cranial measurements, three based on mandibular measurements, and four based on post-cranial measurements; for Japanese there are three based on cranial measurements, one based on mandibular measurements, and 16 based on post-cranial measurements. In addition, for Japanese there are five functions based on a combination of cranial and mandibular measurements and seven based on a combination of cranial and post-cranial measurements; for American Negroes there is one based on a combination of cranial and mandibular measurements. In general, the functions based on post-cranial measurements yield the highest percentages of correct results (93·1 to 96·5 for Caucasians). In spite of this fine showing, Giles concedes that 'it would be misleading to regard sexing by means of discriminant functions as being more accurate than that achieved by a well-trained physical anthropologist' (page 102).

When a physical anthropologist judges the sex of a skeleton by inspection he looks for other things besides the proportional differences reflected in the measurements. One such non-metrical observation, for instance, concerns the form of the dorsal border of the pubic symphysis. If this is irregular and/or shows signs of being undermined by depressions or pits (*Figures 2* and *3*), the individual is almost certainly a female. Scars of parturition, as these bone defects are called, are believed to be due to trauma incurred during childbearing (Stewart, 1957, 1970).

Scars of parturition are, of course, ontogenetically-late pathological changes dependent on childbearing. Otherwise, normally the pelvis undergoes extensive differentiation following puberty as part of the preparation for childbearing. All things considered, the pelvis undoubtedly is the best indicator of sex. It is no wonder, therefore, that non-metric traits related to the normal sexual differentiation of the pelvis have continued to receive attention during the past two decades. The studies of Genovés (1955, 1959) and of Hoyme (1963) along this line unfortunately are not easily summarized. Phenice (1969), on the other hand, has simply focused attention on three normal characters of the pubic bone that by themselves often distinguish females from males: (1) the triangular area on the ventral

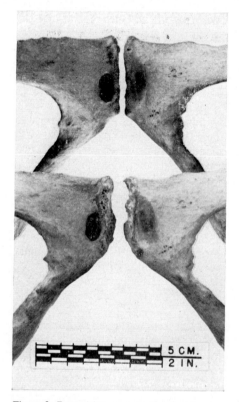

Figure 2. Parturition scars on the dorsal aspect of the pubic symphysis can reach unusual proportions (Terry collection, No. 736, Negro, age 35, number of children unknown). Upper, normal orientation; lower, symphysis opened dorsally to show alterations of articular surfaces

surface of the body at its infero-medial angle; (2) the convexity of the medial border of the inferior ramus where it enters into the pubic arch; and (3) the ridge extending from the inferior end of the articular surface ventro-medially on the inferior ramus. From these characters alone Phenice was able correctly to sex 96 per cent of 275 white and American Negro skeletons.

Pre-adolescent Skeletal Sex Differences

Difficulties in obtaining documented skeletons of pre-adolescents have restricted research on skeletal sexing in this age period to foetuses.

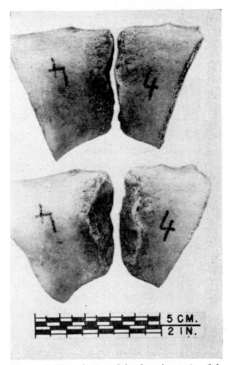

Figure 3. Irregularity of the dorsal margin of the pubic symphysis is often the only evidence of parturition in women given good obstetrical care (Mant's case No. 4, White, age 36, two children). Orientations as in Figure 2
[Reproduced from Stewart (1970) by courtesy of the National Museum of Natural History, Washington]

In 1955 and 1957 Boucher followed up earlier indications and found that a sciatic-notch index yielded a correct indication of sex in 85 per cent of 107 British white foetuses, in 84 per cent of 96 American Negro foetuses, but in only 68 per cent of 33 American white foetuses. This evidence of group difference led Fazekas and Kósa (personal communication) to test the method on 104 Hungarian foetuses. In the process they altered Boucher's measuring technique to permit the use of a sliding caliper and developed several new indices on the basis of which they claim 70–80 per cent success in sexing. The importance of this work is not so much in the area of immediate forensic application—foetal sex is seldom at issue—as in the promise that sexing criteria ultimately will be forthcoming for the rest of the pre-adolescent period where the need is far greater.

AGE AT DEATH

Although the teeth are of major importance throughout the life span for establishing age at death, the remarkable advances in this forensic area will not be considered here. The reader will find them fully covered in Gustafson (1966), Sims (1969), and Johanson (1971).

Variation in Epiphyseal Union

In the past, anatomical texts commonly stated the age of union of an epiphysis as 'about' a particular year. Most physical anthropologists preferred, however, to follow Krogman (1939) in allowing a range of one or two years (four years in the case of the medial clavicle), with females preceding males by up to two years (*see* Stewart, 1954—Figure 113). That the range of variation is far greater than this was revealed when the writer's observations on the American soldiers killed in North Korea were published (McKern and Stewart, 1957; *see also* Stewart, 1963). For example, the proximal epiphysis of the humerus, the union of which Krogman placed at 19·5–20·5 years, was found already united in 21 per cent of 55 soldiers in the 17–18 year age group and still not 100 per cent united in 26 soldiers 23 years of age. It appears, therefore, that Krogman's figures represent what he now (1962—page 33) calls the 'central tendency' and that a range of error of at least ±3 years (±4 years in the case of the medial clavicle) should be added to cover most of the population.

Epiphyseal union has a regular sequence, beginning in the major bones at the distal end of the humerus around 14–15 years of age (males: central tendency) and ending at the medial end of the clavicle around 25–28 years. The sequence, together with individual variation, requires an evaluation of at least a good segment of the total maturational pattern in order to arrive at an acceptable age estimate. For this purpose McKern and Stewart (1957) provide four scoring schemes involving varying combinations ('segments') of joint areas. Table 4 shows the application of one of the simpler schemes to the record of one of the Korean War dead (No. 297 of the Stewart series; age 19 years 1 month and 21 days). The total score given in Table 4 can be interpreted by reference to McKern and Stewart's Table 51 (or Table 23 in McKern, 1970) where the prediction equation for the first part of the score range for this segment (age $= 0{\cdot}0758$ score $+ 16{\cdot}6146$) gives an age of $19{\cdot}34$ years (observed range: 17–22 years).

TABLE 4

Application to a Test Case of a Maturational Score for the Estimation of Skeletal Age*

Maturational features comprising segment III	Score†
Epiphyseal union:	
Humerus, proximal	3
Humerus, med. epicondyle	5
Radius, distal	4
Femur, head	5
Femur, distal	5
Ilium, crest	4
Clavicle, medial	1
Segmental fusion:	
Sacrum, 3–4 centra	5
Sacrum, lateral portions	4
Total score	36

* Assembled from McKern and Stewart (1957), pages 162 and 166–67.
† $1 =$ no union, $2 = \frac{1}{4}$ union, $3 = \frac{1}{2}$ union, $4 = \frac{3}{4}$ union, $5 =$ complete union.

Another of the McKern–Stewart schemes for scoring skeletal maturation involves the articular surface of the male pubis. This operates in the same way as the one just described, except that each of three components of the surface is rated on a scale of 5, for the understanding of which standard casts are provided in addition to printed definitions. The interpretation of the total score again is by means of a Table (Table 27; *see also* Table 24 in McKern, 1970) which gives the corresponding mean ages, observed age ranges and standard deviations.

A female counterpart of the pubic symphysis maturational rating scheme has been worked out for thesis purposes by B. Miles Gilbert of the University of Missouri. Although the details are not yet available, the scheme is said (Gilbert, 1971) to be applicable within an age range of 16–60 years and to be unaffected by the trauma of childbearing.* By contrast, the male scheme is applicable only within an age range of 17–36+ years.

With the cessation of growth the metamorphosis of the joints includes more and more degenerative changes—erosions, lipping, etc. In a study of degenerative changes restricted to the segments of the vertebral column the writer (Stewart, 1958) showed that in white American males such changes tend to intensify from age 40 onward. Note, however, that this is a generalization from one racial group which, until confirmed on other samples, should be cautiously applied to other populations. The same can be said, of course, of all the foregoing ageing procedures.

Before going on to the next subject I will just mention that Boyd and Trevor's doubts about the reliability of suture closure for ageing purposes have been borne out by several other workers (Singer, 1953; Cobb, 1955; Brooks, 1955; McKern and Stewart, 1957; Schmitt and Tamáska, 1970).

Age Changes in Internal Bone Structure

Two of the structural components of the long limb bones—cancellous and cortical tissue—change enough, especially from 30 years of age onward, to offer evidence of age. Prior to 1953 several European investigators, following the example of Wachholz in 1894, reported that the resorption pattern of the cancellous tissue at the upper ends of the humerus and femur is easily observed when these bones are x-rayed, or better still sectioned longitudinally. Schranz (1959) summarized this work, giving special attention to the humerus, which he considers best for the purpose. The main point is that, with the loss of cancellous tissue, the proximal end of the medullary cavity of the humerus assumes a cone shape the tip of which gradually ascends, reaching the surgical neck during the age period 41–50, and the epiphyseal line during the age period 61–74.

Changes in the cortical tissue, being microscopic in scale, are not so easily observed, but by the same token present a more varied presence. Kerley (1965, 1969, 1970) has described for the femur, tibia and fibula a procedure for quantifying four cortical elements—osteons, osteon fragments, lamellar bone and non-Haversian canals—and estimating age therefrom. Ahlqvist and Damsten (1969) have

---

* Gilbert's original study series consisted of one side of the pubic symphysis from each of 82 subjects with parity information. Since announcing his findings he has had the opportunity to examine the 60 bilateral specimens collected by Dr. Mant for the writer (Stewart, 1970) and as a result he realizes that parturition may affect one side more than the other. Consequently, his final report probably will indicate that such damage can lead to more error in age estimation than appeared at first.

confirmed the reliability of the procedure while at the same time simplifying it. This is not to say that the procedure is now so simple that anyone can apply it and quickly arrive at an age estimate. Just the preparation of a suitable cross-section of a bone requires elaborate equipment, careful training, and much time. Yet in 12 forensic cases aged by this method, Kerly achieved an accuracy of age estimate of ± 5 years. Significantly, too, his cases ranged in actual age from 18 to 81 years.

Ageing Foetal Skeletons

Methods for estimating foetal stature from long-bone lengths were discussed on page 198. In continuation of that, I will simply give here a graph (*Figure 4*) and Table 5 for converting statures and/or crown-rump lengths into ages. Since here the age estimate is based on a stature estimate, the former can only be regarded as an approximation.

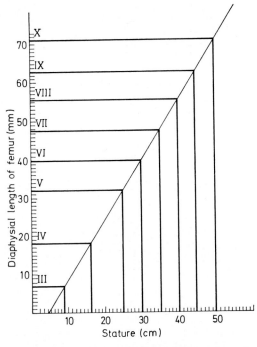

Figure 4. Graph for estimating foetal age from the diaphysial length of the femur and its equivalent stature (after Fazekas and Kósa, 1966)

TABLE 5

Foetal Mean Statures and Equivalent Crown-Rump Lengths by Foetal Months

Foetal month	Mean stature (cm)		Mean crown-rump length (cm)
	Olivier and Pineau (1958)	Fazekas and Kósa (1966)	Olivier and Pineau (1958)
3	—	9·5	—
3½	—	12·3	—
4	—	17·3	—
4½	19·8	22·0	4·0
5	23·8	25·6	4·5
5½	27·4	27·3	5·0
6	30·7	30·6	5·4
6½	33·7	32·6	5·8
7	36·5	35·4	6·3
7½	39·1	37·5	6·8
8	41·6	40·0	7·2
8½	43·8	42·4	7·6
9	46·0	45·6	8·1
9½	48·1	48·0	8·5
10	50·0	51·5	9·0

RACE

The last of the four problems being considered here—race estimation—has received the least attention during the past two decades. In fact, the only contribution to this subject worth mentioning is Howells' (1970) demonstration that multivariate analysis can reveal in an objective manner the racial bent, so to speak, of a skull from a hybrid population; in other words, that a certain combination of cranial measurements is more indicative of one or the other ancestral stock. His immediate concern was with the American Negro population, in which varying combinations of European and African genes predominate.

I will not go into details here, because the method is closely related to that described above for the estimation of sex, and because Howells' exploration of it is still limited. It is important to note, however, that Howells had to approximate the two ancestral stocks as best he could in order to obtain cranial measurements for deriving the discriminant functions. For the generalized European cranial sample he merged Norwegians of mediaeval Oslo and more recent Austrians from the small village of Berg; for his generalized African cranial sample he joined Dogons from Mali in West Africa and Zulus from South Africa. The resulting discriminant functions for males and females, each based on a different set of 15 measurements, produced scores which clearly separate the two ancestral stocks. When in turn the male function was applied to 20 American Negro male skulls (the females were not tested) only seven fell on the white side of the sectioning line. Although one may question whether this is a better result than the trained eye can achieve, any lessening of the subjectivity of the estimate is an important improvement.

Howells is about to produce a book on this subject which will deal with cranial samples from all over the world. After that perhaps someone will extend the method to the post-cranial skeleton (*see* Stewart, 1962).

REFERENCES

Ahlqvist, J. and Damsten, O. (1969). *J. forens. Sci.*, **14**, 205.

Allbrook, D. (1961). *J. forens. Med.*, **8**, 15.

Boucher, B. J. (1955). *J. forens. Med.*, **2**, 51.

— (1957). *Am. J. phys. Anthrop.* (N.S.), **15**, 581.

Boyd, J. D. and Trevor, J. C. (1953). 'Problems in reconstruction—I: Race, sex, age and stature from skeletal material.' In *Modern Trends in Forensic Medicine*, Ed. by Keith Simpson. London; Butterworths.

Breitinger, E. (1937). *Anthrop. Anz.*, **14**, 249.

Brooks, S. T. (1955). *Am. J. phys. Anthrop.* (N.S.), **13**, 567.

Cobb, M. W. (1955). *Am. J. phys. Anthrop.* (N.S.), **13**, 394 (Abstr.). [Also in *Anat. Rec.*, **121**, 277.]

Dupertuis, C. W. and Hadden, J. A. Jr. (1951). *Am. J. phys. Anthrop.* (N.S.), **9**, 15.

Fazekas, I. Gy. and Kósa, F. (1966). *Dt. Z. gericht. Med.*, **58**, 142.

Fujii, A. (1958). *Bull. Sch. phys. Ed. Juntendo Univ.* (*Juntendodaigaku Taiikugakubu Kiyo.* In Japanese with English summary), **3**, 49.

Genovés, S. (1955). *Thesis.* Cambridge; Corpus Christi College.

— (1959). *Publnes Inst. Hist. Univ. nac. auton. Méx.* (1st ser.), 49.

Gilbert, B. M. (Manuscript). *Thesis.* Lawrence, Kansas; University of Kansas.

— (1971). *Am. J. phys. Anthrop.* (N.S.), **35**, 280 (Abstr.).

Giles, E. (1970). 'Discriminant function sexing of the human skeleton.' In *Personal Identification in Mass Disasters*, Ed. by T. D. Stewart. Washington; National Museum of Natural History.

Gustafson, G. (1966). *Forensic Odontology.* New York; American Elsevier.

Hoyme, L. E. (1963). *Thesis.* Oxford; Lady Margaret Hall.

Howells, W. W. (1970). 'Multivariate analysis for the identification of race from crania.' In *Personal Identification in Mass Disasters*, Ed. by T. D. Stewart. Washington; National Museum of Natural History.

Johanson, G. (1971). *Odont. Rev.*, **22** (Suppl. 21)

Keen, E. N. (1953). *J. forens. Med.*, **1**, 46.

— (1955). *J. forens. Med.*, **2**, 190.

Kerley, E. R. (1965). *Am. J. phys. Anthrop.*, **23**, 149.
— (1969). *J. forens. Sci.*, **14**, 59.
— (1970). 'Estimation of skeletal age: after about age 30.' In *Personal Identification in Mass Disasters*, Ed. by T. D. Stewart. Washington; National Museum of Natural History.
Krogman, W. M. (1939). *FBI Law Enforc. Bull.*, **8**, 1.
— (1962). *The Human Skeleton in Forensic Medicine*. Springfield, Ill.; Thomas.
Lorke, D., Münzner, H. and Walter, E. (1953). *Dt. Z. ges. gericht. Med.*, **42**, 189.
McKern, T. W. (1970). 'Estimation of skeletal age: from puberty to about 30 years of age.' In *Personal Identification in Mass Disasters*, Ed. by T. D. Stewart. Washington; National Museum of Natural History.
— and Stewart, T. D. (1957). *Technical Report EP-45* (Environmental Protection Research Division, Quartermaster Research and Development Center, U.S. Army, Natick, Massachusetts).
Müller, G. (1935). *Anthrop. Anz.*, **12**, 70.
Olivier, G. and Pineau, H. (1958). *Arch. Anat. (Sem. Hôp.)*, **6**, 21.
— — (1960). *Annls Méd. lég.*, **40**, 141.
Pearson, K. (1899). *Phil. Trans.*, **A192**, 170.
Phenice, T. W. (1969). *Am. J. phys. Anthrop.* (N.S.), **30**, 297.
Schmitt, H. P. and Tamáska, L. (1970). *Z. Recktsmed.*, **67**, 230.
Schranz, D. (1959). *Am. J. phys. Anthrop.* (N.S.), **17**, 273.
Sims, B. G. (1969). 'Odontology, its forensic applications.' In *Recent Advances in Forensic Pathology*, Ed. by Francis E. Camps. London; Churchill.
Singer, R. (1953). *J. forens. Med.*, **1**, 52.
Steele, D. G. (1970). 'Estimation of stature from fragments of long limb bones.' In *Personal Identification in Mass Disasters*, Ed. by T. D. Stewart. Washington; National Museum of Natural History.
Stewart, T. D. (1954). 'Evaluation of evidence from the skeleton.' In *Legal Medicine*, Ed. by R. B. H. Gradwohl. St. Louis; Mosby. [Revised in 1968 and entitled 'Identification by the skeletal structures.' In *Gradwohl's Legal Medicine*, Ed. by Francis E. Camps. Bristol; John Wright.]
— (1957). *Am. J. phys. Anthrop.* (N.S.), **15**, 9.
— (1958). *The Leech, Johannesburg*, **28**, 144.
— (1962). *Hum. Biol.*, **34**, 49.
— (1963). *J. dent. Res.*, **42**, 264.
— (1970). 'Identification of the scars of parturition in the skeletal remains of females.' In *Personal Identification in Mass Disasters*, Ed. by T. D. Stewart. Washington; National Museum of Natural History.
Telkkä, A. (1950). *Acta. anat. Basel*, **9**, 103.
Trotter, M. (1970). 'Estimation of stature from intact long limb bones.' In *Personal Identification in Mass Disasters*, Ed. by T. D. Stewart. Washington; National Museum of Natural History.
— and Gleser, G. C. (1951). *Am. J. phys. Anthrop.* (N.S.), **9**, 311.
— — (1952). *Am J. phys. Anthrop.* (N.S.), **10**, 463.

REFERENCES

Trotter, M. and Gleser, G. C. (1958). *Am. J. phys. Anthrop.* (N.S.), **16**, 79.
Wachholz, L. (1894). *Friedreichs Bl. gerichtl. Med. SanitPoliz.*, **45**, 210.
Washburn, S. L. (1948). *Am. J. phys. Anthrop.* (N.S.), **6**, 199.

10 Modern Toxicology and Identification Techniques

A. S. CURRY

INTRODUCTION

Tremendous changes have taken place in the last few years in analytical chemistry, as is evident from only a cursory glance at the toxicological literature. The balance, test tubes and paper chromatography of the 1950s gave way in the 1960s to thin-layer chromatography and gas chromatography with a corresponding increase in the capital expenditure required to equip a toxicological laboratory. It appears that the rate of growth requirements will continue to expand for it is already by no means uncommon to find gas chromatography linked to mass spectrometry in many major laboratories, and often data handling facilities are based on a computer.

In the inorganic field the complexity has shown a similar growth, and atomic absorption analyses have replaced the older colorimetric methods for the toxic metals. Mass spectrometry and neutron activation analysis have their own particular place but it would be unrealistic to suppose that the latter techniques at the moment can be other than the province of specialists.

In recent years there has been a complete change in the pattern of work arriving in the laboratory. This has resulted from the pharmaceutical industry's development of new drugs for the treatment of depression, anxiety, pain and insomnia. In addition, the misuse of drugs, particularly the hallucinogens, cannabis and heroin, has materially increased the variety of choice for the toxicologist's menu. Another major change resulting from the increased availability and variety of pharmaceuticals has been the development of polypharmacology where smaller quantities of similar drugs are given in an attempt to diminish side effects but to increase the main desired effect. Unsuspected drug interactions have come to light, some of which are beneficial, others harmful.

As far as criminal poisoning is concerned the variety of agents used by murderers continues to expand. It is still not unknown for such classical agents as arsenic trioxide to be employed but new ones such as insulin and succinylcholine have made their presence felt. Many workers have stressed the high degree of clinical and pathological awareness that must be exercised when thallium salts are used for the purpose of homicide, and Barrowcliffe (1971) re-emphasized only last year how easily even arsenic poisoning could be overlooked despite intensive medical investigations over a period of many months. In his case, the true cause of death was established only when the general practitioner had the courage to rescind his death certificate.

The increased complexity arising from the development of analytical techniques and the number of potential substances that have to be sought in the analysis have placed even more of a burden on the pathologist as far as the collection of samples are concerned. This has followed because of the very high increase in sensitivity that new machines will give. With paper and thin-layer chromatographic techniques, it was necessary to be able to isolate tens of micrograms of a poison from the blood or tissue in order to detect it. Nowadays it is by no means unusual to have a thousand, or perhaps even a million, fold increase in sensitivity over this requirement, with the result that distribution studies of the poison and perhaps many metabolites can be established within a major organ. Selective sampling by the pathologist may be of the greatest importance in the future.

The difference between detection and absolute identification of a suspected poison in relation to sensitivity must be clearly understood and will be discussed in this chapter.

PATHOLOGICAL ASPECTS

The importance of the adequate collection and preservation of specimens for the toxicologist cannot be overemphasized and this applies in both clinical and forensic toxicology. In the living subject clearly the clinical condition of the patient will continue to exert considerable influence on the clinician requesting chemical confirmation of a case of suspected poisoning. There has been a major change in prescribing habits in the last few years and the request for barbiturate analyses on a sample of blood sometimes carries with it the implied suggestion that if the results are negative perhaps a chemical look for all drugs that could produce coma should also be sought. Unfortunately, in the majority of laboratories this is a technical impossibility.

Two factors contribute to this situation. One is the wide range of chemical classifications that make up coma-producing drugs, and the second is the decreasing concentration of drugs that may be responsible for a profound clinical effect. In the past toxic concentrations of bromide were measured in mg/ml; for barbiturates, this decreased to tens of μg/ml, but for the newer tranquillizers, antidepressants, etc., the analyst is required to measure amounts of the order of ng/ml (nanograms per millilitre). It is amusing to compare a nanogram to a gram as a gram to 200,000 five-ton elephants! The very different chemical classifications mean that there is no ubiquitous chemical method of identifying the particular compound responsible for the coma, although a certain degree of suspicion may be invoked by the extraction and examination of the suspected material by gas or thin-layer chromatography. Unfortunately, it is axiomatic that a degree of specificity be included into the analytical procedure and this is a great stumbling block. An examination of a *Pharmacopoeia* or Clarke's (1969) book on the isolation and identification of poisons reveals the great number of compounds, literally many thousands, that may be present in body fluids and which, if a positive reaction was obtained in a case of poisoning, might lead all concerned to suppose that a positive agent had been identified. Unfortunately, it must be recognized that the thin-layer and gas chromatographic procedures are of limited value. Basically, this can be traced back to the fact that there are so many different parameters involved that the choice of system automatically includes rejection of selectivity. In addition, at the very low concentrations of many poisons to be found in blood the separation of the 'signal' from the 'noise' of the co-extracted normal products of the blood leads in itself to difficult interpretation problems.

It must be faced that in clinical toxicology the simple systems for detecting poisonous materials which were described in 1966 by the Association of Clinical Pathologists' Broadsheet (Curry, 1966) have not been materially improved on. Indeed, the only other simple 'spot' test that can be performed by the clinical biochemist is that for paraquat (Tompsett, 1970). It must be accepted that there are no 'spot tests' that can be reliably foreseen to help the clinician in relation to the newer drugs. Specific requests for certain classifications based on clinical findings, e.g. phenothiazines, imipramines, monoamine oxidase inhibitors, methaqualone and the amphetamines, can be met by the laboratory provided it is realized that each classification needs the development of complex procedures, and that it is just not possible for the same analyst to convert from an amphetamine or methedrine case to one involving methaqualone in a matter of minutes. Fortunately, the fact that the analytical findings have, in the majority of cases, little effect on the treatment of the patient has been a saving grace.

SOME FACTORS INFLUENCING THE ANALYSIS OF THERAPEUTIC AGENTS

One feature that has emerged in recent years in the identification of drugs in clinical emergencies has been the recognition that the metabolites may provide an internal marker in the thin-layer or gas chromatographic analyses leading to a pattern which is diagnostic of the drug in question. Indeed, in some cases it has been suggested that the probability of survival can be estimated by the measurement of the continued hydroxylating power of liver microsomes. Sometimes it may be shown that these have been sufficiently damaged that the excretion pattern indicates the patient is unlikely to survive. In cases of paracetamol poisoning it has been found that metabolism is impaired in patients with hepatic injury and that there is a statistically significant correlation between biochemical indices of liver damage and paracetamol half-lives (Prescott *et al.*, 1971). The plasma paracetamol half-life has been found to be the most reliable guide to prognosis and liver damage is to be expected if the half-life has exceeded four hours. Genetic involvement in half-lives has, however, been observed in relation to many drugs, e.g. phenylbutazone, and there is clearly a fascinating story yet to be uncovered on the significance of drug metabolism in drug toxicology.

In discussing the metabolism of drugs the many heterogenic phenomena that may be involved must be considered (McIver, 1967; Herxheimer, 1969). Warfarin may be displaced from its protein binding sites by clofibrate or phenylbutazone, leading to an increase in the anti-coagulant defect. Mepacrine and pamaquine become bound to tissue protein and toxic effects may occur if pamaquine is given after mepacrine due to the high concentration of the latter in the plasma. Another type of reaction leads to decreased concentrations of one of the drugs in the blood; phenobarbitone, for example, increases the metabolism of phenylbutazone, phenytoin, griseofulvin and dicoumarol. This type of interaction is particularly dangerous in the situation where the patient is receiving an anti-coagulant drug. Involvement of drug interaction as contributing to a clinical condition, or indeed death, is an area in which possibilities continue to expand, but in which dogmatism cannot yet be established. Drugs which have been shown to affect mutually their metabolism in animals include glutethimide, meprobamate, chlor-

H

promazine, tolbutamide, phenylbutazone, diphenhydramine, chlor-cyclizine, orphenadrine, testosterone and prednisolone. Similarly, the rate of excretion of a drug may be changed by the simultaneous ingestion of other drugs. The potentiation of hypoglycaemic effects of chlorpropamide and tolbutamide by sulphonamides is known and thiazide diuretics and frusemide can potentiate digitalis prepara-tions by causing potassium depletion. This type of effect is sometimes met in intensive slimming cures (Jelliffe *et al.*, 1967). The anti-depressive drugs and amphetamines may antagonize the hypotensive effects of the guanethidines. Monoamine oxidase inhibitors are well known to be potentially dangerous if taken with foods high in tyramine content and it is clear that the amount of information on potential drug interactions is becoming so large that, without access to computer banks of data, there is a real risk that many cases will go unrecognized. It needs only the example of the problems in the differ-ential diagnosis of ascribing cause and effect in the case of a venous thrombosis of a 'pill'-taking woman to emphasize the situation in which the pathologist may find himself. In many cases the answer must be purely a statistical one.

COLLECTION OF POST-MORTEM SAMPLES

In cases of death following suspected poisoning, one of the major problems that has occurred in recent years has been the recognition that the body at death is still a very efficient chemical factory. Cyanide, carbon monoxide and alcohol have all been shown to be produced in decomposing tissues and there have been many sugges-tions to overcome these most troubling phenomena. The selection of the centre of the brain, away from putrefying tissue on the surface, for analysis has been suggested for cyanide, but little can be done to decide whether a blood alcohol concentration, or a blood carboxy-haemoglobin level in a badly decomposed corpse, reflects anti-mortem exposure or post-mortem production. Fortunately, as far as alcohol is concerned, the increase in specificity and sensitivity afforded by gas chromatographic examinations means that if only a single drop of urine can be collected from the bladder, worthwhile improvements in interpretation can be obtained. It cannot be over-stressed that the collection of several samples of blood from different points of the body, albeit in drop-size samples, is of much greater value now than the collection of a large volume of blood from a single source. If the toxicologist finds that the concentration of such poisons are the same in several samples taken from different parts of the body then he would be on very safe ground in saying that the exposure was extraneous because it has been found that bacterial and chemical decomposition does not occur at exactly the same rate all over the body; indeed, it would be amazing if it were the same. In this context it is highly important that the accuracy and precision of analyses be carefully examined. Toxicologists are used to working to relatively low levels of precision. They are, in the majority of cases, required to determine the difference between a single dose and a fatal dose, usually differing by a factor of ten times or more. In differentiating natural biological systems producing or decomposing cyanide, alcohol and carbon monoxide, the analytical parameters become of much greater importance, but even then the homogeneity of a sample may be a deciding factor. Haemolysis, clot formation, post-mortem diffusion from other body fluids and tissues, coupled with the failure to provide properly preserved samples, may over-ride a superb accuracy and precision obtainable in the laboratory. A typical example of the need for preservation is that concerned with the use of sodium fluoride in blood alcohol determinations. The previously recommended concentration of 0·1 per cent w/v for blood has been shown, in fact, to increase the problem in that it enhances alcohol production rather than reduces it because of bacterial–enzyme interactions (Pleuckhahn and Ballard, 1968). The problem of finding a suitable preservative for urine has also been investigated and to date, although phenyl mercuric nitrate is extremely good for preserving samples suspected of containing alcohol, in cases involving drug analyses the use of 0·1 per cent sodium azide has been recommended (Rutter, personal communication).

The failure of preservative to penetrate a previously formed clot with subsequent alteration in the internal chemistry in the clot, as well as the draining of drugs from the liver into the blood at the base of the jar with a radical change in 'apparent' liver concentrations, are but two illustrations of the problems that can face both the toxicologist and pathologist when it comes to analysing and interpreting post-mortem specimens.

DRUGS OF ABUSE

Intravenous injections of drugs and their abuse have ranged from the classical examples of heroin and morphine to the surprising examples involving abuse of barbiturates and even beer. Pulmonary arterial foreign body granuloma associated with angiomatids have been described particularly in relation to propoxyphene abuse (Butz, 1969). This analgesic, when injected intravenously, has a devastating effect on the veins. In addition, in relation to intravenous use, hepatitis caused by the use of unsterile syringes may be accompanied by severe vascular changes and sepsis is common. Necrotizing angiitis has been noted (Citron, 1970) and even the intravenous injection of cannabis preparations has been observed (King and Cowen, 1969; Henderson *et al.*, 1968). There seems to be no limit to the number of preparations in which the young experimenter will use the syringe. Clinical complications follow and microscopic examination of foreign bodies in the lungs is of obvious value (Johnston, Goldbaum and Whelton, 1969).

The clinical symptoms following intravenous use of modern drugs of abuse is of the greatest value in interpreting the circumstances of any enquiry. The fact that paranoid reactions are to be expected as a natural occurrence of the abuse of amphetamines is of value, especially as users of methamphetamine have been known to take in excess of 1 g every two hours, with the result that they go without sleep for up to five days, gradually getting more paranoid and disorganized (Kramer, Fischman and Littlefield, 1967). Allegations against the police and the doctor are common. Amphetamine intoxication mimicking heat stroke which involved coagulopathy, hyperthermia and reversible renal failure shows the problems of differential diagnosis (Ginsberg, Herzman and Schmidt-Nowara, 1970). The problems of the pathologist in correlating post-mortem findings with possible drug intake are particularly well emphasized by the very wide variety of drugs which are used for hallucinogenic effect and which are referred to by initials, such as DOM, LBJ, STP, etc., and only rarely related to their chemistry. Cases of poisoning from all these drugs have been reported and the nuances of effect are as difficult to categorize as are the chemical tests for their detection. The very recent discovery (Campbell *et al.*, 1971) of pathological changes in the brain that may be seen in cannabis addicts, and possibly related to its effect, dramatizes the absence of knowledge in relation to a drug which has been known for thousands of years. Although clinical evidence of brain damage has been noted over the years, this is the first occasion in which the rôle of the neuropathologist in such cases has been recognized. The fact that crude extracts of cannabis are a mixture of a mass of compounds which undergo further changes when the drug is smoked emphasizes the rôle of the chemist and pharmacologist in such complicated investigations. Although the clinical effect of cannabis is almost certainly due to tetrahydrocannabinol, the congeners have completely different pharmacological effects.

The recognition that addictive drugs can pass via placental transfer into the foetus leading to an addicted neonate, the possibility of teratogenic effects, the observation of chromosomal damage after drug use, the possibility of carcinogenic effects and the balance of clinical effectiveness with side effects in very highly potent drugs, are all relatively recent new factors in the drug scene. It is a feature of the new drugs that are abused that the effective dose is of the order of a few hundreds of micrograms as, for example, in the case of LSD. Indeed, a 'mind-rocking dose' of tetrahydrocannabinol is only 15 mg. It is not surprising, therefore, that at the present time no effective chemical means are available for proving the presence of either material in the blood, tissue or urine of other than the grossest abuser. A dose of 1 mg into a 70 kg 'hippy' could, at the best, lead to an expected concentration of one part in seventy million unless the particular site of the accumulation can be recognized. So far, this cannot be done and cases in which the successful detection and identification of LSD and cannabis compounds in the body have been recorded are very few and far between. Clinical effects of intravenous administration of cannabis solutions involve a brief latent period, severe shaking chills with fever and tachycardia. After one to two hours severe nausea, vomiting and generalized aching pains are experienced which continue for several days.

It is also a factor that when the drug of choice is not available, or is in short supply, abusers tend to take anything that comes to hand.

Another feature of drug abuse is that the normally expected pattern of clinical effects following shortly after the ingestion or injection of the drug is not always followed. With LSD, for example, recurrence of clinical effect following a fairly long period of abstinence is well documented and medical use of LSD in the USA and UK has been severely restricted by self-control. Use of intravenous LSD with subsequent hepatitis has also been noted and I have referred to the phenomenon of abusers taking off their clothes and jumping out of windows as an 'Icarus complex'. There has also been a suggestion that LSD can invoke leukaemia (Leading Article, 1969b).

There have been varying estimates of the severity of the abuse problem in relation to hard drugs in the USA and the UK with estimates of over 500,000 people in the USA abusing barbiturates and amphetamines and an estimated figure of 100,000 heroin addicts in New York City alone; these must be contrasted with the decrease in cases of abuse noted in the UK in 1970 compared with previous years. Statisticians will really have an intriguing time trying to don the astrological hat, but clearly only time will tell what the true pattern will be. The cardiac effects of quinine used as an adulterant in heroin have been described and the pathologist should clearly consider the purity of the alleged drug in coming to his conclusions regarding the possibility of drug involvement when clandestine laboratories may be responsible for the source of the drug. This is a feature to be considered in all investigations because heroin may be 'cut' to a high dilution. Although the presence of morphine in the body may be detected, there is very little information on the relation between tissue levels and cause of death, particularly in addicts, and it could well be that the presence of toxic congeners may have been responsible directly for the cause of death in many cases.

The rôle of urine analysis in screening procedures for large populations either associated with drug abuse or suspected of being involved in drug abuse is becoming widespread. It is not uncommon for populations, such as those of school children and the armed forces, to receive special study and there has been a real need for mechanical aids to assist the toxicologist. These are now available for many drugs such as heroin, morphine, amphetamines and barbiturates (Blackmore *et al.*, 1971), but it must not be thought that a generalized drug screen can be done at the same throughput as can be accomplished by automated machinery. If the nature of a particular overdose is unknown and systematic analysis is required, then each chemical procedure has to be done in exactly the same way as in the 1960s. There are claims that mass spectrometry following chemical isolation can, with the use of computers, lead to rapid and absolute identification of a large number of drugs; I am convinced, however, that if a comprehensive chemical analysis is required then there have been no major advances in automation in the last few years. Major advances have been made in the analytical methodology for a number of specific drugs and indeed I have seen machines analysing urine samples with a high degree of specificity for morphine on 5 ml samples at a rate of 100 per hour. This clearly represents a major advance but, in my opinion, it is but a step on the ladder to what can be expected in drug analysis in the 1970s and the 1980s, provided sufficient money is available.

Very few of the drugs of abuse have been subjected to human studies in relation to the interpretation of the results in cases of death in which they have been involved. This entirely reflects, in my view, the difficulties which the toxicologist faces in his estimation. The chemistry related to such drugs as methadone and pentazocine is of such complexity that a high degree of specialization is required, coupled often with a disproportionate amount of time, before worthwhile findings can be reliably extracted. The sparsity of the data of methadone, for example, is noteworthy, although it has been found that lung tissue concentrations usually exceed that of the liver (Robinson and Williams, 1971). Possibility of the bile being involved has also been suggested and studies on the metabolism of methadone offer great promise.

Levels of pentazocine have been measured but again concentrations in terms of considerably less than $\mu g/ml$ of blood have to be detected (Beckett, Taylor and Kourounakis, 1970). The abuse of heroin is complicated by the different patterns that emerge from geographical variations, and in the UK it is often associated with barbiturates, alcohol and occasionally cocaine, as well as methaqualone. Systematic infections (Briggs et al., 1967), sclerotic veins, ulcerating nodules, and other dermatological complications, must be considered as well as hepatitis (Minkin and Cohen, 1967; Stern, Spear and Jacobson, 1968). Fascinating descriptions of this type of cult have appeared in the literature. The fact that foreign materials are frequently injected by faulty or unclean techniques, and can be found subsequently in the lung and capillary structures, was made above. Talc is the most common contaminant but cotton fibres are not unusual. The need for routine screening of the pulmonary vessels by microscopic examination has been stressed.

Another factor which has frightening implications is the substitution of other drugs for drugs of abuse. Substitution of sodium thiosulphate for cocaine (Kok et al., 1971) has been noted and it requires little imagination to put pathologists on their guard in any case involving alleged death from drug abuse. Indeed, the responsibility becomes greater as time passes because the abuser will undoubtedly have a drug in his tissues but it may well be that the final cause of death was a highly toxic substitute provided by a pusher who wished to get rid of a troublesome client.

The clinical features of drug abuse play a marked rôle in orientating the chemical analyses that are requested by the clinician. Clearly the euphoria of heroin, the stimulation and paranoid inducing features of amphetamines and tryptamines as well as the obvious effects of the hallucinogens are clear cut and require no elaboration, but certain of the other drugs of abuse carry symptoms with them that are of the greatest value to the analyst in deciding his modus operandi in the laboratory. Methaqualone, for example, induces a loss of consciousness with hyper-reflexia, hypertonic clonus, muscle twitching and lowered body temperature (Burston, 1967; Matthew et al., 1968). There is an increased risk of developing cardiac irregularities, haemorrhage and epileptic forms of convulsions. As far as barbiturates are concerned, the significance of bullae has been noted with the characteristic histological appearance (Mandy and Ackerman, 1970) and the fact that the accidental intraarterial injection of barbiturates or hydroxyzine hydrochloride can lead to a partial loss of a limb has been noted (Kratte, Brooks and Rhamy, 1969). The urinary excretion patterns of unchanged barbiturates and metabolites in relation to amylobarbitone is of value in that, as was noted above, some consideration can be given as to possible prognosis or time since the ingestion of the drug (Grove and Toseland, 1971).

ANTIDEPRESSANTS

The benzodiazepines form one of the most widely-prescribed group of drugs for the treatment of depression. So far, no clear case of a toxic overdose leading to death has been described although many cases in which such drugs have been involved have been implicated. It is not unusual for them to be found in cases of alleged impaired driving of motor vehicles and clearly they will be one of the groups of drugs to be studied when a systematic study of the involvement of drugs in accidents is introduced. It is certainly not unusual for one to be asked whether a certain drug level could be responsible for an observed clinical condition associated with this class of drugs. I do not believe the situation is any different from that which used to apply when the barbiturates were involved—in the absence of another clinical condition, clearly the drug must be implicated. Until studies similar to those relating to alcohol and accident involvement have been done the answer must clearly be an inspired, informed guess. A drug which affects behaviour, indeed which is designed to effect behaviour, must have an involvement in accident causation when a complex physical and psychological judgement task is involved. The use of diazepam for the treatment of hallucinogenic crises is of interest in that it has been noted that very few LSD users in a certain locality wished to be without their supply of diazepam when they indulged in psychodelics (Levi, 1971; Solursh and Clement, 1968). Diazepam also acts as an antidote to mescaline and it has been used in the management of heroin withdrawal (Litt, Colli and Cohen, 1971) and in the treatment of strychnine poisoning (Maron, Krupp and Tune, 1971).

The problems of keeping up to date in the toxicological literature are no better demonstrated than in the case of the benzodiazepines which only four years ago were being referred to as a relatively new chemical class, yet by 1971 already numbered 28. The inter-relationship of the metabolites is such that a very large wall chart is needed to even begin to understand and explain them.

The clinical conditions following acute overdoses have been well described although pathological changes are few in the literature. In the case of the phenothiazines a spasm phenomena consisting of a patient who opens his mouth widely, protrudes his tongue, has no abnormal eye movement, but has the characteristic hand tremor with inability to close his mouth, is well known. Spasms of the facial and tongue muscles lasting less than a minute and occurring several times an hour are considered characteristic (Medhurst, 1967). Comments have been made that unless the general practitioner is aware of the problem the patient is treated as an hysteric, but occasionally acute parkinsonism may be encountered; a characteristic tremor of the hands is seen with inability to close the mouth, gradually reaching to a most painful state of spasm.

The distribution of chlorpromazine has been studied with pethidine in maternal, foetal and neonatal biological fluids in samples taken from 220 women who had received 50–100 mg intramuscularly of pethidine, chlorpromazine or promazine, singly or in combination shortly before delivery. Pethidine and norpethidine were found in the amniotic fluid, maternal and foetal plasma. In all, 25 metabolites of chlorpromazine were isolated from the maternal urine and 21 metabolites from the neonatal urine (O'Donoghue, 1971).

As far as imipramine and its chemical analogues are concerned, the clinical effects, and particularly those associated with overdoses in children, seem to be related and characteristic (Steel, O'Duffy and Brown, 1967). A striking feature is the extreme agitation with which patients respond to any stimulants, alternating with periods of drowsiness. Tachycardia persisting during sleep is present in many children, with pupillary dilatation, thirst, dizziness and nystagmus, with vomiting being occasionally found. In severe poisoning convulsions and coma are characteristic, with severe respiratory depression, cardiac arrhythmias, ECG changes and hypotension. Continuous twitching of the limbs, even in deep unconsciousness, with any form of stimulation producing generalized convulsions lasting 30 seconds, is also considered characteristic. The triad of coma, convulsions and cardiac disturbances is the cardinal feature. Again it is unfortunate that autopsy findings are not considered to be specific, with congestion, oedema of the brain and lungs being the only generalized findings. Irritability, restlessness with agitation and abrupt jerking movements have been noted in patients poisoned by the triptylines (Noble and Matthew, 1969). Re-appearance of a tachycardia about 24 hours after admission and, in the latter phase, hallucinations, confusion and drowsiness are also characteristic. These delayed features could therefore indicate a phase of release

223

from tissue binding and certainly the possibility of the metabolites having a pharmacological activity has to be considered.

The interaction of monoamine oxidase inhibitors with tyramine is well known; tyramine may be present in such bizarre substances as bananas, broad beans, beer, cheese, chocolate, cream, game, liver, pickled herrings, Milo, wines, yeast extract and yoghourt! The inhibitors have been described in interactions with depressants, analgesics, phenothiazines, imipramines, anti-hypotensives, anti-parkinsonism drugs, anti-rheumatic, anti-malarial agents, hypoglycaemics and local anaesthetics. The difficulty in detecting routinely many of the MAOI drugs is great unless a degree of suspicion is involved. The compounds based on substituted hydrazine are very unstable and, in addition, very highly sensitive methods of detection have to be employed because of the long-acting effects of the drugs on the body. The fatal reaction may therefore occur when levels of the drug are virtually at the limit of detection; sometimes they may even be beyond it. The use of the enzyme itself, together with a substrate as a spray for thin-layer chromatographic plates on which the extracted drug has been chromatographed, is a novel approach (Curry and Mercier, 1970). Any monoamine oxidase inhibitor stops the reaction proceeding at the position of the drug on the plate. The area of inhibition appears white on a mauve background and this class of drugs can now be detected at about the nanogram level. This particular technique is one that was originally developed for use in the detection of cholinesterase inhibitors but it is clear that the technique of using the inhibition properties of drugs to affect enzyme systems is a subtle method of great potential. The hypertensive interactions between monoamine oxidase inhibitors and foodstuffs have been extensively described in the literature but perhaps the most common interactions are those between the drugs with pethidine and amphetamine-like compounds. Phenylpropanolamine, which is a common constituent of many cough and cold remedies, available without restriction, illustrates how potentially common this interaction can be. The hypotensive agent pargyline and the anti-bacterial drug furazolidone also inhibit monoamine oxidase; pargyline has been shown to cause interactions with dopamine and several foodstuffs, and the latter with tyramine and amphetamine (Cuthbert, Greenberg and Morley, 1969).

The case of the West Indian who experienced a hypertensive crisis after eating green bananas stewed with the skins on is not apophrycal. An overdose of 5 grams of nialamid by a 27-year-old man resulted in great agitation and violent motor activity 12 hours after ingestion (Matell and Thorstrand, 1967). All the muscles of his body seemed to be involved in continual gymnastics and he experienced periods in which he drew himself up into a sitting jack-knife position and then cast himself backward in the bed, throwing his arms and legs about, twisting his fore-legs around in work-like movements and constantly making grimaces and moanings. His jaw vibrated as though he was freezing, but at the same time he sweated profusely. His face was extremely red and this colouring extended downwards over a third of his thorax. There was a stifling sweet odour from his mouth and his eyes were half closed and widely rolling in their orbits. He hallucinated, alternating threats with short toneless laughs and giving an impression of complete disorientation although maintaining a certain amount of contact throughout all this activity. He had hyperthermia and a high pulse rate. At autopsy, with the exception of a slight bronchial pneumonia, there was a complete absence of pathological findings. This particular case is of interest, apart from the clinical manifestations, in the observation of the sweet odour; many of the monoamine oxidase inhibitors have a characteristic smell and the value of the olfactory impression cannot be over-emphasized.

ANALGESICS

The abuse of analgesic drugs has received widespread attention in the last few years. The risk of fatal renal disease following excessive consumption of mixtures containing aspirin, phenacetin and caffeine, as well as the possibility of anaemia, serious gastro-intestinal bleeding or chronic peptic ulcer, has been under intense study. The situation has not been resolved but drug abuse of the analgesics has led to clearly defined clinical descriptions for the 45-year-old woman who appears 10 years older, pale, sickly and slow moving. Suffering from insomnia she takes sedatives, complains tearfully of weakness, weight loss, indigestion and recent vomiting. Her headaches are most oppressive, are virtually continuous and are driving her to thoughts of suicide. Complex medical investigations have led to her hospitalization for depression and possibly a gastrectomy. She complains of nocturia, has experienced loin and colicky lower quadrant pains and in such cases pathologists may well be able to assist with analyses for analgesics in the urine (Gault et al., 1968).

Paracetamol has been indicted in some cases of nephropathy and in fatal cases following acute overdose, gastro-intestinal haemorrhage and acute massive necrosis of the liver have been noted (Maclean et al., 1968).

The incidence of propoxyphene poisoning in the UK has been generally fairly low although it is well established in the Americas. Typical cases involve convulsions, coma and low blood pressure. Very low concentrations of the drug are found in serum. This type of drug illustrates one of the dilemmas of the toxicologist in that a drug widely available to the population must *per se* eventually finish up in the clinical wards as an acute emergency admission. The clinician will then ask the laboratory to determine the blood level and when a drug is taken in very high quantities, possibly many tens of tablets, it is natural to suppose that the laboratory must be able to find an easy and simple answer. Unfortunately, propoxyphene is found in such low values that it is not easily determined and, unless a gas chromatographic system is available, the answer cannot be obtained. Even if gas chromatography can be performed the results may not be obtained for many hours. This dilemma arises from the fact that the classifications of drugs cover such a wide chemical range that it is impossible to have ready for instant use enough gas chromatographs to cover the whole spectrum of drugs. The combinations of column packings, temperatures and detectors required would be phenomenal. The only solution is to have one or two gas chromatographs permanently set up for the very common drugs and to reserve columns which will have to be inserted when a particular need arises. Unfortunately, new columns can take several hours to condition and, indeed, by the time the answer is obtained it is probable that the patient will either be dead or have recovered.

The use of thin-layer chromatography is slightly more advantageous in that using this technique results can be obtained, albeit with much less sensitivity than gas chromatography, in usually much shorter times. Again the technique suffers from the disadvantage that there is no ubiquitous coating material or solvent system. Each analyst usually builds up his own experience based on the type of poisoning particular to his area. Both techniques suffer from the disadvantage that the result at the end is no more than a presumptive positive. By this is meant the fact that if the question is posed 'We believe this person has taken an overdose of X; can you confirm it?' then the answer can be given 'Yes, I have found evidence for it'. Conversely, if the question is posed 'Can you tell us what drug this patient has taken?' then the answer often will be 'I have obtained some evidence for the presence of drug X but the degree of certainty would not provide legal proof'. The question of legal proof is of paramount importance to the forensic toxicologist and in his area of work recourse has to be made to much more sophisticated instrumentation. It is likely that there are very few compounds that can be unequivocally identified using only gas or thin-layer chromatography. Alcohol is an outstanding exception, but it will be noted that this specificity is achieved mainly because alcohol is a simple molecule; the problems of using only chromatographic parameters for more complex molecules are immense.

ANTIHISTAMINES

Antihistamine poisoning is characterized by excitement, agitation, confusion and characteristic hallucinations and hyperactivity with convulsions. Toxic psychosis caused by an overdose of diphenhydramine hydrochloride showed the form of a schizophrenic-like behaviour in a 16-year-old girl apparently following the ingestion of 0·5 g of the drug (Nigro, 1968). This psychotic state included jerky, rapid, coherent but irrational speech, autism, blunted effect with occasional silliness or fear, and visual hallucinations. Later, intermittent disorientation, forgetfulness, dizziness and tremors of the extremities developed. Hypothermia, unconsciousness, with fixed dilated pupils, with unrecoverable cerebral function were noted in a fatal case of a 2-year-old boy who died after the accidental ingestion of 12 tablets of Lomotil. Death occurred after 65 hours with the autopsy showing gross cerebral oedema (Harries and Rossiter, 1969).

OTHER POISONS

In unusual cases of poisoning diagnosis can be extremely difficult and some may require considerable effort before the true cause is discovered. The use of pentachlorophenol for the laundering of diapers and infants' bed linen has given rise to poisoning and adds yet another compound to the number associated with marking inks (*Br. med. J.*, 1970). Toxic effects of carbamazepine have been described (Simpson, 1966) associated with dermatological conditions and hair loss in patients treated with the anti-thyroid drug carbimazole (Papadopoulos and Harden, 1966). Isoniazid poisoning leading to death has also been described with usually a severe metabolic acidosis and clinical signs including deep coma and convulsions (Colombini and Masarone, 1966, 1967; Kristus and Belons, 1967).

Orphenadrine is another drug which occasionally gives rise to acute poisoning following overdose with often a severe initial phase resulting in death (Stoddart, Parkin and Wynne, 1968; Heinonen *et al.*, 1968). The outstanding symptoms include shock and convulsions sometimes requiring drastic therapy by experienced anaesthetists.

Stellate ganglion block as an effective treatment in quinine poisoning has been tried and peritoneal dialysis has been shown to remove significant quantities of the drug (Bricknell *et al.*, 1967). Neuro-toxic effects have been ascribed to piperazine in a case of a girl of 4 years 5 months who received 500 mg three times a day (Savage, 1967). She was afebrile but appeared disorientated and could not communicate. She was quite unable to stand or sit without falling over and could not hold a cup to feed herself owing to frequent myoclonic jerks of the head and limbs.

Considerable interest has been aroused with the availability of radio-immunoassay procedures for the detection of insulin and digitalis glycosides. Methods for use on post-mortem material have been described, greatly facilitating their detection. In clinical work the relationship between effect and body concentration has been and continues to be investigated and in many hospitals there are now routine services to assist the clinician. In fatal cases fortunately the levels are so high that no difficulty is encountered in determining that an overdose has been taken. This is particularly valuable as digoxin in particular is a not uncommon cause of death either because a mistake in dosage has been made or because of an accidental intake by a young child. It may well be that when this technique is introduced routinely into the investigation of elderly patients on such heart drugs, the contribution of the drug to the cause of death can be more accurately assessed. Arrhythmias are said to occur with levels of about 3·3 ng/ml. However, there is clearly a great deal yet to be done on this subject, particularly in the investigation of myocardial–serum digoxin concentration ratios. Average atrial digoxin concentrations are much higher than those in the serum and can average 219 ng/g tissue. No correlation between atrial digoxin concentrations and clinical digitalization has yet been noted.

In the field of agricultural chemicals the great majority have characteristic odours and it is no exaggeration to say that for many compounds the human nose has a greater sensitivity than the best chemical detector. The dog's nose is about one thousand times more sensitive than that of the human and many police forces have found it worthwhile to train dogs specifically for the tasks of detecting certain drugs (such as cannabis) and explosives.

The weed killer paraquat has received great attention because of the number of accidental fatal cases of poisoning in which lung transplantation was used in an attempt at therapy. Simple tests for the detection of the compound in urine are available but the concentration in the blood is extremely low and may be only detectable shortly after ingestion. It has been found extremely difficult to detect any trace of paraquat in peritoneal or haemodialysates. Damage and discoloration of the finger nails by contamination with concentrated solutions of paraquat and diquat have been described (Samman and Johnston, 1969) and the importance of avoiding accidental splashing of dilute solutions into the eye must be emphasized (Cant and Lewis, 1968).

INORGANIC POISONS

Ingestion of corrosives such as hydrochloric acid and formaldehyde have been noted to lead to a linitis plastica type of carcinoma (Kennedy and Bavaki, 1967; Bartone, Grieco and Herr, 1968). As far as inorganic ions have been concerned, peritoneal dialysis has been used in the treatment of a suicide chlorate poisoning (Knight, Trounce and Cameron, 1967), and mental disturbances in the form of an acute psychosis resembling schizophrenia followed potassium thiocyanate ingestion (David and Miketuková, 1967). Thiocyanate was detectable in the urine in very large amounts. The accidental administration of one litre of a 3 per cent boric acid solution into the connective tissue of the pelvis during a bladder instillation led to death from cardiovascular collapse in three days. Histologically, severe acute damage to the renal tubular epithelial cells was found (Hauck and Henn, 1969).

As far as metals are concerned, as was noted above, the introduction of atomic absorption spectrophotometry has revolutionized the analytical investigations that can be made in suspected cases of poisoning. The ability to analyse 10 μl of blood for lead, for example, in a matter of seconds, illustrates the dramatically increased capability. In my opinion, this clearly has great potential in the investigation of sudden deaths because it is now possible to test routinely for a large number of toxic metals such as lead, thallium, mercury, cadium, copper and zinc. Interference with normal metabolism by poisoning may also be reflected in changes in the alteration of concentrations of the normal trace elements, and the possibility of the technique being used diagnostically is surely just round the corner. The technique cannot be used so easily for arsenic but for this element conventional chemical techniques are usually sufficient, except in the case of hair analyses when neutron activation analysis is required.

Significantly, lower plasma zinc concentrations have been found in patients with psoriasis, other dermatoses and venous leg ulcerations (Greaves and Boyde, 1967), and the use of an electron probe micro-analyser has shown a significant difference in the titanium and zinc components of human erythrocytes between normal individuals and patients suffering from lymphoblastic lymphomas (Carroll and Tullis, 1968). Lower concentrations of plasma zincs have been reported in patients taking oral contraceptives and an increase in copper levels in such persons may also be expected (Halstead, Hackley and Smith, 1968). An unusual form of copper intoxication occurred from the use of an unserviced hot water geyser (Nicholas, 1968). Rapid screening methods now exist for the assessment of the severity of the poisoning in accidental overdoses from ferrous sulphate. Deaths from Thoro-trast, which was used as an x-ray contrast medium, continue to occur and an interesting side light is that the *British Medical Journal* found it necessary to comment that it was unlikely that the patholo-gist would be in hazard from the radiation but, equally, found it necessary to emphasize that the code of practice for the safe handling of corpses containing radio-active substance is necessary (*Br. med. J.*, 1967). The radio-isotopes are not usually given to moribund patients but occasionally a patient who has been treated with intraperitoneal gold-198 for metastatic tumour, or even one who has had a high dose of iodine-131 for thyroid carcinoma, may die unexpectedly within a few days of treatment.

Accidental contamination of sausages with barium carbonate led to one death amongst 144 persons, although 19 cases required hospi-talization. In 11 cases paralysis occurred and the respiratory muscles were affected necessitating tracheostomy and artificial respiration (Ogen, Rosenbluth and Eisenberg, 1967). The use of cobalt salts as froth stabilizers in beer led to an unusual series of cobalt cardiomyo-pathic cases amongst heavy drinkers (Leading Article, 1968). The industry is now aware of the possibility of such a relationship and the use of the compounds has been discontinued. Malignant melanoma developing in tattoos was traced to cadmium sulphide in a mercuric sulphide red pigment (Kirsh, 1969). In the last few years a consider-able amount of data has been collected on 'normal' levels in the blood, urine, hair and tissues of what are normally considered toxic metals, for example, arsenic, mercury and even thallium. These have followed directly from the increases in analytical capability and even such diverse findings as the concentrations of arsenic in the blood of people from Taiwan and in Denmark, and in the relationship between such levels in patients suffering from blackfoot disease, have been investigated. Relatively large surveys have been made and there is no doubt that the background of information now available is considerable. The discovery of elevated levels of some metals has led along a fascinating road, even leading to the banning of large consignments of tuna fish from the American market because of high mercury levels. The significance of alkyl mercurials in fish and hence into the food chain is still being debated. Self-administered injection of metallic mercury is a most unusual phenomenon but several cases have been reported within the last few years (Johnson and Koumides, 1967; Chao and Yap, 1967). The ability of the participant to have globules of mercury appear beneath the epidermis makes the phenomenon even more bizarre. Block dissection of mercury deposits in the thighs in one case removed 3·5 g of mercury 12 weeks after the original injections; amazingly no symptoms of acute mercury poisoning were at any time noted (Hill, 1967).

Thallium rodenticides have been described as a social menace in America because of their use as a weapon by the poisoner. The symptoms of poisoning by thallium, like arsenic, can defeat the diagnostic skill of most highly qualified and experienced physicians because of the vague symptoms that poisoning by thallium causes. The astuteness of the forensic pathologist who wondered why the hair of a lady came out during the handling of the head at post-mortem led to the discovery of a recent case in which I subsequently became involved. Staining tissue sections with iodine, which precipitates thallic iodine, resulted in the discovery of dark brown granules in the liver, kidneys and, more outstandingly, in the neurones in the cervical cord (Curry *et al.*, 1969). The microscopical examination of hair roots in cases of suspected poisoning by thallium is another very useful rapid diagnostic aid. Many workers refer to the root containing large deposits of melanin, but in my opinion this may not be melanin but in fact a microscopical artefact, the normal medulla being swollen in the root.

In the last few years there have been significant advances to help the pathologist investigate a suspicious death. These have occurred both in the organic and inorganic fields. The following sections will describe in some detail the basic methodologies, and what can, and what cannot, be expected from them. The evidence for the pathologist can only be gleaned, however, if correct and adequate samples are taken at autopsy. A vast amount of data is becoming available on the distribution of different poisons within the tissues and even sometimes of the biochemical lesions that are involved. It seems likely that the histochemical localization of many drugs and poisons within the tissues may not be too far away. The use of enzymes to detect the drugs has been referred to but it must not be forgotten that there is a great potential for the histochemical demonstration that normal enzyme activity has been lowered or destroyed within a vital cell. This has already been described in relation to cholinesterase and monoamine oxidase inhibitors and the way seems open to expand the diagnostic rôle of enzyme determination in clinical medicine to that of toxicology.

ANALYTICAL TECHNIQUES

Organic

The toxicologist is required to extract the poison from the tissue, to identify it and then quantitate it. These three basic steps require separate consideration.

Extraction

Organic molecules in general are extractable from the tissue with solvents such as ether or chloroform. Occasionally special techniques have to be employed—for example, in the case of the quaternary ammonium compounds—but even some of these can be extracted into organic solvents by the use of ion pairs. The extraction of tubocararine in fatal cases has recently been described using this technique (Stevens and Fox, 1971). It may be that the days of the separator containing blood and chloroform are nearly over in that the use of special resins which have the ability to extract such molecules from aqueous solution have recently been described. The favoured one at the moment is XAD-2 and it shows great promise. Its use has been mainly confined to urine and the procedure is simply that of pouring the fluid down a column containing the resin, washing it with an aqueous solution and then eluting the organic poisons with methanol. This has the advantage that large numbers of samples can be processed in parallel and the technique is obviously of great interest to those involved in screening samples for the presence of drugs of abuse. The use of ion exchange papers has also been extremely well described, although the latter do not seem to be as efficient. Both have been employed in situations where the initial extraction can be performed hundreds of miles away from the laboratory, and the mailing of the resin powder or the ion exchange paper avoids sending urine through the post. It is a feature of the extraction stage that there is no one single recommended method for all drugs. Techniques which will work well for barbiturates may fail completely for phenothiazines, and *vice versa*. This is why it is important for the investigating authority to continue to indicate to the toxicologist the precise examinations that are required. Specifically named drugs can receive attention by the best techniques, but if a request for a search for all poisons is required, then compromises have to be made because of the limited amount of material and time that is available. Hence somewhat inefficient methods may have to be used. The very high sensitivity of the gas chromatographic procedure has, however, enabled some techniques to be developed which avoid the extraction stage altogether. It is possible, for example, to inject very small samples of urine directly onto gas chromatographic columns and for the methods to be made sufficiently sensitive to detect all the barbiturates and several hypnotics provided they are present in sufficient concentrations.

The use of column chromatography for the separation of the small drug molecules has just begun to be applied by using Sephadex; in this procedure the large protein molecules are retained on the column while the small molecules pass through. The subsequent extraction of the drug by organic solvents then proceeds in the usual manner. This technique has been found to be of use in the examination of hypodermic syringes alleged to contain drugs but which are also contaminated with blood (Gomm, 1970).

At the same time as the extraction procedures are being done, there are a limited number of 'spot tests'—direct chemical reactions on body fluids—that will give a preliminary indication as to whether or not the drug is present. Some prefer to work up 100–200 g samples of tissue, such as liver, so that in the subsequent stages of purification relatively large quantities of drug are present. This is because it has been found that when sub-microgram quantities of drugs are being handled, great care has to be taken to avoid their absorption onto glass surfaces and the large-scale procedure avoids many of the problems associated with working with very small quantities of drugs. By working on larger quantities of tissues the necessity of performing a second extraction for identification purposes is avoided but, conversely, a greater period of time is required for the initial extraction. Fortunately, each toxicologist can use the procedure best suited to his needs and undoubtedly the very high sensitivity of the gas chromatograph has resulted in a considerable saving in time and solvents in many toxicological laboratories.

Identification

Every schoolboy will remember the chemical exercise of separating sand from salt; a similar situation occurs in toxicological analysis. A procedure can be designed provided one knows the properties of the material for which one is searching. However, in toxicological analysis the problems are infinitely more complex in that the physical properties of drugs vary by such a minute amount that highly specialized procedures have to be designed for each component. It is still common procedure for a classification to be made first according to the degree of acidity, neutrality or alkalinity of the drug in question. In this way, a high degree of purification can be achieved for particular classes in that the co-extracted unwanted material is spread amongst unwanted fractions. Nevertheless, the high concentrations of cholesterol found in tissues will not be separated from the neutral fraction and indeed the apparent drug purity is reduced in this fraction. A high proportion of purification procedures now make use of one or more forms of chromatography. Paper chromatography was introduced in the late 1940s and has been applied in all aspects of toxicological analysis. As was mentioned above it was relatively insensitive when compared with thin-layer chromatography, but nevertheless many laboratories still retain it for routine procedures. It has the advantage that co-extracted material is much more easily separated when present in large quantities from the wanted drug and interferes less in the running of the chromatogram. In thin-layer chromatography small amounts of fat can materially impede the running of a good chromatogram and can indeed lead to an apparent negative reaction when what is in fact happening is that the drug has been occluded by the natural unwanted material. A vast amount of data has been built up based on paper chromatographic systems and in particular for the alkaloid fraction. A tentative identification—based on the Rf value in the well known butanol –citric acid system on buffered citrated paper, coupled with inspection under 254 nm light and the use of a spray reagent such as iodoplatinate—can often be made. Data is available in many laboratories for many hundreds of alkaloids and much of this is directly transferable to a corresponding thin-layer system based on cellulose plates. The advantage of the thin-layer system is that it considerably reduces the time required for the chromatogram, although there is still a large body of workers who consider that even faster systems offer greater advantages. An inspection of the literature on the chromatography of alkaloids indicates that in many systems results are correlated and some workers are undertaking investigations which materially increase the time required for the analysis without a corresponding increase in specificity. This applies particularly to thin-layer chromatographic examinations for the analysis of LSD in tablets, and an investigation at the Home Office Central Research Establishment showed that the best criteria of identification were to be obtained using acetone as a solvent and plates of Kieselgel and alumina. Correlation in these systems for the ergoline alkaloids is minimal. Thin-layer chromatography is more sensitive than paper chromatography. This is mainly because the size of the small spots is considerably smaller and it is not unusual to be able to detect a few tens of nanograms of material on a thin-layer plate. Commercial devices are also available for scanning thin-layer plates, which enables a reasonable degree of quantitation to be achieved both by visible colorimetry and fluorescence procedures. A good degree of specificity can be obtained using non-correlated thin-layer chromatographic systems, but many workers prefer to elute the spot from the thin-layer plates and to investigate it by mass spectrometry or, if the amount allows, by infra-red spectroscopy. Some compounds are highly resistant to elution and a variety of devices aimed at achieving maximum extraction from the thin-layer plate absorbant have been devised. Great variations are obtained between the compounds and substrates and no firm rule can be laid down. Nevertheless, the attractiveness of combining chemical reactions with the speed of running a thin-layer plate has made the procedure a ubiquitous feature of most toxicological laboratories.

Descriptions of the use of gas chromatography first appeared in the forensic chemical literature in 1955 and it is fair to say that it has gone from strength to strength. The principle of the separation of compounds in the gas phase using either solid or liquid supports is too well known to be reiterated here; sufficient for it to be said that highly efficient separations can be made for compounds that differ by only minor features over a chemical structure. Unfortunately, the basic disadvantage of gas chromatography to the forensic toxicologist is that a considerable length of time may be required to separate all the materials that may be in his extract. In the case of amphetamines, for example, the total length of time the column has to run to clear such co-extracted materials as nicotine is usually in the region of half an hour; more complex separations for perhaps methaqualone, meprobamate, glutethimide, barbiturates or indeed morphine, can take upwards of an hour. This is a highly limiting, rate-determining step when the toxicologist needs to analyse many samples. Nevertheless, the high resolution afforded by gas chromatography in a wide variety of materials makes it also a *sine qua non* of every toxicological laboratory.

Many improvements in technique have taken place since the first discovery of the procedure. The use of capillary columns can make for very high resolutions and also reduce the running time. This has shown itself in many areas, particularly in the chemistry of cannabis. The other useful feature of gas chromatographic separations is that the effluent at the end of the chromatogram can be diverted so that the required material is either trapped in a form that makes it suitable for further investigation by infra-red spectroscopy, or it can be led directly into a mass spectrometer. The combination of gas chromatography with mass spectrometry is perhaps the most potent tool available to the analyst today. The availability of such devices is, however, highly limited and the alternative procedure of derivative gas chromatography is an attractive alternative. In this, use is made of fundamental chemical reactions which are made to occur before chromatography. In this way reactive sites on the molecule can be shown to exist and, whereas 20 years ago organic chemistry consisted of reacting amines to form crystalline acetyl derivatives whose melting point could be measured, nowadays the formation of the derivative is shown by the appearance of a characteristic retention time of a new compound. The extension of this type of reaction to all forms of derivative formation is widely practised in all forms of gas chromatographic analyses. It cannot be stressed strongly enough that, apart from very few exceptions, the identification of a compound by a single gas chromatographic parameter should not be relied upon. Confirmation by the formation of several derivatives must be effected unless the more highly specific tools of infra-red spectroscopy and mass spectrometry can be resorted to. The formation of derivatives in gas chromatography can be made to perform another useful function in that these derivatives can be of halogenated or other forms for which highly sensitive detectors are available, based on such procedures as electron capture. By increasing the number of halogen atoms in the derivative a further increase in sensitivity can be obtained, and Martin's development in the use of chemical multipliers for detectors leads to the promise of a sensitivity which may not be short of amazing.

It is impossible to give detailed instructions for the many hundreds of drugs that have been investigated by gas chromatography. The interested reader will find the information in the list of references (Clarke, 1969; Curry, 1969) given at the end of this chapter and at this stage it is not possible to do more than give a general outline of the methods used for separating drugs from co-extracted materials.

Once the suspected drug has been made as pure as possible by chromatographic techniques, infra-red spectroscopy is of great value to the smaller laboratory which does not have access to mass spectrometers. Techniques have been described which enable excellent curves to be obtained with compounds in as small a quantity as 1 microgram or even less. Computerized average transit can also be applied to give even higher sensitivities, because in this technique repeated runs are made so that the noise tends to cancel itself out, whereas the signal from the drug in question tends to intensify.

Problems do arise in trapping fractions off the gas chromatograph prior to infra-red spectroscopy because cooling of the effluent often results in the formation of fogs or aerosols which are blown out of the trapping area. A host of modifications have been proposed to overcome this and, in general, provided one knows the type of compound for which one is searching suitable arrangements can be made. The transfer of the trapped material to about 0·5 mg of potassium bromide can be made by means of a repeating Hamilton syringe set to dispense the solution of the trapped material on to the bromide held at the end of the tip of the needle (Curry *et al.*, 1968). Providing due regard is made for its purity and for the absence of contamination of all materials and surface areas, first class results can be obtained. There is a vast amount of commercially available literature covering infra-red spectroscopic curves that may be encountered, and once a complete matching of features has been made then the identification may be considered clinched. This is particularly valuable in cases which have to be fought in the courts. One of the problems with this type of investigation is that the procedure is not very sensitive when applied to volatile materials; indeed it is common for them to be lost completely. This is the reason why such procedures as peak shifting by derivative formation have to be applied to such compounds as the amphetamines. Nevertheless, for barbiturates and similar compounds the use of infra-red spectroscopy is particularly attractive.

Mass spectrometry is entering into the toxicological literature as a most useful technique at an exponential rate. Mass spectrometers are available which can be broadly divided into those of high resolution and low resolution. Both can be coupled to the gas chromatograph and a common problem of interfacing the gas chromatograph to the mass spectrometer exists with both. The transfer of a gas chromatographic effluent to the mass spectrometer presents a problem which has been tackled in many ways by the manufacturers. It is not possible to go into details of all the varieties of separators that are available, but all attempt to introduce the drug into the mass spectrometer and yet get rid of the large quantities of carrier gas with which it leaves the exit of the gas chromatograph. All that can be said is that the efficiency varies not only with the device but also with the type of compound with which one is dealing. Not only the plumbing of the equipment is important but also the chemical nature of the drug. The alternative method of introducing the extracted drug by means of a solid probe into the mass spectrometer can also be employed, but this suffers from the disadvantage that the purification stage of the gas chromatograph is not used. This is not often important in the case of high resolution mass spectrometers. Such spectrometers can measure accurate mass numbers of material in question to about 1 to 10 in 10^6 if conditions are right. Provided the molecule does not completely fragment under the conditions of the mass spectrometer, a highly accurate molecular weight can be obtained and this can lead directly to an unequivocal molecular formula for the material in question. An examination of the different fragments produced with various electron bombardment energies is another method of structure determination.

Resolutions of 1 in 1,000 are typical of low resolution mass spectrometers. However, this does mean that fragmentation patterns can be employed and, provided the material is pure enough, useful data can be obtained leading to absolute identification. In general, the quantities required exceed the nanogram scale and, if losses are high in the separator, considerably more than this will be required. Good results can be almost guaranteed for microgram quantities, although the caveat must be made that on occasions a complete loss of material will be effected by the separator. An additional method of providing an insight into the structure of the molecule has recently been revealed by Dutch workers in the study of cannabis products (Vree *et al.*, 1971). They have used mass fragmentography, which uses a controlled series of disintegrations of the molecule by applying a series of different electron energies and times to it. In this way the molecule can be made to disrupt in such a form as to provide an insight to the manner in which its substituent parts are joined together. Most useful information regarding structure of the molecule is therefore obtained by this technique of electron voltage mass fragment intensity graphs. The patterns to be obtained from the breakdown of the molecule when it is investigated by mass spectrometry can be extremely complex and it may not always be possible to get an accurate molecular weight, in that the molecule is so unstable that it breaks down too rapidly. Like infra-red spectroscopy it may be impossible to ascribe a structure to the material from its spectrographic pattern unless a control spectrum is already in the library. The use of computers to analyse and store the data from the mass spectrometer is now commonplace, but the capital costs for the installation of such machines are considerable. In addition, expert mass spectroscropists have to be employed, and clearly their use is limited to all but the largest laboratories. Notwithstanding this, it does appear that their usefulness is so great that, provided capital costs can be reduced, their use in all chemical laboratories will be ensured. Already papers have appeared, by De and Umberger (1970) in New York and by Bonnichsen *et al.* (1970) in Sweden on the use of mass spectrometry applied to practical problems; and at the Home Office Central Research Establishment several instances of its value in operational forensic science have been proved.

In the past year or two an increasing number of papers have been noticed in which use has been made of high pressure liquid chromatography. In this technique, instead of the separation taking place in the gas phase, long columns of liquid are forced through chromatographic material and exchange takes place so as to afford a separation of the compounds under investigation. Because of the length of column required, very high pressures have to be applied but the method shows promise of being useful for purifying small quantities of material. Such columns, as well as high resolution ion exchange columns, have been applied to the analysis of normal components of urine, and many hundreds of compounds can be separated and estimated. Both these techniques unfortunately require a disproportionate amount of time for them to be considered routine instruments in forensic analysis at this stage.

The techniques of ultra-violet spectrophotometry and spectrofluorimetry continue to be of great value to the toxicologist, with an increasing interest being shown in the latter technique. This follows from the availability of commercial instruments. There have been no major advances in ultra-violet spectrophotometric techniques except by the development of microcells, but its use for the identification and quantitation of a very large variety of drugs has been consolidated. Spectrofluorimetry, on the other hand, has shown itself to be capable of achieving very high degrees of sensitivities for certain classes of drugs and for LSD in particular. Unfortunately, like ultra-violet spectrophotometry, it suffers from the disadvantage of a lack of specificity but this is compensated in that it can usually assign a structure to narrow chemical classification. Its use in the analysis of morphine has been described above.

Several techniques have been developed which involve the use of radioactively labelled materials. Radio-immunoassay has been mentioned for the determination of insulin and digoxin (Phillips and Sambrook, 1971; Phillips, Webb and Curry, 1972). In these techniques an antibody protein is raised in animals by injecting into them a chemically bound drug–protein complex. The raised antibody can then be precipitated by a solution of the drug in question. The analysis is arranged so that a limited amount of antibody is used and then this is totally precipitated from solution when a radioactively labelled drug is added to it. If, in the next experiment, the radioactive drug is mixed with the extract under investigation and this extract contains unlabelled drug, the precipitated material will not contain as much radioactivity as before, having been diluted by the unlabelled drug. A measure of the quantity of the drug in the extract can then be made. Similar techniques have been reported as being used for the determination of morphine, and several laboratories are trying to develop similar methods for LSD, cannabinols, etc. Unfortunately, in the initial process of coupling on the drug to a protein a lack of specificity may be introduced and, indeed, with morphine the resultant antibody reacts more efficiently with codeine. A somewhat similar technique has been commercially described using a free radical assay technique (FRAT). In this method electron spin resonance techniques are used to pick up the complex rather than a radiochemical method. A novel reaction introducing a new principle has been described in the analysis of strychnine in which the strychnine is labelled with carbon-14 and thence reacted with a tritium-labelled methyl iodide (Wiley and Metzger, 1967). The resulting double-labelled strychnine methidide has to be purified chromatographically. If subsequently ^{14}C-labelled strychnine is mixed with unlabelled strychnine from the body extract, and this total is reacted with labelled methyl iodine, a lowering of the ratio of ^{14}C to tritium is found. Very sensitive methods of estimation can be achieved. This type of reaction has not been used by toxicologists to any extent up to now, but it gives yet another example of the use of radioactive tracers in toxicology and pinpoints another area where even greater sensitivities may be obtained.

One of the features of toxicology in the last few years has been the need to develop very rapid tests to exercise a statistical degree of control on the drug abuse programme. There are many laboratories that have need to analyse hundreds of samples of urine a day for the major drugs of abuse. This problem has been studied at the Home Office Central Research Establishment and automated machines have been developed which enable barbiturates, amphetamine and morphine to be analysed in small volumes of urine (4–8 ml) simultaneously at a rate of about 20 samples per hour. These devices are based on a continuous flow system in which the urine is segmented with organic solvent and mixed in small mixing coils; after highly efficient extraction, the phases are separated in the machine by a gravity feed principle and the relevant drug-containing extract is purified by pH solvent partitions. Measuring instruments have been attached to the relevant extracts, consisting of ultra-violet spectrophotometers for barbiturates and bases; visible spectrophotometers for colours produced after reaction of morphine with Folin Ciocalteau reagent or amphetamine with a benzene sulphonic acid; and spectrofluorimeters after conversion of morphine to pseudo-morphine with potassium ferricyanide. Very high sensitivities have been obtained which enable these drugs to be easily detected in the urine for many hours after the ingestion of therapeutic doses. The development of automated machines should not be considered solely in the context on the analysis of drugs of abuse. Now that the basic principles have been established involving the automated separation procedures and the development of measuring instruments, using visible ultra-violet and spectrofluorimetry as well as facilities for automated ultra-violet scanning between wide wavelengths, e.g. 220–320 nm, it can be seen that it is possible to automate manual methods for drugs using any of these basic measuring instruments. The calculations as to the sensitivity of the ultimate procedure can now be worked out and the ability to analyse very large numbers of urine samples for any particular drug will have great interest for metabolic studies and kinetic excretion studies. Automated devices have been developed by various manufacturers for the analysis of alcohol in blood using the headspace and internal standard gas chromatographic method and the alcohol dehydrogenase procedures.

Inorganic

It has been stressed above that the technique which has had the greatest impact as far as inorganic analyses for metals has been concerned in recent years has been atomic absorption spectroscopy. All pathologists will be aware of the flame emission techniques used in the measurement of electrolytes such as sodium, potassium and calcium, but atomic absorption works on a slightly different principle which, however, is of the greatest importance. In the use of flame emission a small proportion of atoms are raised by the flame to an excited state and when they decay they give off characteristic light which can be easily measured. The yellow light of sodium is a typical example. In atomic absorption analysis the atoms are aspirated into the flame and in their ground state absorb light of the wavelength of the metal under investigation. The method becomes more sensitive for the vast majority of metals because the problem of raising them to an excited state by heat does not have to be overcome and indeed all of the atoms are in the ground state and hence available for absorption. Because of this, very high sensitivities can be obtained, the only disadvantage being that the lamp has to be changed for each particular metal. In the technique of atomic fluorescence multi-element lamps have been arranged on a rotating device and this technique shows promise of even higher sensitivities with levels of 10^{-15} g already being quoted. Such latter machines are, however,

241

still in their infancy whereas atomic absorption spectrophotometers are now routine instruments in many laboratories. One of the disadvantages in early instruments was that the atoms were aspirated through the flame and hence stayed in the light path for a very short period of time; very high increases in sensitivity have recently been obtained by the design of electric furnaces into which the sample is put and carbonaceous material is burned, leaving the metallic atoms in the light beam for considerably longer periods than with flame aspiration, and consequently with dramatic increases in sensitivity. Already it is possible to measure the concentration of several metals in millimetre lengths of hair, and no doubt this technique will be increasingly employed to follow the growth patterns of metals along lengths of hair, such as has been done in the case of arsenic using conventional techniques and neutron activation analysis.

Neutron activation analysis is a technique in which the sample is put into an atomic reactor and bombarded with what are called thermal or slow neutrons. Certain elements capture the neutrons into their nucleus and become themselves radioactive. By analysing the intensity and energy of the subsequent radiation, as well as its decay time, a measurement of the quantity and identity of certain elements can be established. In biological materials the contribution of sodium is extremely high and consequently it is usual for purification procedures to be applied after the irradiation so that the element in question can be separated and counted separately. This is the technique used in the analyses for such metals as arsenic where, after irradiation, the conventional Gutzeit procedure is followed leading to the liberation of pure arsine which can be trapped, counted and measured. Considerable attention has been paid in recent years to the differentiation of acute and chronic poisoning by the use of hair analyses for arsenic, and some striking correlations with clinical conditions and concentration at different periods of time have been shown by Barrowcliffe (1971).

Fluorine is another element that has received attention following the use of activation techniques suitable for its determination in such samples as bone, and by the development of a fluoride electrode which enables previously highly difficult analyses to be much more easily carried out. Even gas chromatography has been used for the determination of fluoride in urine, serum, saliva and bone in a technique which converts the fluoride to fluorotrimethylsilane which is volatile and hence suitable for gas chromatographic analysis (Fresen, Cox and Witter, 1968). Techniques for the analysis of metals by forming volatile organic complexes is another area which is receiving great analytical attention. Such techniques are extremely attractive in that they avoid the necessity for access to high-cost nuclear reactors.

The availability of inorganic poisons never ceases to amaze me. Artists' materials, for example, can contain iron, cobalt, chromium, barium, cadmium, copper, zinc, mercury, antimony, arsenic and lead compounds—surely as dramatic a toxicological list as one could get. It has also been noted that even the accidental inhalation of talcum powder may have grave consequences (Leading Article, 1969b). Young children playing with a container may spill a fairly large quantity on their face and, if inhaled, signs of respiratory distress, choking, tachycardia, cyanosis, intracostal retraction and signs of bronchitis develop within the hour. Another unusual metal is selenium, and methods for its determination have included neutron activation analysis, fluorimetry and colorimetry. Acute selenium poisoning by selenious oxide has been reported in which death occurred 45 minutes after admission to hospital (Carter, 1966), and miscarriage in laboratory workers handling selenite is not unknown. A very useful methodological technique has been introduced for mercury by the development of a mercury meter. This involves the higher absorption of vaporized metallic mercury atoms at 253·7 nm and carries the name cold vapour atomic absorption analysis. Another general technique for the determination of metals is inorganic mass spectrometry and very high degrees of precision at levels of well below 10^{-9} g can be achieved for virtually any mass number. Its use in the analysis of thallium has already been described but clearly its potential is very great indeed. As with the case of organic mass spectrometry, considerable capital expenditure and a high degree of operator expertise is required.

The histochemical localization of poisons has been referred to both in relation to organic compounds and such inorganic metals as thallium. Another recently developed instrument enables a sliced tissue section to be aligned accurately under the crosswires of a microscope and the chosen area to be vaporized by a laser. The products of this burning rise between the electrodes of an arc emission spectrograph and analysis of the characteristic spectrographic lines enables the presence of many metals to be determined. This technique of laser–arc emission enables areas as low as 20 μ cross-section to be investigated and clearly is going to be of interest in the localization of metallic toxins in cells.

CONCLUSION

Towards the end of an investigation into the suspected case of poisonings all the facts have to be marshalled and the interpretation of the analytical results assume some importance. Unfortunately, it is still a fact that in the majority of cases the biochemical cause–effect relationship between the presence of the poison and the fact of death cannot be established. Recourse has to be made to a statistical evaluation of the clinical effects and the corresponding blood, tissue or urine levels in a large number of people. The degree to which people can become habituated or addicted must also be taken into account. Efforts have been made to determine the possible degree of habituation from differential tissue analyses and by the determination of metabolite to drug ratios. It is impossible in a chapter of this size to deal with virtually the thousands of poisons which may come the way of the toxicologist. Fortunately, several books have been published in the last few years which have attempted to draw together this type of information (Clarke, 1969; Curry, 1969; Sunshine, 1969).

As was intimated at the beginning of this chapter the problems have become more complex because of the very large number of new drugs on the market. The previously unknown hazards, such as those associated with pollution, and with the increasing biological activity of molecules being introduced into clinical medicine and into abuse are increasingly recognized. The analyst now has at his command a vast array of highly sophisticated instruments with which to tackle the problems. These can often only be sited in major centres and, as has been emphasized, they require considerable expenditure on machine and manpower. The hospital toxicologist is still very much in the situation he was five years ago, in that there has been no real development in 'spot-tests'. Gas chromatography must increase in availability and scope and, in the meantime, thin-layer chromatography will no doubt continue to be of the most valuable methods of analysis. Nevertheless, the two problems remaining for the toxicologist both concern the interpretation of results. For the forensic toxicologist the biochemical lesions in poisoning must be established, and for the hospital toxicologist the determination of blood levels must be made to be of assistance to the clinician. Apart from aspirin poisoning, there seems little at the present time that an analytical result will do for the patient, except perhaps to save him from iatrogenic hazards.

REFERENCES

Barrowcliffe, D. (1971). *Med. leg. J.*, **39**, 79.
Bartone, N. F., Grieco, V. and Herr, B. S. (1968). *J. Am. med. Ass.*, **203**, 104.

Beckett, A. H., Taylor, J. F. and Kourounakis, P. (1970). *J. Pharm. Pharmac.*, **22**, 123.

Blackmore, D. J., Curry, A. S., Rutter, E. R. and Hayes, T. S. (1971). *Clin. Chem.*, **17**, 896.

Bonnichsen, R., Maehly, A. C., Marde, Y., Ryhage, R. and Schubert, B. (1970). *J. leg. Med.*, **67**, 19.

Bricknell, P. P., Middleton, H. G., Hollingsworth, A. and Evans, E. M. L. (1967). *Br. med. J.*, **4**, 400.

Briggs, J. H., McKerron, C. G., Souhami, R. L., Taylor, D. J. E. and Andrews, H. (1967). *Lancet*, **2**, 1227.

British Medical Journal (1967), **2**, 331.

— (1970), **2**, 314.

Burston, G. R. (1967). *Practitioner*, **199**, 340.

Butz, B. (1969). *J. forens. Sci.*, **14**, 317.

Campbell, A. M. G., Evans, M., Thomson, J. L. G. and Williams, M. J. (1971). *Lancet*, **2**, 1215.

Cant, J. S. and Lewis, D. R. H. (1968). *Br. med. J.*, **3**, 59.

Carroll, K. G. and Tullis, J. L. (1968). *Nature, Lond.*, **217**, 1172.

Carter, R. F. (1966). *Med. J. Aust.*, **1**, 525.

Chao, T. C. and Yap, C. Y. (1967). *J. forens. Sci.*, **12**, 68.

Citron, B. (1970). *New Engl. J. Med.*, **283**, 1003.

Clarke, E. C. G. (1969). *Isolation and Identification of Drugs.* London; The Pharmaceutical Press.

Columbini, G. and Masarone, M. (1966). *Aggiornaments Pediat.*, **17**, 437. [*Chem. Abstr.* (1967), **67**, 31084.]

Curry, A. S. (1966). A.C.P. Broadsheet, No. 52.

— Read, J. F., Brown, C. and Jenkins, R. (1968). *J. Chromatogr.*, **38**, 200.

— Grech, J. L., Spiteri, L. and Vassallo, L. (1969). *J. Europ. Toxicol.*, **2**, 260.

— (1969). *Poison Detection in Human Organs*, 2nd Ed. Springfield, Ill.; Thomas.

— and Mercier, M. (1970). *Nature, Lond.*, **228**, 281.

Cuthbert, M. F., Greenberg, M. P. and Morley, S. W. (1969). *Br. med. J.*, **1**, 404.

David, A. and Mikětuková, V. (1967). *Arch. Toxikol*, **23**, 66.

De, P. K. and Umberger, C. J. (1970). *Developments in Applied Spectroscopy*, p. 267, Ed. by E. L. Grove and A. J. Perkins. New York; Plenum Press.

Fresen, J. A., Cox, F. H. and Witter, M. J. (1968). *Pharm. Weekbl. Ned.*, **103**, 909.

Gault, M. H., Rudwal, T. C., Engles, W. D. and Dossetor, J. B. (1968). *Ann. intern. Med.*, **68**, 906.

Ginsberg, M. D., Herzman, M. and Schmidt-Nowara, W. W. (1970). *Ann. intern. Med.*, **73**, 81.

Gomm, P. J. (1970). *J. forens. Sci. Soc.*, **10**, 7.

Greaves, M. and Boyde, T. R. C. (1967). *Lancet*, **2**, 1019.

Grove, J. and Toseland, P. A. (1971). *Ann. clin. Biochem.*, **8**, 109.

Halstead, J. A., Hackley, B. M. and Smith, J. C. (1968). *Lancet*, **2,** 278.

Harries, J. T. and Rossiter, M. (1969). *Lancet*, **1,** 150.

Hauck, G. and Henn, R. (1969). *Arch. Toxikol.*, **25,** 83.

Heinonen, J., Heikkila, J., Mattila, M. J. and Takki, S. (1968). *Arch. Toxikol.*, **23,** 264.

Henderson, A. H., Pugsley, D. J., Robinson, A. E., Page, M. R. and Camps, F. E. (1968). *Br. med. J.*, **3,** 229.

Herxheimer, A. (1969). *Prescribers J.*, **9,** 62.

Hill, D. M. (1967). *Br. med. J.*, **1,** 342.

Jelliffe, R. W., Hill, D., Tatter, D. and Lewis, E. (1967). *J. Am. med. Ass.*, **201,** 895.

Johnson, H. R. M. and Koumides, O. (1967). *Br. med. J.*, **1,** 340.

Johnston, E. H., Goldbaum, L. R. and Whelton, R. L. (1969). *Med. Annls.*, *D.C.*, **38,** 375.

Kennedy, S. C. and Bavaki, A. E. (1967). *Br. med. J.*, **4,** 93.

King, A. B. and Cowen, D. I. (1969). *J. Am. med. Ass.*, **210,** 724.

Kirsch, N. (1969). *Archs. Derm.*, **99,** 596.

Knight, R. K., Trounce, J. R. and Cameron, J. S. (1967). *Br. med. J.*, **3,** 601.

Kok, J. C. F., Fromberg, E., Geerlings, P. J., Van der Helm, H. J., Kamp, P. E., Van der Slooten, E. P. J. and Williams, M. A. M. (1971). *Lancet*, **1,** 1065.

Kramer, J. C., Fischman, V. S. and Littlefield, D. C. (1967). *J. Am. med. Ass.*, **201,** 89.

Kratte, E. C., Brooks, A. L. and Rhamy, R. K. (1969). *Radiology*, **92,** 700.

Kristus, L. G. and Belons, D. G. (1967). *Vrach. Delo*, **3,** 154. [Chem. Abstr. (1967), **67,** 9867.]

Leading Article (1968). *Nutrit. Rev.*, **26,** 173.

— (1969a). *Br. med. J.*, **4,** 5.

— (1969b). *Br. med. J.*, **2,** 775.

Levi, R. M. (1971). *Lancet*, **1,** 1297.

Litt, I. F., Colli, A. S. and Cohen, M. I. (1971). *J. Pediat.*, **78,** 692.

McIver, A. K. (1967). *Pharmac. J.*, **199,** 205.

Maclean, D., Peters, T. J., Brown, R. A. G., McCathie, M., Baines, G. F. and Robertson, P. G. C. (1968). *Lancet*, **2,** 849.

Mandy, S. and Ackerman, A. B. (1970). *J. Am. med. Ass.*, **213,** 253.

Maron, B. J., Krupp, J. R. and Tune, B. (1971). *J. Pediat.*, **78,** 697.

Matell, G. and Thorstrand, C. (1967). *Acta. med. scand.*, **181,** 79.

Matthew, H., Proudfoot, A. T., Brown, S. S. and Smith, A. C. A. (1968). *Br. med. J.*, **2,** 101.

Medhurst, M. R. (1967). *Br. med. J.*, **3,** 438.

Minkin, W. and Cohen, H. J. (1967). *New Engl. J. Med.*, **277,** 403.

Nicholas, P. O. (1968). *Lancet*, **2,** 40.

Nigro, S. A. (1968). *J. Am. med. Ass.*, **203,** 301.

Noble, J. and Matthew, H. (1969). *Clin. Toxicol.*, **2,** 403.

Ogen, S., Rosenbluth, S. and Eisenberg, A. (1967). *Israeli J. Med. Sci.*, **3,** 565.

REFERENCES

O'Donoghue, S. E. F. (1971). *Nature, Lond.*, **229**, 124.

Papadopoulos, S. and Harden, R. M. (1966). *Br. med. J.*, **2**, 1502.

Phillips, A. P. and Sambrook, C. A. (1971). Society for Analytical Chemistry Symposium on Liquid Scintillation Counting, Brighton, September 1971.

— Webb, B. and Curry, A. S. (1972). *J. forens. Sci.*, **17**, 460.

Pleuckhahn, V. D. and Ballard, B. (1968). *Med. J. Aust.*, 939.

Prescott, L. F., Wright, N., Roscoe, P. and Brown, S. S. (1971). *Lancet*, **1**, 519.

Robinson, A. E. and Williams, F. M. (1971). *J. Pharm. Pharmac.*, **23**, 347.

Samman, P. D. and Johnston, E. N. M. (1969). *Br. med. J.*, **1**, 818.

Savage, D. C. L. (1967). *Br. med. J.*, **2**, 840.

Simpson, J. R. (1966). *Br. med. J.*, **2**, 1434.

Solursh, L. P. and Clement, W. R. (1968). *J. Am. med. Ass.*, **205**, 644.

Steel, C. M., O'Duffy, J. and Brown, S. S. (1967). *Br. med. J.*, **3**, 663.

Stern, W. Z., Spear, P. W. and Jacobson, H. G. (1968). *Am. J. Roentgenol.* **103**, 522.

Stevens, H. M. and Fox, R. H. (1971). *J. forens. Sci. Soc.*, **11**, 177.

Stoddart, J. C., Parkin, J. M. and Wynne, N. A. (1968). *Br. J. Anaesth.*, **40**, 789.

Sunshine, I. (1969). *Handbook of Analytical Toxicology.* Cleveland; Chemical Rubber Publishing Company.

Tompsett, S. (1970). *Acta. pharmac. toxicol.*, **28**, 346.

Vree, T. B., Breimer, D. D., Van Ginneken, C. A. M. and Van Rossum, J. (1971). *Acta. pharmac. succica.*, **8**, 683.

Wiley, R. A. and Metzger, J. L. (1967). *J. pharmac. Sci.*, **56**, 144.

J

11 Recommended Changes in Death Certification, Cremation Regulations, and Coroners' Procedure

AND SOME OF THEIR IMPLICATIONS

DAVID M. PAUL

INTRODUCTION

This chapter is designed to review the recommended changes in the field of death certification, cremation regulations and coroners' procedure as proposed by the Home Office report of the Committee on Death Certification and Coroners 1971. On 17th March 1965 the then Home Secretary issued a warrant of appointment of a committee to review, first, law and practice relating to the issue of medical certificates of the cause of death and for the disposal of dead bodies and, secondly, the law and practice relating to coroners and Coroners' Courts, the reporting of death to the coroner, and related matters. On 22nd September 1971 the report was completed and submitted to the Home Secretary for his approval, and on 10th November 1971 it was finally submitted to Parliament.

The document contained 114 recommendations relating to various aspects within the terms of reference of the Committee. A bald re-statement of these recommendations would serve no useful purpose in this chapter, and the intention, therefore, is to look at each part of the report, define the present situation relating to that section, précis the recommended changes, and then discuss their implications. A list of the recommendations, under the same headings as the text, is included at the end of the chapter.

MEDICAL CERTIFICATION OF THE CAUSE OF DEATH

The first statute requiring registration of death was the Births and Deaths Registration Act 1836, which came into force on 1st July

1837. This Act provided for the registration of every death which occurred in England and Wales and it was primarily designed to facilitate legal proof of death and to provide accurate mortality statistics. Although the prescribed form included a space for the cause of death, the Act did not require that this information be provided by a medical practitioner.

The Births and Deaths Registration Act of 1874, as well as introducing penalties for the failure to register a death, placed a duty on any registered medical practitioner in attendance during a patient's last illness to deliver to the registrar a written statement setting out the cause of death to the best of his knowledge, unless he knew that an inquest was to be held. The 1874 Act also made it an offence to bury the body of any child without either a medical practitioner's certificate of cause of death or a certificate of stillbirth.

Unfortunately, neither the 1836 nor the 1874 Act required registration of death to precede disposal of the body and, despite the recommendations of the Parliamentary Select Committee in 1893 and other recommendations in 1903 and 1904, no statute corrected this grave omission until the Births and Deaths Registration Act of 1926.

The 1926 Act made it unlawful to dispose of the body before either a registrar's certificate or a coroner's certificate had been issued. The 1926 Act also required registration of stillbirths and it imposed restrictions on the disposal of bodies of stillborn children. This same Act imposed certain controls on the movement of bodies into and out of England and Wales.

The provisions of the 1926 Births and Deaths Registration Act, running in harness with the provisions of the Coroners (Amendment) Act of the same year, were aimed at ensuring that the medical cause of death was registered in every death in England and Wales. The two Acts together ensured that no body would be disposed of without the authority of the registrar or a coroner, and that such authority would be granted only when the medical cause of death was certified by a registered medical practitioner. The intention of these two Acts was that the medical cause of death be firmly established in every case.

In practice the above intentions were not fulfilled for a variety of reasons. The statutes did not require the certifying registered medical practitioner to see the body before issuing a certificate; neither did the Act specify the type or extent of any external examination after death and prior to the signing of the certificate. As a result of these two omissions, it was possible for a certificate to be issued in the name of a person still alive, and it was even more possible for signs of injury or poisoning to escape notice.

The Acts did require the certifying doctor to be in attendance during the last illness and within 14 days of death, but they failed to define the word 'attendance'. The combination of these factors resulted in the faint possibility of a living person being named on a death certificate; the real possibility that many unnatural deaths due to trauma or overdose could escape notice of the attending physician; and the certainty that the diagnosis of the cause of death would be inaccurate in many cases. The risk of undetected homicide, though ever-present, was probably not the most important result of the lax regulations regarding certification of death.

Recommendations

First, to ensure that only the more experienced medical practitioners should be allowed to certify the cause of death in hospital patients, the Brodrick Committee recommend that only fully registered medical practitioners should be qualified to issue such a certificate.

Secondly, they recommend that no doctor should be qualified to sign a certificate unless he has attended the deceased person at least once during the seven days preceding death. This 'seven day rule' is suggested in preference to any definition as to the meaning of 'attendance' but it is implied that the attendance was for the condition which resulted in the subsequent death.

Thirdly, they suggest that the certifying doctor should inspect the body of the deceased person prior to issuing any certificate.

Once a registered medical practitioner has inspected the body after death and has fulfilled the 'seven day rule', the Committee recommends that he shall issue a certificate of the fact and cause of death only if:

(1) He is confident on reasonable grounds that he can certify the medical cause of death with accuracy and precision.

(2) There are no grounds for supposing that the death was due to or contributed to by any employment followed at any time by the deceased, any drug, medicine or poison, or any violent or any unnatural cause.

(3) He has no reason to believe that the death occurred during an operation or under or prior to complete recovery from an anaesthetic or arising out of any incident during an anaesthetic.

(4) The cause or circumstances do not make the death one which the law requires should be reported to the coroner.

(5) He knows of no reason why in the public interest any further enquiry should be made into the death.

If he is not satisfied on these five points, the doctor must report the death to the coroner as soon as possible, and such a report shall be in the first instance an oral one, followed as soon as possible by a written report on a new form of certificate, and shall include such matters as: (*a*) the National Health Service number of the deceased; (*b*) other major morbid conditions present which have not caused or contributed to death; (*c*) information about surgical operations performed within three months of death, and information of serious accidents occurring within twelve months of the death.

Discussion

There can be no doubt that these recommendations would produce some improvement in the statutes regarding certification.

The 'seven day rule' would certainly be helpful in increasing the accuracy of diagnosis of the mortal condition, and the speedy and compulsory notification to the coroner would precipitate prompt investigation of those cases where the physician is not qualified to issue a full certificate.

The use of the word 'inspection' after death, rather than the word 'examination' is quite deliberate. The Committee did not consider that an external examination should be carried out, and this inspection may still allow such things as bruises, ligature marks, capsular and tablet debris in the mouth, and other signs of injury to escape notice. Without an examination it would appear impossible for any physician to be satisfied under paragraph 2 above that 'there are no grounds for supposing that the death was due to, or contributed to by, any employment followed at any time by the deceased, any *drug*, *medicine* or *poison* or any *violent* or *unnatural cause*'. It would appear that the entire value of this condition of certification would be minimized.

There is not a coroner, pathologist or medical practitioner who at some time in his career has not had a case where a patient suffering from a known mortal condition has hastened the end by overdose or some other means. A routine external examination of the body would undoubtedly help in the early detection of such an occurrence, and would lead to increased accuracy in the cause of death statistics. The value of such an examination is obvious in the field of infant and child death in relation to the abused child syndrome, and would reduce still further the risk of the undetected homicide.

The external examination is even more important when the method of disposal of the body is to be cremation, and this facet will be referred to later, when the cremation regulations are discussed.

The report refers to the difficulties of conducting adequate external examination of the body in the deceased's own home with bereaved

251

relatives nearby, and possibly poor lighting conditions. It would seem that these difficulties are rather exaggerated, for just such an examination is an integral part of the cremation regulations in force at the present time, and as this method of disposal was the method of choice in 56 per cent of all deaths in 1970, it follows that a routine external examination should have been carried out in all these cases.

The requirement of full registration as a qualification for the certifying physician is an attempt to ensure that only the more experienced hospital doctors would be charged with the responsibility of certification of death. This is undoubtedly an ideal recommendation, but it must be obvious that such a regulation in many National Health hospitals would result in a delay in the issuing of a certificate of the fact and cause of death. In many hospitals under the National Health Service, the house physician and the house surgeon are pre-registration practitioners, and they are often the only medical staff present when patients die. If no certificate can be issued until a doctor or senior house officer of registrar grade is in attendance delays are bound to occur. In very many cases it is the pre-registration physicians who have had the intimate contact with the patient during the previous seven day period, and by virtue of this fact it would seem that they are the only medical practitioners who are qualified to sign the death certificate under the 'seven day rule'.

CERTIFICATION OF PERINATAL DEATHS

The term perinatal death was recommended by the World Health Organisation some ten years ago, and the Committee recommend that this term shall be used for all stillbirths and deaths in early infancy.

At the present time the law governing certification of death of the human foetus depends on the duration of the pregnancy, and whether the foetus has ever breathed and had a separate existence. A foetus can be (a) a miscarriage if the pregnancy is less than 28 weeks, and in which case no registration of death is required; (b) a stillbirth if the pregnancy has lasted 28 weeks or over, and if the foetus has then never breathed or had a separate existence; (c) a live birth which does not depend on the duration of the pregnancy but only on whether the child has been completely expelled from the mother's body and has breathed and had a separate existence.

As has been stated there are no statutory requirements for the registration of a miscarriage with the Registrar of Births and Deaths. Under the Births and Deaths Registration Act of 1926 a stillbirth must be registered and a certificate, issued by either a physician or a state certified midwife who has either attended at the birth or has examined the body after the birth, must be presented to the Registrar within 42 days of the birth. If no qualified person is present then the informant is required to make a declaration to that effect. In point of fact a stillbirth is regarded more as a birth than as a death.

A live birth which dies in the immediate post-delivery period is considered as an ordinary death, and must be registered with the normal certificate of cause of death signed by a medical practitioner.

Recommendations

The Committee recommend no change in the 28-week gestation period which separates the miscarriage from the stillbirth.

The main recommendation is the use of a single form of certificate to cover both stillbirths and deaths in the immediate delivery period up to seven days from delivery. The theory underlying this recommendation is that frequently the same pathology is responsible for the death in late pregnancy as for death in early infancy.

The time interval of up to 42 days allowed for the registration of a stillbirth under the 1926 Act would obviously be too long in cases where the certificate covers both stillbirths and deaths in the first seven days. The Committee recommend that the interval of 42 days be abolished and that perinatal deaths should be considered in the same way as ordinary adult deaths and must be registered within five days.

The Committee also recommend that the qualifications of the doctor who may issue the perinatal death certificate must be the same as the doctor who may issue an ordinary certificate of cause and fact of death, i.e. the physician must be a fully registered practitioner who has been in attendance during the previous seven days before death.

In the case of a stillbirth the Committee still recommends that a midwife is qualified to give a certificate of perinatal death, but it recommends that such a certificate should be given by a midwife or a doctor only if:

(1) The certifier is confident on reasonable grounds that he or she can certify the fact and the medical cause of stillbirth with accuracy and precision.

(2) There are no grounds for supposing that the stillbirth was due to, or contributed to by, any employment followed at any time by the mother, any drug, medicine or poison, surgical operation, any administration of an anaesthetic, or any other violent or unnatural cause.

(3) The certifier knows of no reason why, in the public interest, any further enquiry should be made into the stillbirth.

In any case where neither a doctor nor a midwife is present at the birth, an alleged stillbirth should be reported to the coroner.

The Committee further recommend that the Registrar of Births and Deaths should be under an obligation to report a stillbirth, or an alleged stillbirth, to the coroner in the three sets of circumstances:

(1) When he is unable to obtain a certificate from a doctor or midwife in respect of a stillbirth which has been reported to him by another informant.

(2) When he has reason to believe that the stillbirth should have been reported to the coroner by the certifying doctor or midwife.

(3) When it is suggested to him by any person that a product of conception certified as stillbirth may have been born alive.

Discussion

The main effect of these recommendations would be to create better correlation for research into the causes of stillbirth and deaths in early infancy. Indeed, there is a suggestion that autopsies on stillbirths and deaths in early infancy should be performed in hospital mortuaries where a pathologist specially qualified in paediatric pathology is available, and that the post-mortem examination should be designed to go much further than merely establishing cause of death.

There can be no doubt that this is an admirable concept, as is the recommendation to reduce the time for notification of stillbirths from 42 to 5 days. Both these recommendations would further the research in the important field of perinatal mortality, as well as expediting the coroner's investigation of any deaths in this category which cannot be properly certified by the attending physician or midwife.

DISPOSAL BY CREMATION

Disposal of a dead body by cremation has only been legal in England and Wales since 1884, following the direction of the Judge in the case of R. v Price, although the Cremation Society, founded in 1876, had petitioned to have cremation made legal for some years prior to that date.

It was the Cremation Society's own restrictions and regulations which form the basis of the cremation regulations that are in force today. The Cremation Act of 1902 authorized the Home Secretary to make regulations governing the practice of cremation and provided penalties for the non-compliance of these regulations. Regulations were issued in 1903 and these closely followed the restrictions imposed by the Cremation Society. They were designed to reduce to a minimum the risk of cremating a body and destroying evidence of murder by violence or by poison.

In its early days, cremation was considered a bizarre method of disposal of the dead and in 1885, the year after R. v Price, only 3 cremations were carried out. Sixteen years later in 1901 some 427 cremations were carried out, and over the following years this figure increased enormously. In 1930 4,281 cremations were carried out or 0·9 per cent of all registered deaths. In 1950 the figure had reached 81,576 and represented 16·3 per cent of all registered deaths. In 1970 some 325,552 cremations, representing 56·7 per cent of all registered deaths, were performed. From these figures it is obvious that cremation can no longer be considered an unusual form of disposal, and if this trend continues earth burial will soon be the unusual method of disposal of the dead body.

The regulations governing cremation at the present time are the Cremation Regulations of 1930 (as amended by the regulations of 1952 and 1965). Included in these regulations is the procedure which has to be followed in every case for cremation. This consists of a certificate known as Form A, which is an application for cremation. In all cases where death has not been reported to the coroner, Form A must be supported by two medical certificates on the prescribed forms, one of these—known as Form B—to be completed by the ordinary medical attendant and the other—known as Form C—by a doctor quite unconnected with the physician signing Form B. Forms A, B and C are then sent to the medical referee of the crematorium who, if he is satisfied with the details given on these three certificates, will issue a Form F, which he will send to the superintendent of the crematorium authorizing the cremation to take place. After cremation the superintendent of the crematorium completes a Form G which is the register of cremations.

Cases which have been referred to the coroner are dealt with by the issue of a Form E, issued by that officer, which takes the place of the medical certificates B and C in other cases, and which will be accepted by the medical referee. Once Form E has been received the medical referee will again issue his Form F and the cremation will take place. After cremation Form G will again be completed in the normal way.

In some cases the medical referee will accept a Form D. This is a certificate after autopsy by either the medical referee or by a pathologist appointed by the crematorium. As in the other cases Form D will allow cremation to take place and after cremation Form G will be completed.

The physicians signing Forms B and C are supposed to satisfy themselves by questioning persons present at the death, and by conducting an external examination of the body, that the death is not due to violence, poisoning, privation, or any other suspicious circumstances. The medical referee must satisfy himself that the regulations of the Cremation Act and Regulations have been complied with, and the cause of death has been definitely ascertained. He must also be quite satisfied that there is no apparent reason for further examination of the body or investigation into the circumstances of the death.

Recommendations

The Committee recommends the abolition of all the Forms other than Form G (the Register of Cremations). The argument to support this recommendation is that by improving the standard of certification of the fact and cause of death the need for Forms B and C will be abolished. The perusal of the documentary evidence by the referee will be replaced by the perusal of the new certificate of the cause of death by the registrar. Form F, the authority to cremate issued at the moment by the medical referee, will be replaced by the authority to dispose of the body issued by the registrar.

The Committee believe that the safeguards in the new certificate of fact and cause of death, such as the 'seven day rule', the inspection of the body after death, and the mandatory reporting to the coroner of all cases where the precise medical cause of death is not known, are such as to make the multiplicity of certificates and forms under the present cremation regulations quite unnecessary.

Discussion

It is undoubtedly true that to look upon cremation as an unusual and bizarre method of disposal of the dead now has no basis, but it is equally true that cremation could destroy all evidence of homicide, poisoning or trauma.

If the recommendations of the Committee in regard to certification of the fact and cause of death included a defined external examination of the body, rather than a mere 'view' to establish identity and fact of death, it could be held that there were added safeguards against traumatic deaths, and if this examination were combined with the documentary investigations by some form of referee, be he crematorium medical referee or coroner, the risk of cremating bodies which had died as a result of trauma would indeed be reduced.

The referral of all cases of cremation to the coroner is not a new concept, and is already in use in certain medical examiner systems in the United States of America, and in certain coroner's jurisdictions in Canada, although it is true that in these countries the percentage of cremations is very much lower than it is in England and Wales.

Cremation is certainly a more permanent method of disposal than earth burial. This being the case, it would be prudent to maintain some additional safeguards in relation to this method. The minimum safeguard required would seem to be a careful external examination of the body by the doctor issuing the certificate of the fact and cause of death and a review of the documentary evidence in that certificate by some independent referee.

THE CORONER

Today the appointment, duties, procedure and power of the coroner is controlled by a number of statutes and rules which have gradually evolved over the 800-year history of the office.

Generally speaking the coroner is most affected by the Coroners Act of 1887 which consolidated in statute form all previous acts, and the Coroners (Amendment) Act of 1926. These two Acts form the basis of coroners' practice, and are modified by the Coroners Rules of 1953, the Coroner (Fees and Allowances) Rules of 1955, and the Coroners (Indictable offences) Rules of 1956, which incorporate some of the recommendations of the 1936 report of the Department Committee under the Chairmanship of Lord Wright.

Under existing statutes it is the responsibility of the local authority to advertise, short-list, interview and appoint a coroner, should a vacancy arise. The local authority also have the duty of providing court and mortuary accommodation, and paying the coroner's salary and expenses. Applicants must be qualified either in medicine or law, and must have at least five years' seniority in their profession. The office is either whole-time or part-time, and one of the recommendations of the 1936 Departmental Committee Report was to increase the size of the coroners' jurisdictions by the amalgamation of small jurisdictions as they became vacant.

In England and Wales today there are 271 coroners' jurisdictions, of which only 16 are full-time. To illustrate the work-load, in 1969 131,639 deaths were reported to coroners in England and Wales. Of this number 116,104 autopsies were performed, and 25,130 deaths were investigated at inquest. It is of note that out of this total some 30 per cent were investigated by the 16 full-time coroners.

The coroner is bound by law to enquire into:

(1) All deaths where the attending physician is unable to issue a certificate of the medical cause of death.

(2) All deaths due to trauma, poison or privation, even when the clinical cause of death is known.

(3) The death of any person in prison after sentence or on remand.

(4) All deaths due to industrial disease.

In all cases where the cause of death is not natural disease the coroner has to hold an inquest. This is a hearing in open court, where all evidence is taken on oath or on affirmation, and where interested parties may be represented at the coroner's discretion. The coroner has by law to sit with the jury when he is investigating death that has resulted from vehicular incidents, industrial incidents, industrial disease, the deaths of persons in prison from any cause, and deaths that may involve homicide. The coroner may choose to sit with the jury in any other case when he considers that this is in the public interest. It is no part of the coroner's duty to ensure that witnesses whose conduct may be in question at the inquest are legally represented.

The Coroner's Court at an inquest acts as a court of record, and by statute has to record the four facts involving a death. It must record the identity of the deceased, the date and place where death was certified, the medical condition which caused the death, and the circumstance in which the fatal condition was acquired. This last point is known as the verdict.

The verdict must not record any opinion regarding liability, but if the evidence presented at the inquest reveals a dangerous situation likely to cause similar fatalities, the coroner, or coroner's jury, is allowed to add as a rider to the verdict any suggestion designed to prevent a similar incident from occurring.

The coroner is an independent judicial officer, solely responsible, but subject to the requirements of the law. He is completely independent of the local and central Government, and cannot be directed, called to account, or instructed to review his decisions, by any minister.

It would not be correct to state that there is no appellate procedure against a coroner's verdict, but the present procedure is extremely complicated and includes an application to the High Court to have the inquisition quashed and a new inquest ordered, on the grounds of: (a) absence of view by the coroner; (b) irregularity in the proceedings at inquest; or (c) insufficient enquiry leading to a wrong verdict.

It does not necessarily follow that a different verdict would be returned at the second inquest.

Recommendations

The Committee heard evidence from a large number of organizations and individuals concerned with coroners' investigations, including members of the general public who were probably the most affected and least well informed.

Based on the evidence they heard, the Committee made 79 recommendations in respect of the reform and development of the coroner's service. Some of these recommendations are in reality only putting into statute what has been 'coroners' case law' for many years; others are radical in their proposals.

For convenience the recommendations will be considered under separate headings.

Qualification of Coroners

The effect of the Committee's recommendation on the certification of death will be to increase the number of deaths reported to the coroner. The exact increase is hard to assess, but it is the writer's opinion that this may well be as high as 30 per cent on the existing case-load. If all the recommendations in that regard are implemented, together with the Committee's recommendations in relation to the enquiry which the coroner must perform in all deaths, there will be a vast increase in the number of cases where the main concern of that officer will be the determination of the medical cause of death.

The Committee, having recognized these factors, perversely recommends that only barristers or solicitors of at least five years' standing in their profession should be eligible for future appointment as coroners, deputy coroners and assistant deputy coroners. They further suggest that it is desirable that, before appointment to a full-time post, a coroner shall have had some previous experience as a deputy or assistant deputy.

Appointment and Retirement of Coroners

At the present time once a coroner is appointed by a local authority he is appointed for life. Certain authorities write into the contract of employment a retirement clause on the grounds of age, but apart from this a coroner can only be removed from office by the Lord Chancellor on grounds of inability or misconduct in the discharge of his duties.

It follows that one authority is responsible for appointing and paying the coroner, and another authority is responsible, within certain limits, for his subsequent actions.

The Committee recommend that, as the Lord Chancellor is already responsible for the appointment of legally qualified persons to public duty of a judicial character, he is well placed to appoint coroners. They therefore suggest that the Lord Chancellor should in future make the appointments of coroner after appropriate consultation with local authorities, and that he should also have the power to remove a coroner from office not only on the grounds of incapacity or misbehaviour in the execution of his office, but for any incapacity or misbehaviour which, in the Lord Chancellor's opinion, renders the coroner unfit to continue in office. As the Lord Chancellor would be acting judicially in complaints regarding the coroner's conduct, it would be inappropriate for him to have the duty to investigate such complaints as well. It is therefore suggested that investigation responsibility should be allocated to another minister—most appropriately, in the Committee's view, the Home Secretary.

Under existing statutes, coroners appointed to county jurisdiction are required to reside within the district to which they are appointed or within two miles of it. The reason underlying this statute was to ease communication with the coroner, but in these modern days of improved facilities in communication this residential requirement appears to be unnecessary. The Committee therefore recommend that a residential requirement for the coroners be abolished and in its place an assurance that the coroner, or in his absence his deputy or assistant deputy, should be readily available at all times to undertake the duties.

The Committee found it undesirable that coroners should be appointed for life. They recommend that the normal retiring age for coroners should be 65, and that the Lord Chancellor should have the power to extend a coroner's appointment of office annually in appropriate cases up to a ceiling age of 72. They further recommend that these conditions should also apply to deputy coroners and assistant deputy coroners.

Salaries

As has already been stated, coroners' salaries are paid by the local authority which appoints them. This salary is determined by agreement between the authority and the coroner, but either side may appeal to the Home Secretary, who has power to fix the salary at such rate as he thinks proper. Since 1967 most part-time coroners have been paid in accordance with the national agreement reached between the Local Authority Associations and the Coroners' Society of England and Wales, which established a scale of salary based on the number of deaths reported. The salary of whole-time coroners is related to the salary of the third grade in a major department of local authority, and this relationship does not produce uniformity of the salary since the same appointment may carry a different salary according to the size of the local authority concerned.

The recommendations of the Committee are aimed at producing a more uniform type of coroners' service. For this reason the Committee recommend that there be a uniform salary structure for whole-time coroners, and that these officers should be paid standard salaries which may well relate to the salary of a stipendiary magistrate. The Committee have no recommendation to make regarding the salary of part-time coroners, and suggest that the present arrangement of work-load criteria should be continued. It is not clear in the report as to whether the Committee recommend that the local authority is still responsible for the payment of the coroner, or that such payment shall come from some central fund.

Deputy Coroners, Assistant Deputy Coroners and Supporting Staff

At present all preliminary enquiries in a case referred to the coroner are made by the coroner's officer. This person may be either a civilian attached to the coroner, a serving police officer permanently seconded to the coroner, or, in some rural areas, the first police officer on the scene of any incident.

In many of the larger jurisdictions, the coroner's officer is a serving police officer permanently seconded to work with the coroner in the preliminary investigation of cases. Police officers nearly always work in plain clothes, have had previous experience as deputy coroners' officers, and are well able to interview the bereaved relatives, medical practitioners, hospital staff and witnesses. By virtue of the fact that they are 'in the job' they are able to get great co-operation from police stations and police forces with whom they come into contact.

Some of the evidence heard by the Committee indicated that bereaved relatives and doctors resented being interviewed by a police officer investigating a death in which there was no suspicion or criminality. Other evidence indicated that it was a waste of police manpower to use trained and disciplined police officers to investigate cases in which the possibility of criminality is remote.

The Committee therefore concluded that the duties of a coroner's officer could be effectively performed by properly trained civilian employees in the coroner's office, and recommend that police officers should no longer serve in the capacity of coroner's officer. They suggest that the coroner himself should continue to be responsible for recruiting staff for administrative work and to help in investigation into the circumstances of death, thus ensuring the independence of the coroner's staff from both the local and central Government, and they recommend that every coroner should be provided with the services of a civilian coroner's officer and, where necessary, the services of a secretary.

The civilian coroners' officers responsibility would be in the field of collating medical and police reports, preparing cases for the coroner's decision, arranging for the removal of bodies for autopsies, and for inquests. He would also be responsible for communicating with witnesses and relatives, paying expenses to witnesses, and for liaison with the Press. The secretary would have to be responsible for the normal range of office tasks, but would also include within his sphere of responsibility the taking down of particulars of death as they are reported, giving simple advice to relatives, making enquiries of doctors on the coroner's behalf, and possibly providing inquest transcripts. At present the coroner's officer actually attends at the scenes of most deaths. Since 90 per cent of reported deaths are investigated only by post-mortem and do not proceed to inquests, it is unusual for the coroner's officer to make much enquiry into the circumstances, as opposed to the medical cause of the death. In the remaining 10 per cent of the cases the coroner's officer is the first officer to make any enquiry into the circumstances of death, and a properly trained and observant officer may well start the enquiry as a result of his own observations, later handing over to the police authority. In the opinion of the Committee the need for this 'field work' would be greatly diminished as a result of their recommendations. The recommendation that doctors should be under a statutory obligation to report certain deaths to the coroner, and that whenever possible an initial telephone report supplemented by a written notification should be made, together with a new form of certificate of the fact and cause of death, would abolish the need for any field visit in the great majority of cases. In the remaining cases the Committee recommend that the police authority is asked to undertake the field investigations, and rationalize this decision on the grounds that if the total demand from coroners for police assistance is reduced, chief officers of police would be willing to make available for the coroner an officer with the rank and experience commensurate with the difficulty of the particular investigation. In addition to police officers investigating the field circumstances of any death, the Committee recommend that the local authority should be able to assist the coroner in some of the field work by using health visitors and representatives of the social workers and welfare departments. These suggestions are in line with the Committee's intention that the coroner's work should become more 'medico-social' in character than 'medico-legal'.

The present statute demands that every coroner shall appoint a

Deputy, and that at his own discretion a coroner may also appoint an Assistant Deputy. The names of the deputy and assistant deputy must be submitted to the local authority for their approval. The Committee recommends that the appointment of Deputy Coroners to full-time jurisdictions should in future be made by the Lord Chancellor after appropriate consultation with local authorities. They further recommend that the appointments of Deputy Coroners to part-time jurisdictions, and of Assistant Deputy Coroners to all jurisdiction should continue to be made by the coroner, but that in these instances the names should be submitted to the Lord Chancellor for approval.

Coroners' Areas and Territorial Jurisdictions

At present every coroner holds an independent territorial jurisdiction by virtue of his appointment by local authorities. Resulting from this method of appointment there are a large number of small part-time coronerships, many having very few cases reported each year. Indeed nearly 50 of the part-time coroners deal with less than 100 cases each year. The average case load of the part-time coroner is somewhere in the region of 350 cases a year.

The 1936 recommendations regarding the amalgamation of these small part-time jurisdictions have not been fulfilled in more than a very few cases. The Wright Committee, in 1936, expressed the view that the system of whole-time appointment was 'a goal to be aimed at', and the same Committee went on to say that 'many part-time coroners, because of the smallness of their district, have little experience or prospect of experience in the conduct of their duties' and, further, that 'the problem of the smaller coronerships can only be satisfactorily solved by a radical readjustment of coroners' districts'.

With the impending reorganization of local Government due to take effect on 1st April 1974, and the proposed reorganization of the National Health Service with the creation of new Local Health Authorities, the Committee have concluded that the time is now ripe for a reorganization of coroners' areas.

They recommend that in future the new County and Metropolitan authorities should be statutorily required to submit for approval by the Home Secretary proposals for the organization of the coroner's service in their area, and should have to give detailed reasons to justify the creation of any part-time coroners' districts. Before submitting any such proposal for a part-time jurisdiction, the authority concerned should statutorily be required to consult with the authorities controlling the areas bordering on the proposed part-time jurisdiction, with a view to enlarging that jurisdiction to whole-time status by inter-authority adjustment of coroners' district boundaries.

The Committee envisage that the boundaries of jurisdictions would be largely determined by: (a) the desirability of creating a whole-time jurisdiction; (b) the distribution of population and locality trends; (c) communication and transport facilities; (d) the likely mobility of the coroner and his staff; (e) the availability of mortuary, pathological and other relevant services; and (f) the accessibility of registrars of deaths.

The ultimate aim of these recommendations is to secure a distribution of coroners to the advantage of the service, and to ensure that future legislation should be formulated in such a way that coroners need not be bound by their territorial jurisdiction and, if required, could move into another territorial area and give assistance should there be a major disaster or something of that nature.

The enlarging of a coroner's territorial jurisdiction, and the suggested overlap of territorial jurisdictions, would facilitate the coroners' powers of calling as witnesses persons who are not resident within his own strictly defined territory, and this aspect will be referred to later when changes in inquest procedure are being discussed.

Coroners' Accommodation

In most full-time jurisdictions coroners are provided with permanent office accommodation by the appointing authorities, but in some part-time jurisdictions coroners are forced to use their own private accommodation, sometimes without any financial contribution from the authorities for this purpose; in many parts of the country a room in a police station or a hospital is used as a coroner's court. Ideally, the administrative offices, court premises, postmortem facilities, and possibly the offices of the registrar of deaths, should all be contained in a single complex.

The Committee propose that in future the Home Secretary should be placed under a statutory duty to secure the provision of suitable staff and accommodation for the performance by the coroner of his various statutory functions, which would include the holding of such inquests as are necessary. The proposals establish that although the Home Secretary would be statutorily obliged to secure such accommodation, he should be empowered to make arrangements for other persons to act as his agents and pay for expenditure incurred by them as his agents.

This means that the coroners themselves would be able to recruit certain groups of staff, or local authorities to provide staff, office and other accommodation or to come to some arrangement with those responsible under the Courts Act 1971 for the provision of staff and accommodation. In this way the staff would come under the new administration court service, and office and court accommodation would become the responsibility of the Department of the Environment.

CHANGES IN INQUEST PROCEDURES

The present law demands that a coroner hold a formal inquest in all unnatural deaths. The Committee heard that a formal court hearing in many cases of simple accidental deaths, and suicides, was obviously unnecessary, served no useful purpose in the public interest, and often caused additional distress to bereaved relatives. They heard how the public at large equated the word verdict, referring to the circumstances in which a fatal condition was acquired, with implied criticism of some person or authority.

It became obvious that in certain cases the extent of enquiry at inquest was limited by the coroner's power only to summon those witnesses who lived within his territorial jurisdiction. They heard evidence of complaint in such matters as the right to representation, the publication of court lists, the possible implied criticism in coroners' riders, the standard of record keeping, and the availability of court records.

The Committee also heard evidence regarding the existing function of the coroners' juries in those cases where by present statute the coroner is obliged to sit with a jury when considering certain classifications of death.

The Committee define the responsibility and duties of the coroners of the future as being:

(1) To establish the medical cause of death when, for whatever reason, the cause of death has not been certified by a medical practitioner.

(2) To make enquiries into the circumstances in which some deaths occur, irrespective of whether or not the medical cause of death is already known.

As has been stated the Committee envisages that each jurisdiction will increase in size as the trend to whole-time office develops. They suggest that the strict territorial boundaries can be waived in cases where the death and the incident which caused it take place in separate jurisdictions, or if a competent court orders an inquest or a fresh inquest to be held.

Under present statutes, besides the duty to enquire into death, coroners have certain other duties, each of them more or less an historical survivor. The Committee recommends that the coroners' jurisdiction over treasure trove be retained, but that jurisdiction of the Coroner of the City of London over fires which do not cause death be abolished.

Having recommended certain changes in the certification of death by a registered medical practitioner, the Committee intend to establish the coroner's office as a recipient office for reports, rather than as a 'seeker' of reports. Under this heading, they have recommended certain additional statutory duties to report deaths to the coroner. These recommendations affect people who are deprived of their liberty, either permanently or temporarily. The present statute lays down that the death of any person in prison either after trial or on remand, be reported to the coroner even if that death is known to be natural. By definition this statute excludes persons who are being held in police stations, and persons who are being held under order in hospitals for nervous disorders.

In future persons in charge of prison service establishments, similar institutions maintained by the armed forces, approved schools and remand homes would continue to be required to report the deaths of inmates to the coroner. In addition there should be a statutory obligation upon the officer in charge of the police station to report a death to the coroner if a person dies in police custody. The Committee further recommends that it should be statutory for the death of a compulsorily detained psychiatric patient to be reported to the coroner, and the obligation to make this report should be placed on the person in administrative charge of the hospital in which the patient is detained.

When a death is reported to a coroner who has a territorial jurisdiction, he should have a duty first to determine the identity of the deceased and the fact and cause of death; secondly to make such enquiries as will allow him to decide whether a post-mortem examination or an inquest or reference to other authority (or any combination of these) is required in order that he may determine such matters as are his concern; and thirdly to send a certificate incorporating the results of his enquiries to the registrar of deaths of the district in which the death occurred.

Under these recommendations the coroner will be able to issue a certificate of the cause of death: (a) on the basis of the information provided for him by a doctor with knowledge of the deceased's last illness; or (b) after he has seen the results of the post-mortem examination and is satisfied that no further enquiries are necessary; or (c) after he has held an inquest with or without a post-mortem examination.

The Committee recommends that the coroner should always be responsible for certifying the medical cause of death in every certificate that he issues, whether a post-mortem has been performed or not. This recommendation abolishes the main differences between the present 'pink Form A' and 'pink Form B' procedures. Accordingly, the Committee recommend a new form of certificate for use by the coroner which will be used in all reported cases whether autopsy has been performed or not, and whether inquest has been held or not. This new certificate will consist of seven parts.

Part I is concerned with such matters as particulars of identification which for the first time would include the deceased's National Health Service number.

Part II will show the medical cause of death and the approximate period between the onset of disease and death.

Part III will contain such supplementary information as will assist the Registrar General in his statistical analyses and will refer to other morbid conditions present, to surgical operation performed within 28 days of death, and to any accident suffered by the deceased within three months of death.

Part IV will classify the death in categories of accident, suicide or other, and will contain an annotation as to whether the papers regarding the case had been referred to the Director of Public Prosecutions.

Part V relates solely to accidental death and gives the details of the accident including the place where it occurred, the details of how it happened, the type of injuries sustained, the parts of the body injured, and the interval between injury and death.

Part VI records other findings relating to the circumstances of the death.

Part VII, which is to be completed in all inquest cases, records the occupation of the deceased, whether the inquest was held with or without jury or whether it was adjourned under Section 7 (2) of the Visiting Forces Act of 1952, and the marital state of the person concerned.

The introductory part of this new form contains a statement by the coroner that: (a) I am satisfied that neither autopsy nor inquest is necessary and the cause of death was as shown below; or (b) having received a report of an autopsy I am satisfied that an inquest is unnecessary and that the cause of death was as shown below; or (c) an inquest was held on the body on a certain date and that the cause of death and other findings are shown below. The single form is designed to do away with the pink Forms A and B, and with the coroner's certificate after inquest.

The Committee heard some evidence alleging that there was delay in certain cases between a death and the subsequent issuing of a death certificate, particularly in inquest cases where the hearing was long adjourned after the death. Under certain circumstances this delay could cause grave inconvenience to the family of the deceased in such matters as insurance. At the present time most coroners issue a letter on their headed paper, certifying to all whom it may concern that they have, on a certain date, opened an inquest on the body of the named individual, but many insurance companies will not act on such an informal letter. Accordingly, the Committee recommend the introduction of a coroner's interim certificate of the fact of death which will be used in such cases as require further investigation, and thereby make the full coroner's certificate of the fact and cause of death unavailable. This new form of interim certificate will give details of identification and date of death, and in inquest cases will give either the medical cause of death, or a statement that the precise medical cause of death has yet to be established. All insurance companies and other interested organizations will be bound by statute to accept and act on the interim certificate.

The future rôle of the coroner is to establish the medical cause of death when, for one reason or another, certification by a doctor is impracticable or inappropriate, and to initiate enquiries into the circumstantial causes of death where this seems desirable in the public interest. To fulfil that rôle coroners' enquiries should extend as far as, but no further than, is necessary to enable them to complete the task of establishing the cause of death.

Within these boundaries, the Committee recommends that a coroner should have complete discretion as to the form which his enquiries may take after a death has been reported to him. The only exceptions being that he must hold an inquest in all deaths on suspected homicide, deaths of persons deprived of their liberty by society, and deaths of persons whose bodies are unidentified. This recommendation will give a coroner wide discretionary powers in the use of inquest procedure. The Committee recognizes that such discretionary powers, exercised by a single individual, may often give rise to complaint from relatives or from other interested parties that proper investigation into a death has not been held. Accordingly, they recommend certain appellate procedures to be used in such instances, and this is referred to under the sub-heading of Appeals on page 292.

To assist the coroner in making a proper investigation, the Committee recommend that he have a statutory power to require a post-mortem to be carried out, or to have an exhumation made. In addition he should have statutory powers to take possession of a body; to enter and inspect the place or area where the body was found, and any place from which the body was moved, or any place from which there is reasonable grounds to believe that the body was moved before it was found; and to enter and inspect the places or areas in which the deceased person was, or the places in which there is reason to believe the deceased person was, prior to his death. The coroner should have the right to enter into any place, to inspect and receive information from any records or writings relating to the deceased and to reproduce and obtain copies of them; and to take possession of anything that he has reasonable grounds for believing is material for the purpose of his investigation, and to preserve it until the conclusion of his investigation, when it is his duty to restore that thing to the person from whom it was taken, unless he is authorized or required by law to dispose of it in some other way.

The Secretary of State for the Home Office should have the power to direct that an inquest be held in the absence of a body, and that an application for such an inquest to be held can be made by the coroner, by the next-of-kin of the presumed deceased, or by any other interested parties.

At present the exact nature of coroners' jurisdiction to enquire into a death which has occurred outside England and Wales, and where the body is subsequently brought into the country for burial, has not been clear. The problem used to arise in the case of people who had died on the Continent on holiday, or on business, and whose bodies were flown into the United Kingdom or brought back by sea, and in cases of death on board ship outside territorial waters where the bodies were subsequently landed at English ports. In more recent years the presence of near offshore drilling rigs have increased the perplexity of this problem. According to strict statute, if the coroner is informed that there lies within his territorial district a body of a person who is believed to have died a violent or unnatural death, he must hold an inquest regardless of where the death occurred.

The implied suggestion in the report is that the coroner need not act if judicial enquiry has been made in the country where death occurred, but should act if the death has occurred on board ship or aircraft. At present if a death occurs outside England and Wales and the body is not available, for example a death followed by burial at sea, the coroner has no power to act since there is no body, and the Home Secretary has no power to order an inquest to be held unless there is reason to believe that the death occurred near the coroner's district. To deal with this situation, the Committee recommend that the coroner's jurisdiction should be extended to cover cases where the death occurred outside the country and the body has been disposed of or lost.

The Committee recommend that as the modern practice of medical investigation and autopsy is an integral part of all coroners' investigation, and that the identity of the deceased is nearly always established prior to inquest by someone who knew him well, the view no longer serves any useful purpose. They therefore recommend that the view of the body by the coroner should no longer be required to give him jurisdiction.

Having made the recommendation that a formal Court inquest serves no useful purpose in many unnatural deaths, the procedure to be followed in these categories of death had to be reconsidered. The Committee propose therefore that there be three alternative procedures open to the coroner at his discretion.

First, the coroner may investigate unnatural deaths by means of history taking, autopsy and reports submitted to him by the investigating authorities. This documentary evidence could be studied in private, and an administrative decision as to the fact, medical cause and circumstances of death could be made. This decision should be recorded on the new form of certificate already described.

Such a procedure could be followed in simple accidents in the home; in deaths due to chronic alcoholic poisoning; in certain cases of suicide; and in certain medical or surgical misadventures.

Secondly, the coroner could investigate certain unnatural deaths by means of a documentary inquest. This would be a hearing in open court, but witnesses would not be required to attend, and all evidence would be in the form of statements and documents. The coroner's findings upon this documentary evidence would be made public in open court and would again be recorded on the coroner's certificate. These 'short inquests' could be used to investigate many violent deaths resulting from road traffic incidents, industrial incidents, industrial disease, and those domestic accidents, suicides, and medical and surgical mishaps, which it would be inappropriate to deal with by perusal of the documentary evidence in private.

In the case of these 'short inquests' any interested party should have the right to request that the hearing be a full inquest with the attendance of any witnesses whom they may wish to cross-examine.

Thirdly, the coroner should have the choice of hearing in open court the evidence of witnesses to any incident. Such an inquest should be mandatory in the investigation of persons who have died whilst in custody, in prison, in approved schools, or under order in a psychiatric institution, or cases of suspected homicide.

The Committee recommend that the coroner need no longer

summon a jury to investigate with him deaths resulting from vehicular, industrial or homicidal incidents, but suggest that the coroner should retain the power to summon the jury in any case where he considers that there are special reasons for so doing. In those cases where a coroner chooses to sit with the jury, the jury should be summoned in accordance with the same rules as are used by the High Sheriff in summoning juries for other courts.

Because of the implied criticism in the term verdict, the Committee recommend that in future the coroner's conclusion with regard to any case investigated at inquest should be termed 'findings'. If, in the course of his enquiry to ascertain the circumstances that led to a death, the coroner discovers certain dangerous practices that may cause similar incidents, he should retain the right to draw attention to them. The Committee recommends, however, that this right should no longer be exercised by the addition of a rider to his findings, but instead he should refer the matter to the appropriate expert body or public authority, and in inquest cases he should announce that he is doing so.

Under present statute the coroner only has the power to summon witnesses to appear at inquests if they live within his territorial jurisdiction. The Committee recommend that this power should be extended to enable the coroner to summon witnesses from anywhere in England and Wales. The witnesses, when being informed about the arrangements for an inquest, should also be told that as properly interested persons they are entitled to legal representation should their conduct be open to question.

The present procedure, where properly interested parties have the privilege of cross-examination at the coroner's discretion, should be changed. The current definition of a properly interested party depends on the coroner's discretion, and the Committee suggest that certain categories of persons must be given the absolute right to be present at an inquest and to ask relevant questions. This category of person includes: (*a*) the next-of-kin of the deceased; (*b*) the parents, children and personal representatives of the deceased; (*c*) any beneficiary of a policy for insurance on the life of the deceased and any insurer having issued such a policy; (*d*) any person whose act or omission on the part of himself, his servants or agents, irrespective of whether it may give rise to civil liability, may be thought to have caused or contributed to the death of the deceased; (*e*) the chief officer of police; (*f*) any person appointed by a Government department to attend the inquest. In addition to these special categories, the coroner should retain the discretionary right to allow any other person to appear, and he should have the discretionary power

K

to waive the requirement that the police may only appear at an inquest by legal representation. The right of the trade union representative to examine the witness in any case of industrial injury or disease should be retained.

There are certain cases in which it is highly desirable that certain parties at an inquest are legally represented, but in which, because of financial circumstances, such representation is unavailable. To counter this difficulty, the Committee recommend that the scope of the Legal Aid Advice Act of 1949 be extended to cover certain enquiries in the coroner's court and they hope that whatever technicalities are required in this matter will be expedited so as to impose a minimum of delay in the hearing of these cases.

The Committee recommend that every coroner should be required to exhibit a list of the inquests which he proposes to hold, together with a list of witnesses to be called to each, on a notice board outside his office and outside the place or places most commonly used as a coroner's court, and that at least 48 hours' notice of his intention to hold a 'short' inquest should be given.

At present the use of shorthand writers and tape recorders varies from one coroner's jurisdiction to another. Only in cases of murder, manslaughter or infanticide, is the coroner required by law to take formal depositions at inquests. In all other cases, the only requirement is that the coroner should make notes of the evidence, and the contents of these notes is left to his own discretion. He is expected to make fairly comprehensive notes in cases where there is a likelihood that the inquest will be followed by other legal proceedings. The Committee have recommended that a full transcript should be taken at every inquest.

At present the coroner is responsible for employing and paying, out of his expenses allowance, all secretarial help. He is also responsible for providing all necessary office furniture such as tape recorders, photocopiers, typewriters and paper. The Committee's recommendation, already referred to in the text, that a coroner should be provided with a secretary, will undoubtedly assist in the preparation of notes of evidence and transcripts of inquest evidence. It would seem from the report that the coroner will still have the right to charge for copies of notes of evidence requested by properly interested parties. The Committee recommend one change in the existing practice, namely that the general practitioner only be entitled to a free copy of the post-mortem report upon request.

The historic duty of the coroner's jury to commit for trial in cases of murder, manslaughter or infanticide was unanimously considered as an archaic institution serving no useful purpose in the modern day and age. The Committee therefore recommend that the duty of a coroner's jury to name a person responsible for causing a death and the coroner's subsequent obligation to commit that person for trial be abolished. In its place the coroner should have the right, at any stage in an inquest, to adjourn the enquiry and refer the papers to the Director of Public Prosecutions. In cases where this step is taken, the Director should be obliged to notify the coroner of his decision where no further court action ensues, and the coroner should make public the Director's decision. Under these circumstances there would be no need for the coroner to reopen the inquest.

In other cases of homicide, where the person suspected of the offence is dead, the coroner should be required merely to record a finding of homicide and should no longer be under the legal obligation to name the person responsible.

To support such a finding the coroner should have evidence, either documentary or oral, from a senior officer of police indicating that there is no further purpose in enquiries. Such a suggested procedure would obliterate the coroner's duty to name as a murderer a person who has subsequently died with the attendant distress to his relatives that such a duty may cause.

The current machinery for reversing a coroner's verdict is complicated and cumbersome, and the right to new inquests is restricted to a very few types of case. The Committee recommend quite sweeping changes in the methods of appeal against inquest findings. Because of the extent of the recommended changes in inquest procedure, and the wide discretionary powers regarding the need to hold an inquest, there would be a need for an appellate procedure both against the findings of an inquest, and against the coroner's decision not to hold an inquest.

The Committee recommend that the rights of appeal should be exercised locally by application to a High Court Judge sitting at a major centre outside London, but that the existing right of an aggrieved party to go to the Divisional Court should be preserved.

A coroner's decision not to hold an inquest on a death that has been reported to him must be open to rapid challenge, for in these cases time is the essence, and these appeals should be determined by a High Court Judge outside London who should have the power to order an autopsy and to suspend any burial or cremation until the results of the autopsy are known.

As far as the rights to appeal against the findings of an inquest are concerned, the Committee have two recommendations to make. First, that the right of appeal should be based on *any* error in *any part* of the record of the findings in the coroner's court, including the

273

findings as to the medical and circumstantial causes of death. An appeal based on these grounds would, if successful, result in a fresh inquest being held.

Secondly, the right to appeal against the findings of a coroner's inquest when there is no error in the record would be at the discretion of a High Court Judge outside London who would have to designate a Judge not lower in status than a Circuit Judge to hear the appeal. Under these circumstances it would be for the Circuit Judge to decide whether the re-hearing should be a complete oral re-hearing of the witnesses, or merely a study of the transcript of evidence of the inquest.

Neither of these recommendations should abolish the right of an aggrieved individual to apply to the Divisional Court but would in fact be complementary to that right and would bring local decisions within the jurisdiction of High Court Judges operating locally.

Discussion

There can be little doubt that expertise and efficiency depend on experience and that, in the field of coroners' investigation, experience must depend on case-load. The suggestion of the 1936 Wright Committee to increase the size of coroner's areas by the amalgamation of smaller jurisdictions was never implemented. The Brodrick Committee recommendations that these amalgamations proceed in association with the reorganization of Local Government, and of the National Health Service, will do much to increase the professionalism and the expertise of coroners.

The concept of a single employing and paying authority is also in line with increased efficiency and the establishment of a constant standard. Provided that the complete political independence of the office of coroner is maintained, there would seem to be no objection in the Lord Chancellor's Department taking over this duty, and it would seem only right that a coroner should be removed from office for any incapacity or misbehaviour which renders him unfit to continue in office.

It is the fact that many of the coroner's decisions as to the advisability of autopsy, or of inquest, are judicial ones, that cause the Committee to recommend that in future the qualification for office should be a legal one. This argument appears to be falacious in some respects, for many of the decisions involving whether or not autopsy should be performed, and of interpreting medical histories from attending physicians, are matters in which understanding of medicine

274

is vital. In such matters it would appear that a medically qualified coroner would be in a better position to make this primary assessment. The argument that in the eyes of the lay public a medical coroner is (a) likely to favour the medical profession in his decisions, and (b) completely in touch with all recent advances in medicine and surgery, is equally falacious. Indeed, regarding the first of these points, the medically qualified coroner is often much harder on his professional brethren than is the legally qualified coroner, and in regard to the second it must be the duty of any judicial officer to keep abreast, at least superficially, with recent advances and decisions in his field.

There are very few successful practising lawyers, whether solicitors or barristers, whose earnings are so low as to allow them to be attracted to a full-time coroner's jurisdiction, even if this were paid in line with a stipendiary magistrate. This fact raises doubt as to the calibre of those lawyers who would be prepared to enter into the 'coroners' service'. It is a sad reflection on our modern times, that the remuneration of medical practitioners, even those of consultant grade, lags far behind the remuneration of the able and successful lawyer, and this fact alone creates a pool of high calibre applicants.

There can be little doubt that the most important qualifications for the office of coroner are those of clear thought, humanity and previous experience as deputy. It is doubtful whether the first two of these qualifications are more likely to be found in lawyers than in doctors.

The recommendations of the Committee regarding deputies and supporting staff to the coroner contain several points of interest. There can be little doubt that future whole-time coroners will be drawn from the ranks of deputy coroners in other whole-time jurisdictions. It is therefore logical that the same appointing authority should make the appointment of the deputy coroner to whole-time jurisdictions as makes the appointment of coroner, and the suggestion they should be appointed by the Lord Chancellor has much to support it. Such a step would create a 'career structure' and would do much to establish a uniform system. It would seem a logical step to extend this proposal to cover the appointment of assistant deputy coroners to full-time jurisdictions as well, and that these appointments be made by the Lord Chancellor after consultation with the coroner. As the ultimate aim of the Committee's recommendations appears to be the abolition of the part-time jurisdiction, the temporary retention of a part-time coroner's right to appoint his own deputy and assistant deputy would seem to be a sensible arrangement.

The recommendation that police officers should no longer be

used as coroner's officers is open to considerable discussion. The advantages of a disciplined and trained police officer conducting the preliminary enquiries in cases of sudden death are great, and have been referred to earlier in the text. They include the willing co-operation of police authorities in the coroner's investigation, and the vital contribution that an 'on scene' investigation by a trained observer can make to any enquiry. Although the Committee envisage a situation where the number of 'field' investigations will be considerably reduced, and that, where such an investigation is necessary, a police officer of rank commensurate with the complexity of the investigation will be made available, and that other field investigations will be made by members of the local authority welfare service, it is reasonable to suppose that such 'piece meal' investigation will lack the effectiveness of a single, well co-ordinated, investigating officer.

The importance of just such an officer is already well recognized by most police forces, in as much as a 'scenes of crime' officer is now in common use at all investigations.

Unless trained criminal investigation officers are to attend the scene of any unexpected death in the home, the abolition of field enquiries by a coroner's officer would seem to create a lacuna in the entire investigating system. It is very doubtful whether trained civilians would be able to undertake this on scene investigation. The concept of civilian coroner's officers sitting in the coroner's administration building and answering queries on the telephone, receiving reports from other investigating authorities, and arranging for the removal of bodies, does not appear to be one which will increase the efficient operation of the coroner's jurisdiction.

The provision of efficient secretarial help and the recommended use of modern methods of recording evidence are recommendations with which no one could quarrel, as are the recommendations concerning the coroner's accommodation.

In practice police officers in charge of police stations already notify the coroner of any death of a person in a police cell, and the recommendations to include such notification in statute does no more than consolidate what is already 'case', and the extension of this principle to include the death of patients under order in psychiatric units will minimize the risk of allegations of ill-treatment or neglect being made some months after the death of any such patient.

The abolition of formal inquest in open court in many simple domestic, industrial and classic incidents, as well as in many suicides, should give rise to no opposition. The freely available appellate procedure should ensure that no coroner will dispense with an inquest

276

in cases where it would be in the public interest, or in the interest of next-of-kin, for such enquiry to be held.

With the right of interested parties to insist on oral evidence and cross-examination of witnesses should it be needed, the proposed short documentary inquest will expedite many coroner's investigations without adding the extra anguish of a court appearance for bereaved relatives. The mandatory full inquest in cases of suspected homicide, cases where the identity of the deceased is unknown, and in the cases of death in custody, should safeguard the public interest in these matters, and the discretionary right of the coroner to hold full inquest in all other cases where the public interest is involved, should minimize the risk of any allegations of 'whitewashing'.

The proposed definitions of 'properly interested parties' in their right to appear and to question witnesses can only be welcomed, as can the recommendations that legal aid be made available to those people who should be legally represented at inquest but who for financial causes are unable to retain a lawyer.

The abolition of the duty of the coroner's jury's to name a person responsible for a homicide, whether it be to commit him for trial or not, will be welcomed by all concerned. Whether the proposed procedure of adjournment and referral of the papers to the Director of Public Prosecutions will serve as an efficient 'back stop' or not is arguable, but the fact that the Director's decision in any case will be made public by the coroner would help to increase the efficiency of the suggested procedure.

The proposed abolition of the jury's rider, and the substituted procedure of notifying directly the appropriate authority, has much to recommend it; it will dispense with any implied criticism such as may be contained in a jury's rider, and it will ensure that the appropriate authority is informed of the circumstances.

The proposed appellate procedure both in regard to the coroner's decision not to hold an inquest, and against the findings of his enquiry, can only be welcomed, for such an appellate procedure will help to enforce a constant standard of practice throughout the country, and this will be further reinforced by the proposal that a transcript of evidence shall be taken at every inquest.

The coroner's right to order autopsy, to hold an inquest in the absence of a body, and to investigate death occurring outside England and Wales, together with his statutory power to make an order for exhumation, are all integral portions of a comprehensive system for the investigation of sudden death, and the proposal that the coroner shall have the right to summon a witness living outside his territorial jurisdiction can only improve the efficiency of the system.

The proposed powers of investigation, including as they do the right of possession of the body, of entry and search, and of possession of material exhibits, also reinforce the efficiency of the system.

PATHOLOGICAL AND RELATED SERVICES

In 1969 in England and Wales 116,104 autopsies were performed on the instructions of coroners out of the total of 159,024 autopsies. Violent deaths constitute about 4·2 per cent of this total, and it follows that the remaining cases involved natural disease of some sort. These figures reflect the increasing trend of reporting deaths to coroners because the medical cause of death was in doubt rather than because the circumstances of the death were suspicious. If the recommendations of the Brodrick Committee regarding the certification of death are accepted, the number of cases in which a doctor feels that he cannot accurately certify the cause of death will increase and the percentage of natural deaths investigated by autopsy will also increase.

In London and in many other areas of heavy population there are university departments of forensic pathology. In these areas it has been the trend for coroners to employ forensic pathologists wherever possible to undertake their autopsies. The reason for this preference is twofold:

(1) When the investigation involves the death of a patient in hospital, it is advantageous to employ a pathologist who is not connected with the hospital where the death occurred. In this way the relatives of the deceased can be assured that the examination is being performed by a doctor completely independent of the hospital and that any allegations of bias would be unfounded; the same independence ensures that a consultant on the staff of a hospital would never be placed in the invidious position of having to imply criticism of a consultant colleague.

(2) A forensic pathologist, by training and experience, has a higher threshold of suspicion and is often able to recognize injuries that do not fit in to the normal pattern of accidental trauma. There are many cases involving the abused child, for instance, where the significance of the multiplicity of injury and the characteristics of certain injuries have escaped the notice of hospital morbid anatomists and have only come to light when the body has been subsequently studied by a forensic pathologist.

Unfortunately the expansion of forensic pathology has been severely hindered for years by the absence of any clear-cut career structure in that field, and young men and women have been loathe

278

to devote some five years of training in general pathology followed by an equally extended period of training in forensic pathology in the absence of any certainty for the future. This short-sighted policy, pursued by almost all the university departments in England and Wales, has led to a severe shortage of qualified people in this field.

Because of this shortage the great majority of coroners' work outside London and the major centres of population is carried out by hospital pathologists working on a fee per case basis for the local coroner. It is interesting to note that in London for the quarter 31st October 1968 to 31st December 1968 6,274 post-mortems were carried out on coroner's orders, and of that number 4,889 were performed by either whole-time forensic pathologists or consultant pathologists with special forensic experience and interest. In the same period in the County of Lancashire some 3,123 autopsies were ordered by the coroner, and out of this total only 453 were performed by pathologists with forensic experience, and in Nottinghamshire in that quarter 615 autopsies were ordered by the coroner and only 174 of these were performed by pathologists with forensic experience.

The gross autopsy is not the end of the story, for the efficiency of the pathological investigation must depend on good ancillary services in the laboratory. This country is one of the very few in the western civilized world where the development of forensic science institutes has been completely ignored. Even in the coroner jurisdictions in the United States such institutes have developed, with morbid anatomy, toxicology, ballistics, criminalistics, histology, serology, and the coroner's court and administration all housed in the same building, and with adequate funds made available by the local authority. In England and Wales the departments of forensic medicine attached to universities in the main lead lives of glorious isolation, and are entirely dependent upon the hospitals in which they are housed for many of these back-up services, and are dependent upon the forensic science laboratories of the Home Office for assistance in the matters of ballistics, etc.

Morbid anatomists, working from National Health Service hospitals, have immediately available in their own departments histologists, bacteriologists, haemotologists, and usually toxicologists.

The responsibility at present for arranging an autopsy rests with the coroner himself and, in choosing the doctor whom he will direct or request for the examination, he is controlled by the coroners' rules of 1953 to take into consideration the following matters:

(1) The post-mortem examination should be made, whenever practicable, by a pathologist with suitable qualifications and experience and having access to laboratory facilities.

K*

(2) If the coroner is informed by the chief officer of police that a person may be charged with the murder, manslaughter or infanticide of the deceased, the coroner should consult the chief officer of police regarding the legally qualified medical practitioner who is to make the post-mortem examination.

(3) If the deceased died in a hospital, the coroner should not direct or request a pathologist on the staff of, or associated with, that hospital to make a post-mortem examination, unless the obtaining of another pathologist with suitable qualifications and experience would cause the examination to be unduly delayed, nor if: (*a*) the pathologist does not desire to make the examination; (*b*) the conduct of any member of the hospital staff is likely to be called in question; or (*c*) any relative of the deceased asks the coroner that the examination be not made by such a pathologist.

(4) If the death of the deceased may have been caused by pneumoconiosis, the coroner should not direct or request a legally qualified medical practitioner who is a member of the pneumoconiosis medical panel to make a post-mortem examination.

The Committee heard evidence from numerous witnesses on these points: some witnesses challenged the wisdom of the coroner's choice in the selection of pathologist; clinical pathologists criticised the diverting of autopsies to forensic pathologists, and forensic pathologists in their turn criticised the involvement of clinical pathologists. The Committee propose that the responsibility for selecting the appropriate pathologist or pathologists to investigate any particular death should cease to rest with the coroner. They recommend that the provision of a pathologist service for coroners should become the responsibility of the National Health Service, and that the appropriate National Health Service authority should designate for each coroner a senior pathologist (or, failing this, a senior medical administrator) among whose responsibilities it would be to receive requests from each coroner for pathological examination, to select the pathologist to carry them out, and to satisfy himself that facilities were available for their purposes.

The Committee envisage that the future rôle of the forensic pathologist will be to assist the police solely in cases where there is reason to believe that criminality is involved in the death, and that this service in forensic pathology should be firmly based in the National Health Service.

Discussion

It can be argued that with the non-medically qualified coroner in office, a suitably qualified authority should be available to select his pathologist for him, and that such a method of selection of the pathologist would put an end to any allegations of 'patrimony' in the coroner's selection of his pathologist.

If this premise is accepted, the qualification of the suitable authority must be very closely looked at. Although it is obvious that the majority of coroner's autopsies involve cases where there can be no suspicion of unnatural death, such a possibility must always be considered. One of the essentials of investigation of sudden death is the speed at which the investigation gets under way. Any delay in nominating a pathologist and carrying out an autopsy can have far-reaching results in the consequent investigation of suicide, accident or crime. Deaths do not occur constantly during the working hours of senior administrative officers and it is not too difficult to envisage cases where a delay of 10 hours or more may occur should the death take place between, say, the hours of 6 p.m. and 10 a.m. on a working day, with much longer delays if an unfortunate person comes to his or her death after 5 o'clock on a Friday evening. It would again seem an anomaly to remove the choice of pathologist from a lay coroner's hands and to place it in the hands of a lay medical administrator.

The initial decision as to whether to employ a forensic pathologist or a hospital morbid anatomist must be made very rapidly, and must be made solely on the basis of the history of the incidents leading to death. By virtue of their training, forensic pathologists are probably able to appreciate more readily suspicious circumstances in a history than are their hospital colleagues. It could, therefore, be argued that in each coroner's jurisdiction there should be a forensic pathologist who would be responsible for the selection of the pathologist required to undertake any particular autopsy. He would be in a position, by studying the history of a particular case, to decide whether this case should be autopsied by a hospital morbid anatomist, or by a pathologist with special training in forensic pathology, and it could be established that in any case where there are no suspicious circumstances in the history, a hospital pathologist backed by suitable laboratory facilities should undertake the post-mortem. In cases where there are suspicious circumstances a forensic pathologist should not only undertake the autopsy, but should also visit the scene of the incident before the body is moved.

The selection of the grade of hospital pathologist requested to carry out coroner's autopsies would also need considerable care. The findings of the coroner, in any incident, whether it be investigated at inquest, investigated purely administratively in the office, or investigated merely by autopsy for the cause of death, are a judicial finding and as such are open to challenge. If coroner's autopsies are to be entrusted to junior members of National Health Service pathology departments, there is a very real risk that their post-mortem findings will be strongly challenged by interested parties who have been advised by more senior and experienced pathologists.

The teaching of forensic medicine in England and Wales leaves much to be desired. Such teaching as takes place is in the hands of the departments of forensic medicine at the various universities, and these departments are almost invariably staffed only by forensic pathologists. Forensic pathology is but one part of the full picture of forensic medicine, which by definition must include matters of clinical medicine, toxicology and allied subjects. The viability of any academic department of forensic medicine rests on the numbers and calibre of the forensic physicians in that department, and any measures to reduce their number, or to reduce the very high standard of training, will still further reduce the general standard of teaching of forensic medicine as a whole.

My dictionary defines forensic medicine as 'the science which applies the principles in practice of medicine to the elucidation of questions in judicial proceedings'. The Committee defines the coroner as an independent judicial officer, and by this definition alone implies that all coroner's investigations are judicial proceedings whether they result in a court hearing at a coroner's court, or a hearing in any other criminal or civil court. It would seem to be a gross anomaly under these circumstances to remove the forensic pathologist from a position of primary responsibility in all coroner's investigations.

CONCLUSION

After a gestation period of some six years, the Committee on Death Certification and Coroners has finally been delivered of its report. Many parts of this report are viable and excellent; some parts appear to be grossly pathological.

There can be little doubt that in the fields covered by the terms of reference by the Brodrick Committee there was urgent need for reform. Prompt consultation and discussion between the various bodies concerned in the recommendations of this report will decide whether it develops into a 'lusty new statute' or ends up as the subject of one of its own recommended perinatal certificates.

SUMMARY OF RECOMMENDATIONS
Medical Certification of the Cause of Death

(1) Before a doctor is allowed to certify the fact and cause of death for registration purposes he must: (*a*) be a fully registered medical practitioner; and, (*b*) have attended the deceased person at least once during the seven days immediately preceding death.

(2) If a doctor who is called upon to certify the fact and cause of death is qualified under the terms of proposal (1) above to give a certificate, he should be obliged to: (*a*) inspect the body of the deceased person; and, (*b*) either send a certificate of the fact or cause of death to the registrar of births and deaths, or report the death to the coroner.

(3) The Secretary of State for the Social Services should have the power to make regulations, which may be national or local in their application, prescribing certain categories of death as 'reportable deaths,' and a doctor should be obliged to report to the coroner any death which he has reasonable cause to believe falls within one of these categories.

(4) A qualified doctor should issue a certificate of the fact and cause of death only if:

(*a*) he is confident, on reasonable grounds, that he can certify the medical cause of death with accuracy and precision;

(*b*) there are no grounds for supposing that the death was due to, or contributed to by, any employment followed at any time by the deceased, any drug, medicine or poison or any violent or unnatural cause;

(*c*) he has no reason to believe that the death occurred during an operation or under or prior to complete recovery from an anaesthetic or arising out of any incident during an anaesthetic;

(*d*) the cause or circumstances do not make the death one which the law requires should be reported to the coroner; or

(*e*) he knows of no reason why in the public interest any further inquiry should be made into the death.

(5) Any doctor who is not qualified to give a certificate of the fact or cause of death and who, in the course of his professional duties, is informed of the death of a person who he has previously attended, or who attends someone whom he finds to be dead, should be obliged to report the fact of death to the coroner, together with any information which may assist the coroner's enquiries. He should not report a death to the coroner without first seeing the body and establishing the fact of death.

(6) A doctor should be obliged to report a death to the coroner as soon as possible after he has decided that a report is necessary. An oral report should be followed up as soon as possible by the issue of a certificate. The certificate which the doctor sends to the coroner should be a new certificate of the fact and cause of death. In future this should be sent either to the registrar of deaths or to the coroner, as appropriate.

(7) In relation to the certification of the medical cause of death, the registrar of deaths should retain his present function, and in drawing up his instructions to registrars the Registrar General should have regard to the specific categories of 'reportable deaths.'

283

(8) The new certificate should specify the circumstances in which the doctor should report to the registrar and to the coroner.

(9) The new certificate should have space for:

(a) the National Health Service number;

(b) the recording of major morbid conditions which have not caused or contributed to death;

(c) the provision of information about surgical operations performed within three months of death; and

(d) the inclusion of details of serious accidents occurring within 12 months of death.

(10) The time allowed for registering of stillbirths should, in future, be the same as the time allowed for registering a death.

(11) A single certificate of perinatal death should be introduced for the use of stillbirths and the death of children within seven days of birth.

(12) The qualification of a doctor to give a certificate of perinatal death should be the same as a doctor giving a certificate of the fact and cause of death.

(13) A doctor (or midwife in the case of a stillbirth) who has attended at the birth should be obliged to give a certificate of perinatal death or to report the stillbirth to the coroner, but a certificate should only be given if:

(a) the certifier is confident on reasonable grounds that he or she can certify the fact and the medical cause of stillbirth with accuracy and precision;

(b) there are no grounds for supposing that the stillbirth was due to, or contributed to by, any employment followed at any time by the mother, any drug, medicine or poison, any surgical operation, in the administration of an anaesthetic, or any other violent or unnatural cause; or

(c) the certifier knows no reason why, in the public interest, any further enquiry should be made into the stillbirth.

(14) In every case where neither a doctor nor a midwife is present at the birth, an alleged stillbirth should be reported to the coroner. An obligation to make this report should be placed first on any doctor or midwife who has called to see the body and then on any person present at the moment of stillbirth.

(15) The registrar of births and deaths should be obliged to report a stillbirth, or alleged stillbirth, to the coroner in three sets of circumstances:

(a) when he is unable to obtain a certificate from a doctor or midwife in respect of a stillbirth which has been reported to him;

(b) when he has reason to believe that the stillbirth should have been reported to the coroner by the certifying doctor or midwife; or

(c) where it is suggested to him by any person that a product of conception certified as a stillbirth may have been born alive.

MEDICAL CERTIFICATES FOR THE DISPOSAL OF DEAD BODIES

(1) The procedure for the disposal of stillbirths should be the same as for dead bodies.

(2) A disposal certificate either issued by a registrar of deaths or by a coroner to whom a death has been reported should be sufficient authority for disposal by any method.

(3) The existing cremation forms and certificates and the office of medical referee should be abolished.

(4) Should any of the proposed changes have to be deferred for a considerable period, the Committee recommend that the cremation form C (the confirmatory certificate) should be abolished without delay.

(5) Preservative treatment should in future never be started before either:

(a) a death has been registered on the basis of the certificate given by a doctor qualified to issue such a certificate; or

(b) if the death has been reported to the coroner, the consent of the coroner has been obtained.

(6) The registrar should be responsible for issuing the certificate for the disposal of the dead body in all cases except where an inquest is held.

(7) In every case in which a coroner holds an inquest he should be obliged to issue a disposal certificate to a person who appears to him to be responsible for arranging the disposal of the body.

(8) When a body of someone who has died outside this country is brought back for disposal, the certificate authorizing disposal of the body should be issued by the registrar of deaths, unless the death is one on which the coroner has decided to hold an inquest.

(9) When a review of the registration service is next arranged, special studies should be given to the question of whether a closer degree of integration could or should be sought between the two services.

(10) Consideration should be given to the appointment of an advisory committee representative of coroners, doctors and other relevant interests.

QUALIFICATION OF CORONERS,
RESIDENTIAL REQUIREMENTS AND RETIREMENT

(1) Only barristers or solicitors of at least five years' standing in their profession should be eligible for future appointment as coroners, deputy coroners and assistant deputy coroners. In order to preserve flexibility for the future, this new qualification should be prescribed by regulation rather than by statute.

(2) Appointments of all coroners and deputy coroners to whole-time posts should be made by the Lord Chancellor, after appropriate consultation with local authorities.

(3) Appointments of deputy coroners to part-time posts and of assistant deputy coroners should be made by the coroner with the approval of the Lord Chancellor.

(4) Coroners who are appointed to county jurisdictions should no longer be required to reside within the district to which they are assigned, or within two miles of it. Instead, it should be a condition of appointment

that a coroner, or in his absence his deputy or his assistant, should be readily available at all times to undertake coroner's duties.

(5) Unless special circumstances necessitate an early retirement, a coroner should normally retire at the age of 65; the Lord Chancellor should have power to extend the coroner's tenure of office annually in appropriate cases up to the age of 72. These conditions should also apply to deputy coroners and assistant deputy coroners.

(6) The power of removal should lie solely with the authority having the power of appointment, i.e. the Lord Chancellor.

(7) The power of removal should be exercisable only for incapacity or misbehaviour.

(8) The Lord Chancellor should be able to remove a coroner for any incapacity or misbehaviour which, in his judgment, renders the coroner unfit to continue in office.

(9) Investigation of the grounds for removal from the office of coroner should be carried out on behalf of the Lord Chancellor by the Home Secretary.

(10) Whole-time coroners should be paid standard salaries. An appropriate analogy to follow would be the salary of the stipendiary magistrate.

Coroners' Areas

(1) The new county and metropolitan authorities should be statutorily required to submit for approval by the Home Office proposals for the organization for coroners' service in their area.

Before submitting any proposals for a part-time jurisdiction the authority concerned should be statutorily required to consult the authority of the areas bordering on the part-time jurisdiction with a view to enlarging that jurisdiction, if possible to full-time status, by inter-authority adjustment of the coroner's district boundaries.

The authorities should be under a statutory obligation to keep the distribution of coroners' districts under review and to consider any proposals made by the Home Secretary for alteration of district; and to facilitate central oversight they should be statutorily obliged to send to the Home Office information or reports on the work in individual coroners' districts as the Home Secretary may from time to time request.

The Home Secretary should have power to approve or reject proposals submitted to him; power, after consultation with the local authority or local authorities affected, to amend the proposals for coroners' districts, and power to propose and impose alteration from time to time to any coroners' districts that seem to him to be unsatisfactory in size for the efficient working of the service.

(2) As a transitional measure provision should be made in the forthcoming legislation on local government for coroners in England and Wales outside the metropolitan areas to be appointed by the new county authorities in the metropolitan areas by the council of the new metropolitan areas.

SUPPORTING STAFF FOR CORONERS

(1) Police officers should no longer serve in the capacity of coroner's officer. They should be 'phased out' gradually and should be withdrawn by chief officers of police only after the closest consultation with the coroner, local authorities, hospital and, where appropriate, other bodies.

(2) Every coroner should be provided with the services of the civilian coroner's officer and, where necessary, the services of a secretary.

(3) The Home Secretary should be placed under a statutory duty to secure the provision of suitable and sufficient staff and accommodation for the performance of coroners of their statutory functions (including the holding of inquests). He should be empowered to make arrangements for other persons or bodies to act as his agents to pay for the expenditure incurred by them on his behalf.

THE CORONER'S FUTURE RESPONSIBILITIES

(1) Persons in charge of prison service establishments, similar institutions maintained by the armed forces, approved schools and remand homes should continue to be required to report the death of inmates to the coroner.

(2) There should be a statutory obligation upon the officer in charge of a police station to report a death to the coroner when a person dies in police custody.

(3) It should be a requirement of the law that the death of compulsorily detained psychiatric patients should be reported to the coroner and the obligation to make such a report should be placed on the person in administrative charge of the hospital in which the patient was detained.

(4) Intentional failure by any person to comply with an obligation to report a death to the coroner should be an offence punishable by a fine.

(5) If the coroner in the area where the death occurred has grounds for believing that an enquiry should be made into the circumstances of death, and that it could more appropriately be made in the area where the incident leading to death occurred, he should be able to refer the death to that other coroner and the latter should then have a duty to accept jurisdiction over the death. It should not be necessary to move the body for this purpose.

(6) When a competent court orders an inquest, or a fresh inquest, to be held, it should have power to direct any coroner (regardless of the area of his territorial jurisdiction) to hold the inquest.

(7) When a death is reported to a coroner who has territorial jurisdiction over the death he should have a duty:

(a) to determine the identity of the deceased and the fact and cause of death;

(b) to make such enquiries as will allow him to decide whether a post-mortem examination or an inquest or a reference to some other authority (or any combination of these) is required in order that he may determine the matters referred to in (a) above; and

287

(*c*) to send a certificate incorporating the results of his enquiries to the registrar of deaths in the district in which the death occurred.

(8) The coroner should have the statutory power to require a post-mortem examination to be carried out, to open an inquest or to make the reference referred to in (7) above.

(9) The coroner, or any person acting with his authority, should have an express power:

(*a*) to take possession of a body and to enter and inspect the place or area where the body was found, and any place from which the body was moved, or any place from which there is reasonable grounds to believe that the body was moved, before it was found;

(*b*) to enter and inspect the places or areas in which the deceased person was, or the places or areas in which there is reason to believe the deceased person was, prior to his death, if in the opinion of the coroner, the entry and inspection of such places or areas is necessary for the purposes of his investigation;

(*c*) to enter into any place to inspect and receive information from any records or writings relating to the deceased and to reproduce and retain copies therefrom; and

(*d*) to take possession of anything that he has reasonable grounds for believing is material for the purposes of his investigation and preserve it until the conclusion of his investigation. When his investigation is complete, the coroner should have a duty to restore that thing to the person from whom it was taken unless he is authorized or required by law to dispose of it in some other way.

(10) The Secretary of State should continue to have the power to direct that the inquest be held in the absence of the body.

(11) If, for a particular reason, a second inquest into a death is held, the finding of the second inquest should automatically replace the finding of the first, but where the second inquest is conducted in the knowledge that an earlier inquest has already been held, the coroner conducting the second inquest should have power to take into account the evidence given at the first inquest.

(12) The Home Office should keep a register of cases in which the Secretary of State has directed an inquest to be held in the absence of a body, and coroners should consult the Home Office in cases where a body is found in circumstances which suggest that it may reasonably be thought to have been lost.

(13) For the avoidance of doubt it should be provided that a coroner has discretion whether or not to act in any case where he is informed that there is within his area a body of a person who has died overseas in circumstances which, had they occurred in this country, would have given him jurisdiction to act.

(14) There should be legislation to provide that the death on an off-shore installation of any person ordinarily resident within the United Kingdom whose body is, for any reason, not brought into the jurisdiction of the coroner, should be reported to a coroner so that the latter may be in

a position, if he thinks it desirable and practical, to make enquiries to ascertain fact and cause of death and, if he wishes to hold an inquest, to seek the Secretary of State's authority for this.

(15) The coroner should have the statutory power to make an order for exhumation.

(16) Coroners should continue to exercise the duty of enquiring into finds of treasure until comprehensive legislation is introduced to deal with the whole question of antiquities.

(17) The City of London Fire Inquest Act of 1888 should be repealed.

Coroner's Procedure When a Death is Reported to Him

(1) Coroners should be recipients, not seekers, of reports of death which call for their investigation, and their enquiries should extend as far as, but no further than, is necessary to enable them to complete the task of establishing the cause and, where necessary, the circumstances of death.

(2) The coroner should retain the right to accept the cause of death given to him by a doctor, but having done so he should take the responsibility of certifying the cause of death. He should send the certificate to the registrar on the basis of the information which the doctor has provided.

(3) The coroner should be obliged to open an inquest when he is informed of: (a) a death from suspected homicide; (b) deaths of any person in legal custody (including persons who are compulsorily detained in hospital); and (c) deaths of persons whose bodies are unidentified.

(4) Except in those cases mentioned in paragraph (3) above, the coroner should have complete discretion as to the form which his enquiries may take after a death has been reported to him.

(5) The restriction which precludes the coroner from returning any verdict which may appear to determine any question of civil liability should be retained.

(6) It should no longer be obligatory for the coroner to view the body prior to an inquest.

Inquests

(1) A coroner should have authority to summon a witness from anywhere in England and Wales.

(2) When witnesses are told about the arrangement for an inquest, they should be told also that, as properly interested persons, they are entitled to legal representation.

(3) If a properly interested party asks to be kept informed of the inquest arrangements and has supplied a telephone number or address at which he can be contacted, then the coroner should be obliged to inform him of the arrangements which he makes.

(4) A coroner should be required to exhibit a list of the inquests which he proposes to hold (together with a list of the witnesses to be called to each) on a notice board outside his office and outside the place or places most commonly used as the coroner's court.

(5) Coroners should not change the declared time of an inquest without giving adequate notice to the persons concerned.

(6) If for any reason the nearest surviving adult relative whose existence is known to the coroner is not present at the inquest, the coroner should be obliged to notify him of the findings of the inquest, and to inform him that a certificate can be obtained from the registrar of births and deaths to whom the coroner's own certificate has been sent.

(7) A transcript of the evidence should be taken at every inquest.

(8) Coroners should be required to complete and deliver to the next of kin an interim certificate of the fact of death in cases where the conclusion of an enquiry is likely to be delayed. This certificate should be acceptable to third parties, e.g. insurance companies, as evidence of the fact of death.

(9) Coroners should continue to record in inquest cases medical cause of death and sufficient information about the circumstances of the death to enable the Registrar General to ascribe the death to a statistical category.

(10) The term 'verdict' should be abandoned and replaced by 'findings.'

(11) The mandatory requirement to summon a jury for inquest on certain categories of death should be abolished, but the coroner should retain the power to summon a jury where he considers there are special reasons for doing so.

(12) When a coroner decides to sit with a jury, it should be summoned in accordance with the same rules as are used by the High Sheriff in summoning juries to other courts.

(13) The right to attach a rider to the findings of the coroner's court should be abolished; the coroner should confine his enquiry to ascertaining and recording the facts, both medical and circumstantial, which caused or led up to a death, and, where he thinks that action should be considered to prevent recurrence of the fatality, he should have a right to refer the matter to the appropriate expert body or public authority, and he should announce that he is doing so.

(14) The coroner should not be prevented from commending the conduct of an individual or an institution, provided that this can be done without prejudice to others.

(15) The following categories of properly interested persons should be given an absolute right to be present at an inquest and to ask relevant questions either by themselves or through their legal representative:

(*a*) the next of kin of the deceased;

(*b*) the parents, children and personal representatives of the deceased;

(*c*) any beneficiary of a policy for insurance on the life of the deceased and any insurer having issued such a policy;

(*d*) any person whose act or omission on the part of himself, his servant or agents, irrespective of whether it may give rise to civil liability, may be thought to have caused or contributed to the death of the deceased;

(*e*) a chief officer of police; or

(*f*) any person appointed by a Government department to attend the inquest.

In addition the coroner should retain a discretionary right to allow any other person to appear.

(16) In cases of industrial injury or disease, the existing right of the trade union representative to examine the witness at an inquest should be preserved.

(17) A coroner should have a discretionary power to waive the requirement that the police may only appear at an inquest by legal representation.

(18) Legal aid should be made available to enable interested parties to be represented at an inquest.

(19) Subject to the same right of objection for properly interested persons as listed under the present law, coroners in future should have a general discretion to accept documentary evidence from any witness at an inquest.

(20) A 'properly interested person' should have the right, and be given the opportunity, to object to the holding of an inquest based exclusively on documentary evidence.

(21) Once an all-documentary inquest has been opened a properly interested person should have the same right as he now has in relation to any inquest where documentary evidence is admitted to require that the inquest be adjourned so that a particular witness may give oral evidence.

(22) A coroner should be obliged to give at least 48 hours' notice of his intention to hold a 'short' inquest.

(23) Such notice should be given in two ways, by display on notice boards outside his office and outside the place or places most commonly used as the coroner's court, and by written notice to the person to whom he proposes to issue a certificate for disposal of the body.

(24) A coroner should continue to arrange for post-mortem examinations to be made whenever suspected pneumoconiosis death is referred to him, and these post-mortem examinations should be carried out by a pathologist attached to specialist thoracic centres, and that relevant pathological material should continue to be made available to the nearest pneumoconiosis panel.

(25) Before giving consent to the use for transplant purposes of the heart of a victim of an accident whose death has been reported to him, the coroner should ascertain that the deceased has been the passive victim of violence.

CORONERS' CERTIFICATES AND RECORDS, AND DISCLOSURE OF DOCUMENTARY INFORMATION

(1) There should be a new coroner's certificate of the fact and cause of death; it should be completed by the coroner in every case.

(2) Coroners should be required to make and retain a copy of the new certificate as the formal record of their action in respect of every death reported to them.

(3) The Registrar General should prescribe by regulation the information which the registrar of deaths should be obliged to copy into his register.

(4) A coroner should have a wide discretion to make documents available whenever he thinks fit, within the general framework of guidance to be provided by the Home Office.

(5) The coroner should be obliged to supply a copy of a post-mortem report to the deceased person's family doctor on request and no charge should be made for this service. The supply of copies of this report to other doctors and other persons who may ask for it should continue to be a matter for the coroner's discretion.

Assessment of Guilt and Committal for Trial

(1) The duty of a coroner's jury to name the person responsible for causing a death, and the coroner's obligation to commit a named person for trial should be abolished.

(2) There should be express provision for the coroner to refer his papers to the Director of Public Prosecutions, should he consider it necessary to do so, at whatever stage in the inquest seems to him to be the most appropriate.

(3) The coroner should avoid making any statement directly implying that a dead person thought by the police to be a murderer was, in fact, responsible for a death.

(4) In a case where a coroner sends his inquest papers to the Director of Public Prosecutions, the Director should be obliged to notify the coroner of his decision where no further court action ensues, no matter for what reason, and the coroner should publish a statement to the effect that the Director of Public Prosecutions is satisfied upon the evidence presently available that there is no case for any criminal proceedings.

(5) The coroner should be responsible for notifying the registrar of deaths of the results of any criminal proceedings or the results of further enquiries made by the Director of Public Prosecutions or by the police on behalf of the Director.

(6) If, during the course of an inquest, evidence is produced for the first time which suggests that an offence which has a bearing on the cause of death may have been committed, the coroner should make a report to a responsible public authority and announce in neutral terms that he is doing so.

Appeals

(1) There should be wider rights of appeal against the findings of an inquest: an error in any part of the record of findings of the coroner's court (including the findings as to the medical and circumstantial causes of death) should constitute a ground for an application for a fresh inquest.

(2) These rights should be exercisable locally by application to a High Court Judge sitting at a major centre outside London; the existing right of an aggrieved party to go to the Divisional Court should be preserved.

(3) A coroner's discretion not to hold an inquest on a death that has been reported to him should be open to rapid challenge and the matter should be capable of determination by a High Court Judge outside London.

(4) In such a case the High Court Judge should have power to order an autopsy and power to make an order suspending the operation of any burial or cremation order until the results of the autopsy are known.

PATHOLOGICAL AND RELATED SERVICES

(1) Responsibility for selecting the appropriate pathologist or pathologists to investigate a particular death should cease to rest with the coroner; instead it should be entrusted to another authority, familiar with the services and resources which could be made available to assist the coroner and familiar also with the needs of coroners and the circumstances of their work.

(2) The provision of a pathologist service to coroners should become the responsibility of the National Health Service.

(3) The appropriate National Health Service authority should designate to each coroner a senior pathologist (or failing this a senior medical administrator) among whose responsibility it would be to receive requests from each coroner for pathological examination, to select the pathologist to carry them out, and to satisfy himself that facilities, e.g. mortuary and laboratory facilities, were available for their purpose.

(4) The designated officer should:

(*a*) be prohibited from asking any member from a pneumoconiosis panel to carry out a post-mortem examination on behalf of the coroner in any case where pneumoconiosis is supposed to have caused the death; and

(*b*) do what he can in such a case to encourage the closest liaison between the pathologist acting on behalf of the coroner and the pneumoconiosis panel members.

(5) A service in forensic pathology for the police (like the pathology services for coroners) should be firmly based in the National Health Service.

(6) The general training framework for forensic pathology should be based on National Health Service practice.

(7) The principal training schools in forensic pathology should continue, as at present, to be located in universities.

(8) The general supervision of postgraduate training in forensic pathology should primarily be the responsibility of the Royal College of Pathologists.

(9) The requirements for a national service in forensic pathology should be determined only by consultation between the Home Office, police authorities and regional hospital boards or similar authorities.

(10) The Home Office should take responsibility for initiating discussions referred to in the previous paragraph, for representing the police requirements, and making a financial contribution in respect of the provision ultimately made.

Index

Acid phosphatase, histochemistry of, 75
Acid picro-Mallory stain, 70
Adenosine deaminase in paternity testing, 59
Adenylate kinase in paternity testing, 59
Adrenal gland investigations, cot deaths, and, 15
Ag group system in paternity tests, 56–59
Age at death, estimation from skeletal remains, 204–208
  changes in internal bone structure, 206
  epiphyseal union variation, 204
  foetal, 207
Aircraft accidents, investigation of, 171
Alkaline phosphatase, histochemistry of, 75
Amino acid disorder, cot deaths, and, 15
Aminopeptidase, histochemistry of, 75
Ammunition for firearms, refinements and variations of, 123–129
Amphetamine poisoning, 218
Analgesic drugs, poisoning, 225–227
Analytical techniques in toxicological identification, 232–243
  atomic absorption spectroscopy, 241

Analytical techniques—*contd.*
  column chromatography, 233
  gas chromatography, 235
  high pressure liquid chromatography, 239
  inorganic, 241–243
  mass spectrometry, 237
  organic, 232–241
  paper chromatography, 234
  radio-immunoassay, 239
  spectrofluorimetry, 239
  thin-layer chromatography, 234
  ultra-violet spectrophotometry, 239
Antidepressant drugs, poisoning, 222–225
Antihistamines, poisoning, 227
Atomic absorption spectroscopy, 116, 241

Bacteria, involvement in cot deaths, 12
Battered baby syndrome, 19–42
  burns in, 36
  clinical data, 23–25
  definition, 21
  frequency, 20–23
  incidence,
    age, 22
    race, 22
    sex, 22
  injuries, 25–36
    head, 25
    liver, 36
    long bone, 34

Battered baby syndrome—*contd.*
  injuries—*contd.*
    rib, 34
    sexual, 36
    visceral, 36
  management, 40–41
  pathology, 36–40
  perpetrator of, 22
  socio-economic factors, 22, 23
Benzodiazepines, poisoning, 222
Blood
  grouping, paternity, techniques
    in, 43–63
    Ag groups, 56–59
    chance of exclusion, 61–63
    dissimilar twins, 49–50
    Gc groups, 54–56
    Gm blood serum polymor-
      phism, 52–53
    likelihood of paternity, 44–47
      methods of calculation, 45
    red cell enzyme groups, 59–61
    second order exclusions, 47–49
    serum haptoglobins, 53–54
    variant haemoglobins, 50–52
  importance in criminal investi-
    gation, 113
  pigments, wound histopathology,
    in, 73–74
Body, examination of
  buried, 105–107
  decomposed, 102–105
Bone
  injuries, histopathology of, 86–89
    haemorrhage, 86
    medullary callus, 87
    necrosis, 86
    osteogenic granulation tissue,
      87
    traumatic inflammation, 87
  structure, internal, age changes
    in, 206
Bottle-feeding, cot deaths, and, 14
Breast-feeding, cot deaths, and, 14
Burns
  battered baby syndrome, in, 36
  histopathology of, 84–86

Cannabis poisoning, 218
Carbamazepine poisoning, 227
Cervical spine epidural haemorrhage, cot deaths, in, 11
Chlorpromazine poisoning, 223
Collagen, formation of, 69
Column chromatography technique, 233
Connective tissues, histochemistry
  of, 68
Coroner, recommended changes in
  procedure of, 257–265
  accommodation, 264
  appointment, 259
  areas, 263
  deputies, 261
  inquest procedures, changes,
    265–278
  qualifications, 259
  retirement, 259
  salary, 260
  supporting staff, 261
  territorial jurisdiction, 263
Cot deaths, 1–18
  bacteriological studies, 12
  bottle-feeding, and, 14
  breast-feeding, and, 14
  case procedure, 2–3
  forensic aspects, 15–16
  hypersensitivity in, 14–15
  incidence
    age, 3–4
    season, 4–5
    sex, 3
  maternal factors, 6
  mode of death, 7–8
  pathology, 8–11
  premonitory symptoms, 7–8
  serum gamma globulin in, 12–13
  socio-economic status, and, 6–7
  suffocation in, 13–14
  time of, 5–6
  upper respiratory infection in, 7
  virus isolation in, 11
Cow's milk hypersensitivity, cot
  deaths, and, 14

Cremation, recommended changes for, 254–257

Criminal investigation, pathologist's role in, 93–119
blood, 113
buried body, examination, 105–107
decomposition of body, procedure, 102–105
equipment, 117
examination at scene, 97–100
fingerprints, 109
footmarks, 107
casts, 109
lifting, 109
photography, 108
glass fragments, 116
hair, 114
Locard's exchange principle, 94
mortuary examination, 100–102
paint, 116
procedure, 94–95
scientific techniques, 107–117
temperature recording, 95–97

Cytochrome oxidase, histochemistry of, 75

Death certification, recommended changes in, 248–252

Dehydrogenase, histochemistry of, 75

Digoxin poisoning, 228

Diphenhydramine poisoning, 227

Drugs of abuse, toxicological identification of, 217–222

Ehlers–Danlos syndrome, battered baby syndrome, and, 30

Elastic tissue in wound healing, 72–73

Electron microscopy in wound histopathology, 82–84

Embden–Meyerhof pathway, 74

Enzyme histochemistry in wound histopathology, 74–80
acid phosphatase, 75
alkaline phosphatase, 75
aminopeptidase, 75
cytochrome oxidase, 75
dehydrogenase, 75
esterases, 75

Epiglottitis, acute, cot deaths, in, 11

Epiphyseal union variation in estimating age at death from skeletal remains, 204

Esterases, histochemistry of, 75

Exclusion of paternity
chance of, 61–63
second order, 47–49

Fibrin in wound healing, 70–71

Fingerprints, importance in criminal investigation, 109

Firearms injuries, 120–138
ammunition, 123–129
physical evidence, 132–134
research, 135–136
weapons, 120–123
wounds, 129–132

Foetal skeletons, estimating age at death from, 207

Foetal stature, estimation of, 198

Footmarks, importance in criminal investigation, 107
casts, 109
lifting, 109
photography of, 108

Gas chromatography technique, 235

Gc group system in paternity tests, 54–56

Glass fragments, examination in criminal investigation, 116

Gm blood serum polymorphism in paternity tests, 52–53

Haematoxylin and eosin stain, 70
Haemoglobin variants in paternity tests, 50–52
Haemorrhage in bone fractures, 86
Hair, importance in criminal investigation, 114
Haptoglobins in paternity tests, 53–54
Head injuries in battered baby syndrome, 25
Heroin poisoning, 220, 221
High pressure liquid chromatography, 239
Hip joint
  central fracture dislocation of, 159
  posterior fracture dislocation of, 158, 160
  tolerance of, knee injuries and, 150, 160
Histopathology of wounds, 64–92
  bone injuries, 86–89
  burns, 84–86
  early morphological changes, 66
  elastic tissue, 72–73
  electron microscopy, 82–84
  enzyme histochemistry, 74–80
  epithelial regeneration, 66
  fibrin, 70–71
  histochemistry, 67–69
    collagen formation, 69
    connective tissues, 68
  immunofluorescence techniques, 80–82
  mucopolysaccharides, 69–70
  pigments, 73–74
  platelets, 71–72
  standard laboratory examination procedure, 89–90
Hurler's syndrome, battered baby syndrome, and, 30
Hypersensitivity in cot deaths, 14–15
Hypogammaglobulinaemia in cot deaths, 12
Hypoventilation syndrome in cot deaths, 10

'Icarus complex', 219
Imipramine poisoning, 223
Immunofluorescence techniques in wound histopathology, 80–82
Inflammation in bone fractures, 87
Inorganic poisons, 229–232
  analysis, 241–243
Inquest procedures, recommended changes in, 265–278
Insulin poisoning, 213, 228
Isoniazid poisoning, 227

Laser arc emission spectrography, 116
Liver injuries in battered baby syndrome, 36
Lomotil poisoning, 227
Long bone injuries in battered baby syndrome, 34
Lysergic acid diethylamide (LSD) poisoning, 219

Marfan's syndrome, battered baby syndrome, and, 30
Martin's scarlet blue stain, 70, 71
Mass disaster, investigation of, 170–192
  accident reconstruction, 189
  accident site, at, 172–177
  aircraft accidents, 171
  autopsy room facilities, 178
  definition, 170
  dental evidence, 183
  elimination of causes, 173
  external examination of body, 181
  full internal autopsy, 182
  identification form, 187
  identification of bodies, 173, 174
  mortuary accommodation, 177
  mortuary procedures, 177–187
  photographic record, 181
  radiographic examination, 182
  reconstruction of accident, 174
  review of evidence, 189
  transportation of bodies, 175

Mass spectrometry, 116
technique, 237
Maternal factors in cot deaths, 6
Medullary callus in bone fractures,
87
Metabolism of drugs, 215
Methaqualone poisoning, 221
Microgroove system in rifles, 120
Mirror, car interior, injury from,
155
Monoamine oxidase inhibitors,
poisoning, 224
Micropolysaccharides in wound
healing, 69–70

Nasopharynx, obstruction in cot
deaths, 10
Necrosis in bone fractures, 86
Neutron activation, 116
analysis, 132, 242
Nialamid poisoning, 224

Organic analysis, 232–241
Orphenadrine poisoning, 227
Osteogenic granulation tissue in
bone fractures, 87

Paint, examination in criminal investigation, 116
Paper chromatography technique,
234
Paracetamol poisoning, 215, 225
Paraquat poisoning, 228
Parcel tray, injury from, 156
Paternity blood grouping, techniques in, 43–63
Ag groups, 56–59
chance of exclusion, 61–63
dissimilar twins, 49–50
Gc groups, 54–56
Gm blood serum polymorphism,
52–53
likelihood of paternity, 44–47
methods of calculation, 45
red cell enzyme groups, 59–61
second order exclusions, 47–49

Paternity blood grouping—contd.
serum haptoglobins, 53–54
variant haemoglobins, 50–52
Pathological services, recommended changes in, 278–282
Pathologist, role in criminal investigation, 93–119
blood, 113
buried body, examination, 105–
107
decomposition of body, procedure, 102–105
equipment, 117
examination at scene, 97–100
fingerprints, 109
footmarks, 107
casts, 109
lifting, 109
photography, 108
glass fragments, 116
hair, 114
Locard's exchange principle, 94
mortuary examination, 100–102
paint flake, 116
procedure, 94–95
scientific techniques, 107–117
temperature recording, 95–97
Pedestrian injury, 154
Pentachlorophenol poisoning, 227
Percentage method of calculation
in paternity testing, 45
Perinatal death certification, recommended changes in, 252–
254
Phenothiazines, poisoning, 223
Phosphoglucomutase in paternity
testing, 59
Phosphotungstic acid haematoxylin
stain, 70
Piperazine poisoning, 228
Platelets in wound histopathology,
71–72
'Polychoke' extensions for shotgun
muzzle, 120
Post-mortem specimens, toxico-
logical identification from,
216–217

Propoxyphene poisoning, 226
Pubic symphisis in judging sex from skeletal remains, 201
Pyrolysis gas chromatography, 116

Quinine poisoning, 228

Race, estimation from skeletal remains, 208–209
Radio-immunoassay technique, 239
Red cell enzyme groups in paternity tests, 59–61
Retinal haemorrhage in battered baby syndrome, 26
Rib injuries in battered baby syndrome, 34
Road traffic accident injuries, investigation of, 139–169
  data recording and analysis, 153
  experimental work, 148–153
  procedure, 140–145
    accident enquiry, 142
    impact, direction of, 142, 143
    medical investigation of casualties, 140
    vehicle examination, 142
  purpose, 139–140
  results, 145–148

Safety belts, road traffic accident research, 162
Second order exclusions in paternity tests, 47–49
Sephadex, 233
Serum gamma globulin in cot deaths, 12–13
Serum haptoglobins in paternity tests, 53–54
Sex
  determination from skeletal remains, 199–204
  pre-adolescent differences, 203
  injuries, battered baby syndrome, and, 36

Skeletal reconstruction, 193–211
  age at death, 204–208
  race, 208–209
  sex, 199–204
  stature, 194–199
Socio-economic status in cot deaths, 6–7
Spectrofluorimetry, 239
Stature estimation from skeletal remains, 194–199
  equations for, 195
  foetal, 198
  fragmentary bones in, 197
  long limb bones in, 195–197
Status thymicolymphaticus, 9
Subhyaloid haemorrhage in battered baby syndrome, 26
Succinylcholine poisoning, 213
Suffocation in cot deaths, 13–14

Temperature recording for estimation of time of death, 95–97
Thallium salts poisoning, 213, 231
Thin-layer chromatography technique, 234
Toxicological identification techniques, 212–247
  analgesics, 225–227
  analysis of therapeutic agents, 215–216
  analytical techniques, 232–243
  antidepressants, 222–225
  antihistamines, 227
  drugs of abuse, 217–222
  inorganic poisons, 229–232
  pathology, 213–215
  post-mortem sample collection, 216–217
  urine analysis, 220
Twins, dissimilar, paternity tests, 49–50

Ultra-violet spectrophotometry, 239
Upper respiratory infection in cot death, 7

Urine analysis in toxicological screening, 220

Victoria blue stain, 70
Virus isolation in cot deaths, 11
Visceral injuries in battered baby syndrome, 36

Weigert's fibrin stain, 70
Wounds
  firearm, 129–132
  histopathology of, 64–92
    bone injuries, 86–89
    burns, 84–86
    early morphological changes, 66

Wounds, histopathology—*contd.*
  elastic tissue, 72–73
  electron microscopy, 82–84
  enzyme histochemistry, 74–80
  epithelial regeneration, 66
  fibrin, 70–71
  histochemistry, 67–69
    collagen formation, 69
    connective tissues, 68
    mucopolysaccharides, 69–70
  immunofluorescence techniques, 80–82
  pigments, 73–74
  platelets, 71–72
  standard laboratory examination procedure, 89–90